ALCOHOL and the FAMILY

Research and Clinical Perspectives

R. LORRAINE COLLINS
KENNETH E. LEONARD
JOHN S. SEARLES

Editors

Foreword by Edward Kaufman

THE GUILFORD PRESS
New York   London

© 1990 The Guilford Press
A Division of Guilford Publications, Inc.
72 Spring Street, New York, NY 10012

Printed in the United States of America

This book is printed on acid-free paper

Last digit is print number: 9 8 7 6 5 4 3 2 1

Library of Congress Cataloging-in-Publication Data

Alcohol and the family / edited by R. Lorraine Collins, Kenneth E.
  Leonard, John S. Searles
      p.   cm.—(The Guilford substance abuse series)
    Includes bibliographical references.
    ISBN 0–89862–169–0
    1. Alcoholism.   2. Alcoholics—Family relationships.   3. Family
psychotherapy.   I. Collins, R. Lorraine.   II. Leonard, Kenneth E.
III. Searles, John S. (John Steven), 1946–   IV. Series.
RC565.A394   1990
362.29'23—dc20   89–37204
                                                    CIP

ALCOHOL AND THE FAMILY

The Guilford Substance Abuse Series

EDITORS

HOWARD T. BLANE, Ph.D.
Research Institute on Alcoholism, Buffalo

THOMAS R. KOSTEN, M.D.
Yale University School of Medicine, New Haven

ALCOHOL AND THE FAMILY: RESEARCH AND CLINICAL
PERSPECTIVES
  R. Lorraine Collins, Kenneth E. Leonard, and John S. Searles, Editors

CHILDREN OF ALCOHOLICS: CRITICAL PERSPECTIVES
  Michael Windle and John S. Searles, Editors

GROUP PSYCHOTHERAPY WITH ADULT CHILDREN OF
ALCOHOLICS: TREATMENT TECHNIQUES AND
COUNTERTRANSFERENCE CONSIDERATIONS
  Marsha Vannicelli

PSYCHOLOGICAL THEORIES OF DRINKING AND
ALCOHOLISM
  Howard T. Blane and Kenneth E. Leonard, Editors

ALCOHOL AND BIOLOGICAL MEMBRANES
  Walter A. Hunt

ALCOHOL PROBLEMS IN WOMEN: ANTECEDENTS,
CONSEQUENCES, AND INTERVENTION
  Sharon C. Wilsnack and Linda J. Beckman, Editors

DRINKING AND CRIME: PERSPECTIVES ON THE
RELATIONSHIPS BETWEEN ALCOHOL CONSUMPTION
AND CRIMINAL BEHAVIOR
  James J. Collins, Jr., Editor

Foreword

This volume presents a very scholarly and up-to-date review of the three major aspects of the relationship of the family to alcoholism: genetics, family processes, and family oriented treatment. It is particularly relevant since it arrives at a time when there has been a widespread move to exclude the input of many different types of professionals from the treatment of alcoholism. Fortunately, family therapists have been historically more welcome in the treatment of substance abusers than most professional disciplines. It is time, however, that the family therapy field had a sound scientific foundation on which to build its critical role in a comprehensive, therapeutic approach toward alcoholics. This book has taken a giant leap forward in that direction.

Genetic studies of alcoholics have been helpful to clinicians in several critical ways. They have provided support for the disease model of alcoholism, contributed to the identification of a group that is at high risk for the disease, and helped to direct prevention efforts to vulnerable individuals. Genetic studies have also helped to confirm a diagnosis of early alcoholism in those individuals with family histories of the disease. They point to the need for abstinence as a primary goal for those with histories of early, out of control drinking, who also have strong genetic loading. The important discovery of two specific types of alcoholism, one with and one without genetic loading, is well documented and discussed in this first section.

Yet the authors wisely interject a cautionary note in viewing genetic studies to date. Caution is necessary for three reasons: (1) the alcohol researcher's lack of knowledge of behavior genetic analyses and heritability, (2) the tendency of biological reductivity to ignore psychological variables, and (3) the lack of emphasis on the interaction between genes and environment.

The search for individual trait markers for alcoholism has certainly been heightened over this past decade. For this reviewer, who has placed little credence in most of this work to date, it was helpful to see these markers so effectively summarized. These trait markers become critical if inherited vulnerability to specific effects of alcohol, such as brain damage or cirrhosis, can be demonstrated.

The chapters dealing with basic aspects of behavioral genetic methods will certainly be of great value to any alcohol researcher who undertakes genetic studies, while a clinician such as myself can gain valuable information from the family processes and therapy sections. It was rewarding to see discussions of developmental, marital, and family contributions to alcohol abuse in the section on family processes. The valuable longitudinal work begun by researchers such as Brock, Kandel, Jacob, and Jessor was funded by the NIDA and NIAAA during the time I was a member of and consultant to several grant review panels.

In the family processes section, several sets of findings emerged as interesting. For example, high levels of parental support and contact, with moderate levels of control and minimal rejection, are emphasized as protective factors in the development of adolescent alcohol abuse. Additionally, substance use by older siblings constitutes a strong risk for abuse by younger siblings. Sibling order has long been an interest of mine. As early as 1976, I observed that male substance abusers tended to be the youngest or only children. There were several reasons for this, including the need on the part of some parents to hold on to the youngest child so that they would always have a baby around to nourish, often at the neglect of meeting each other's spousal needs.

Another set of thought provoking findings is presented in the review of the many variables in parental drinking that affect the children of alcoholics. Generally, the research reviewed in the family processes section is important to the future of prevention, and answers many questions for practitioners, researchers, and parents who seek to prevent substance abuse in children.

The highly scientific section on family therapy summarizes the theory, research, and practice of behavioral family treatment of alcoholics in a manner that will be of practical and theoretical help to both researchers and clinicians. The related issue of coping skills is covered in depth. These chapters set the background for the excellent follow-up research of the Stanford group. Their work definitively debunks the myth of the alcoholic's wife as one who benefits from her husband's drunkeness, and decompensates when he gets sober. Differences between intermittent and steady drinkers, another long ignored aspect of this problem, is also well developed.

Each of the three sections of *Alcohol and the Family* demonstrates the many differences among alcoholic families, scientifically explores these variations, and describes how to understand and deal with them therapeutically. It's about time we had a book that dealt with these issues in a rigorous way. *Alcohol and the Family* fills the bill.

EDWARD KAUFMAN, M.D.

Preface

The earliest seeds for this volume were sown by presentations made at a Research Institute on Alcoholism seminar series on "Alcohol and the Family." The burgeoning research and clinical literature in this area indicated that a host of issues, ranging from the role of genetics in the development of alcoholism to the move to involve family members in treatment, were important in theoretical and applied formulations of alcoholism. With the growth in empirical data on various aspects of the family's role in alcoholism, we felt that further exploration and presentation of the "state-of-the-art" was warranted and so invited the distinguished authors herein to contribute to this edited volume.

The favorable response from those we approached as well as the positive reactions of our colleagues offered further support for the decision to pursue this project. The book that evolved from our meetings and invitations to contributors is presented here. The chapters represent the work of investigators who have made significant contributions to this area of research. The book is organized into three sections: Genetics, Family Processes, and Treatment. Each chapter is designed to present either a review of a particular area or a program of research. The book is intended for both researchers and clinicians who have an interest in alcoholism and/or family-related issues. We hope that the issues raised in the chapters presented in this volume will stimulate further developments in research and clinical endeavors on alcohol and the family.

Part I presents the research on the genetics of alcoholism, which has direct implications and practical applications for family issues. The consequences of alcoholism almost always negatively affect family functioning. The promise of the genetic research agenda is the identification of individuals at risk for developing certain alcoholic disorders and the possible amelioration or arrest of incipient alcoholic-type behaviors. However, as the chapters in this section indicate, a genetic predisposition may not inevitably lead to the expression of alcoholism. Although one current focus in extant research is the identification of genetically transmissible markers, very little attention has been afforded environments that may either enhance or inhibit alcoholism. Even less notice has been paid to complex interactions between genetic and environmental factors. Part of the problem in investigating such complex interrelationships is the unfamiliarity with higher level statistical and methodological concepts that allow the simultaneous consideration of several components. Rowe's chapter on behavior genetic models illustrates some of these methods and offers substantive suggestions as to how they may be applied to current research paradigms. This chapter offers both researchers and clinicians an introduction to some of the new and powerful multivariate statistical techniques which when correctly employed with appropriate data may aid in untangling the intricacies of critical etiological factors in alcoholism.

The general review chapters by Searles and Cadoret offer a unique opportunity to view basically the same literature from two different perspectives. Searles' chapter implies that the evidence supporting a genetic basis for alcoholism may be too flawed to draw any firm conclusions at this time. He also offers suggestions for incorporating environmental and gene-environment correlation effects in order to more completely and precisely specify etiologic models. Cadoret, whose adoption studies have had a major impact in generating the current intense interest in the genetics of alcoholism, concludes that there is convincing evidence of an active genetic component in the development of some types of alcoholic disorders. However, he also suggests that environmental factors may have a significant effect.

In the third chapter in this section, Tarter, Moss, and Laird review and summarize the literature pertaining to putative markers for alcoholism. Since much of the seminal research in this area has been conducted by these scientists and their colleagues at the University of Pittsburgh, their insights are particularly relevant and timely. Their viewpoints are especially appropriate now because the identification of persons at high risk to develop alcoholism is an area that is attracting substantial theoretical attention and research funding.

Taken as a whole, the section on genetics presents a cautiously optimistic view of the current research endeavor and the prospects for methodological and technical refinements in future efforts. It will be clear after reading this section that the behavior genetics of alcoholism encompass genetic factors, environmental effects, and the influences arising from the combination of the two.

Part II focuses on family processes. Since environmental factors exert an influence on the development of alcoholism, it is likely that family processes will be a major environmental factor placing an individual at risk. Disruption of normal family processes, or the occurrence of deviant family processes, can be expected to exert a major influence on both individual and family development. Alcoholism can represent: (1) a disruption of family processes, (2) a marker for the occurrence of deviant processes, as well as (3) an outcome of the disruption of family processes. As a disruption of family processes, alcoholism exerts a more or less chronic impact on family functioning including both marital and parental roles. The precise family processes affected may differ among families; they may be as subtle as a lack of consistency in parenting or as marked as continual conflict and violence. As a marker of deviant processes, alcoholism is associated with factors that may have an independent impact on the family. Most notable in this regard is the presence of psychopathology in either the alcoholic or his/her spouse. As an outcome of family processes, alcohol use and alcoholism may be seen as arising from specific parent–child interactions. Alternatively, alcoholism may result from the interplay of parental alcoholism and family interactions. Finally, alcoholism may be maintained and perpetuated by family processes that reinforce drinking or fail to reinforce sobriety. As such, Part II includes chapters in which the interrelationship between alcoholism and different family processes are explored.

Barnes focuses on parent–child interactions that relate to alcohol use and problems in adolescence. This chapter reviews the importance of a variety of family factors, including parental warmth and control in the development of drinking in adolescence. Johnson's chapter describes psychosocial deficits in children of alcoholics, many of which occur presumably as a result of the specific impact of an alcoholic parent on child development. Johnson argues that an understanding of the psychosocial deficits of children of alcoholics requires a developmental perspective that recognizes the potential for different developmental trajectories of psychosocial maladaptation. In Bennett and Wolin's chapter, both family of origin and current marital processes which relate to the transmission of alcoholism from parents to offspring are discussed. In particular, they describe one process, the ability to maintain family rituals in the face of escalated drinking, as a protection against the development of alcoholism in the offspring. Another process, deliberateness in the development of family rituals among married couples, also appears to protect the members from developing alcoholism. Next, Leonard's chapter focuses on the marital relationships and interactions of different subtypes of alcoholics. After reviewing the research on marital interaction of alcoholics, a series of studies by Jacob and his colleagues addressing marital interaction differences among episodic and steady alcoholics is described. Finally, O'Farrell's chapter describes the impact of alcoholism on sexual functioning (and related aspects of marital functioning) in couples. The evidence described in his chapter suggests that the sexual functioning of alcoholics is impaired, in part as a result of the effects of chronic alcohol abuse, but also as a result of psychosocial and interpersonal factors associated with their drinking.

Part III focuses on family-oriented treatment. The inclusion of family members in alcoholism treatment is receiving growing attention in research and clinical arenas. While this step represents a logical extension of research on the role of environmental factors in the etiology and maintenance of alcoholism, considerably more research is necessary before the efficacy of family-oriented treatment can be firmly established. Nonetheless, conceptual and methodological developments in this area offer promise for improving the lives of alcoholics and their families.

Collins' chapter presents an overview of research on the behavioral and family-systems approaches to family treatment. Empirical research in this area is in its infancy and as such offers many opportunities for further development. Collins describes and evaluates the research to date, makes recommendations for improving research methodology, and suggests directions for future research. Following this, the work of Moos and colleagues at the Social Ecology Laboratory in Palo Alto, California is described in the chapter by Cronkite, Finney, Nekich, and Moos. This chapter presents a program of research, within a stress and coping framework, which spans the past decade. Cronkite et al. outline the processes of remission and relapse following alcoholism treatment as they impact generally on the family and specifically on spouses and children. They conclude by citing future directions for assessment, diagnosis, and treatment. McCrady's chapter focuses on research on the marital relationship during alcoholism treatment. She examines research on the nature of the marital relationship, the efficacy of marital therapy, and the relationship between marital functioning and treatment outcome, along with an overview of her own research in this area. Rychtarik's chapter begins with a review of research on the coping skills of spouses of alcoholics. He goes on to describe the development and testing of a new measure of spouses' coping skills, the Spouse Situation Inventory. While spouses of alcoholics are being included in treatment there is a paucity of research relevant to the development and evaluation of spouse-oriented interventions. The Spouse Situation Inventory provides improved methodology for conducting research and clinical assessment in this important area. In sum, the chapters in this section provide a comprehensive presentation of the range of research and clinical issues related to family-oriented interventions for alcoholism.

We wish to thank the authors who have contributed to this volume. Their willingness to share their expertise was essential to the realization of this project. We would like to thank Brenda Miller for her valuable contributions at the initiation of this project and her continued involvement throughout its development. Finally, our thanks to Howard Blane for his leadership in creating the collegial and intellectually stimulating environment that exists at the Research Institute on Alcoholism and for his support of this volume.

R. LORRAINE COLLINS
KENNETH E. LEONARD
Buffalo, New York
JOHN S. SEARLES
Philadelphia, Pennsylvania

Contributors

GRACE M. BARNES, Ph.D., Research Institute on Alcoholism, New York State Division of Alcoholism and Alcohol Abuse, Buffalo, New York

LINDA A. BENNETT, Ph.D., Department of Anthropology, Memphis State University, Memphis, Tennessee

REMI J. CADORET, M.D., Department of Psychiatry, The University of Iowa Psychiatric Hospital, Iowa City, Iowa

R. LORRAINE COLLINS, Ph.D., Research Institute on Alcoholism, New York State Division of Alcoholism and Alcohol Abuse, Buffalo, New York

RUTH C. CRONKITE, Ph.D., Social Ecology Laboratory and Far West Health Services Field Program, Stanford University, and Veterans Affairs Medical Center, Palo Alto, California

JOHN W. FINNEY, Ph.D., Social Ecology Laboratory and Far West Health Services Field Program, Stanford University, and Veterans Affairs Medical Center, Palo Alto, California

JEANETTE L. JOHNSON, Ph.D., Committee on Child Development Research and Public Policy, National Research Council/National Academy of Sciences, Washington, DC

SUSAN B. LAIRD, B.S., Department of Psychiatry, University of Pittsburgh, Pittsburgh, Pennsylvania

KENNETH E. LEONARD, Ph.D., Research Institute on Alcoholism, New York State Division of Alcoholism and Alcohol Abuse, Buffalo, New York

BARBARA S. McCRADY, Ph.D., Center of Alcohol Studies, Rutgers—The State University of New Jersey, Piscataway, New Jersey

RUDOLF H. MOOS, Ph.D., Social Ecology Laboratory and Far West Health Services Field Program, Stanford University, and Veterans Affairs Medical Center, Palo Alto, California

HOWARD MOSS, M.D., Department of Psychiatry, University of Pittsburgh, Pittsburgh, Pennsylvania

JAMIE NEKICH, M.A., Social Ecology Laboratory and Far West Health Services Field Program, Stanford University, and Veterans Affairs Medical Center, Palo Alto, California

TIMOTHY O'FARRELL, Ph.D., Alcohol and Family Studies Laboratory, Veterans Affairs Medical Center, Brockton, Massachusetts, and Harvard Medical School, West Roxbury, Massachusetts

JON E. ROLF, Ph.D., School of Public Health and Mental Hygiene, Department of Maternal and Child Health, Johns Hopkins University, Baltimore, Maryland

DAVID C. ROWE, Ph.D., Division of Family Studies, University of Arizona, Tucson, Arizona

ROBERT G. RYCHTARIK, Ph.D., Research Institute on Alcoholism, New York State Division of Alcoholism and Alcohol Abuse, Buffalo, New York

JOHN S. SEARLES, Ph.D., School of Medicine, University of Pennsylvania, Philadelphia, Pennsylvania, and Department of Veterans Affairs Medical Center, Philadelphia, Pennsylvania

RALPH E. TARTER, Ph.D., Department of Psychiatry, University of Pittsburgh, Pittsburgh, Pennsylvania

STEVEN J. WOLIN, M.D., Center for Family Research, Department of Psychiatry and Behavioral Sciences, George Washington University Medical Center, Washington, DC

Contents

PART I

GENETICS

1

The Contribution of Genetic Factors to the Development of Alcoholism: A Critical Review

JOHN S. SEARLES

Results of recent research seem to suggest that at least one form of alcoholism has a substantial genetic basis (Cloninger, Bohman, & Sigvardsson, 1981; Goodwin, 1976, 1979; Petrakis, 1985). It has been described by Goodwin (1979) as having an early onset, severe symptomatology, and requiring extensive and early treatment. It is always confined to males and often associated with an antisocial personality (Tarter, Alterman, & Edwards, 1985). Schuckit (1973) and Cadoret, Troughton, and Widmer (1984), however, maintain a distinction between the primary alcoholic and the sociopathic alcoholic, with alcoholism being a secondary characteristic of the latter. In addition, there is some evidence that alcoholism and sociopathy may be a subset of a "character spectrum disorder" under substantial genetic control (Akiskal, Hirschfeld, & Yerevanian, 1983).

The following review of the major methods and significant studies that have converged on these findings will help to place the research in proper context. There have been only a few objective critical appraisals of work in this area (Lester, 1988; Murray, Clifford, & Gurling, 1983; Peele, 1986)[1] for several interrelated reasons. First, although many of the methods used

The material contained in this chapter is a revised version of: Searles, J. S. (1988). The role of genetics in the pathogenesis of alcoholism. *Journal of Abnormal Psychology, 97*, 153–167. Copyright 1988 by the American Psychological Association. Adapted by permission of the publisher.

have been available since the time of Francis Galton, the behavior genetic approach has only recently been formalized (Fuller & Thompson, 1960; Jinks & Fulker, 1970), and most alcohol researchers are unfamiliar with the theoretical models, methodologies, and increasingly sophisticated statistical techniques employed in behavior genetic analyses, which puts them at a disadvantage in evaluating this body of research.

Second, because of this unfamiliarity, the concept of heritability (h^2) has been widely misinterpreted and misunderstood. The heritability statistic (h^2) is that part of observed phenotypic variance that can be accounted for in terms of genetic influence ($h^2 = V_g/V_p$).[2] There is an analogous "environmentality" statistic ($e^2 = V_e/V_p$) that represents all environmental influences of observed phenotypic behavior (Fuller & Thompson, 1978). Methodologically, h^2 is usually estimated from behavioral genetic data and e^2 is what remains ($e^2 = 1 - h^2$). There are three important considerations that follow from this explication: (1) The heritability statistic is sample dependent and, therefore, is *not* an immutable figure. (2) Environmentality is not generally measured directly. (3) Environmentality subsumes all nongenetic variance including errors of measurement (unreliability).

Third, this misunderstanding has led some scientists to view the behavior genetic approach as offering pseudoscientific support for racist, nonegalitarian, and oppressive policies (Kamin, 1974; Lewontin, Kamin, & Rose, 1983). Lewontin has gone so far as to suggest that behavior genetic research is fundamentally racist and should be suppressed (Wilson, 1978).

Fourth, the highly publicized "Burt Affair" in which Sir Cyril Burt created both research assistants and data to support his genetic theory of intelligence has served as a stimulus for many to dismiss *all* behavior genetic studies (Hearnshaw, 1979). Finally, many psychosocial researchers object to what appears to be a biological reductionist position that ignores important psychological and sociological variables such as expectancy, modelling effects, and family dynamics.

The cumulative effect has been to minimize or at least impede the impact of the behavior genetic perspective in general, with several important exceptions such as the area of personality development (Bouchard, 1982), certain psychiatric syndromes (Weissman, et al., 1986), and alcoholism. Recent reconceptualizations of alcoholism as multidimensional, consisting of distinct types of alcoholism and alcoholics, have included at least one form that is highly heritable in nature as described above. A genetic basis for alcohol abuse would seem to offer support for the disease model of alcoholism currently in vogue, and the subject of an acrimonious debate (see Peele, 1987, and Roizen, 1987, for excellent summaries of the controversy).[3] This may partially explain why research in the genetics of alcoholism has been so readily and uncritically accepted.

GENE × ENVIRONMENT INTERACTION

The behavior genetic model is based on phenotypic variability and assumes that this variability can be decomposed into basic components attributable to genes and environment. The approach has been heavily criticized for what appears to be ignoring the obvious; that is, behavior is also a function of some complex gene × environment interaction (Lewontin, et al., 1983).[4] However, despite an active analytical search in the data from the Colorado Adoption Project, Plomin and DeFries (1985) have been unable to uncover any gene × environment interactions of significance that account for even a modest amount of variance. Plomin (1986) suggests that this may be due to the age of the subjects (infants) and/or the quality of the measures, but he also points out that the search for meaningful gene × environment interactions in other areas (specifically, aptitude × treatment) has also proved fruitless despite long-term research efforts.

The empirical viability of gene × environment interactions was spurred primarily by the early positive results of animal studies of "maze bright" and "maze dull" strains of rats interacting with enriched and impoverished environments (Cooper & Zubek, 1958). Specifically, Cooper and Zubek (1958) reported that maze errors were a function of strain *and* rearing environment. While this study has been featured in virtually every introductory psychology textbook as evidence of gene × environment interaction, there are several problems of interpretation that are rarely mentioned:

1. The terms "maze bright" and "maze dull" imply some sort of intellectual or cognitive ability on the part of the rat. However, it is not at all clear what exactly mediates the differences between the two strains; differences in curiosity, activity level, emotionality, fear of open spaces, and fear of mechanical devices could (and, in some cases, have) led to the same outcome. While this does not obviate the obtained interaction, it does question its applicability to human intellectual functioning.

2. In situations where animals were exposed to highly motivating situations (life-threatening), learning was a function of genetic factors; environmental and gene × environment interaction had little impact (Henderson, 1972).

3. Cooper and Zubek (1958) themselves qualify the results in the following manner: "The ceiling of the test may have been too low to differentiate the animals; that is, the problems may not have been sufficiently difficult to tax the ability of the bright rats. . . . It might also be suggested that it is relatively more difficult for the bright animals to reduce their error scores, say from 120 to 100, than for the dull animals to reduce theirs from 160 to 140" (p. 162).

4. The most serious problem with the study is one of cross-species generalizability. It would be difficult to find such pure genotypes or extreme environmental conditions as obtained in the Cooper and Zubek (1958) study available for human research.

With respect to alcoholism, Cloninger et al. (1981) have reported what appears to be a genuine interaction between genetic predisposition to alcoholism and an alcohologenic environment. However, this finding may be artifactual, as will be demonstrated in a detailed examination of this study below. Although Cadoret, Cain, and Crowe (1983) have reported a significant gene × environment interaction in the development of antisocial behavior which has sometimes been associated with alcohol abuse (Tarter et al., 1985), this same group (Cadoret, O'Gorman, Troughton, & Heywood, 1985) was unable to find any evidence for gene × environment interactions for alcoholism. It should be stressed that current measures of the environment are relatively unsophisticated and undifferentiated compared to measures of phenotypic expression of personality. For example, the "environment" as measured by Cadoret et al. (1985) consisted of dichotomous indicators (present/absent) of rated alcohol, antisocial, or other psychiatric problems of the adoptive parents and siblings as well as gross measures (also dichotomous) of parental health, marital stability, and socioeconomic status, and neighborhood. It may be that with more refined instruments, gene × environment interactions which are intuitively appealing but empirically elusive will be found.

There has been a recent increase in both the theoretical and empirical effort in elucidating meaningful gene × environment interactions. Zucker and his colleagues (Zucker, 1987; Zucker & Lisansky-Gomberg, 1986; Zucker & Noll, 1987) have been active in suggesting and implementing innovative research approaches to assess the impact of gene × environment interactions in the development of alcohol and drug abuse. Bergeman, Plomin, McClearn, Pedersen, and Friberg (1988) recently reported several significant gene × environment interactions gleaned from data on 99 monozygotic (MZ) twin pairs reared apart. Although the effects were relatively small (no single interaction accounted for more than 7% of the total variance) this study is the first scientific account of significant gene × environment interactions. In addition, the mean age of the sample was approximately 59 years providing some important, albeit retrospective, information on the influence of early environments on later personality development.

GENE–ENVIRONMENT CORRELATION

Much more theoretical and research effort has gone into the notion of gene–environment (g–e) correlation (Jensen, 1976; Plomin, 1986; Plomin, DeFries, & Loehlin, 1977; Plomin, Defries, & McClearn, 1980; Scarr & McCartney, 1983). Three distinct types of g–e correlations have been proposed (Plomin, DeFries, & Loehlin, 1977):

1. *Passive.* This refers to the fact that children are exposed to environments that are not independent of their inherited genes. Thus, highly educated, intelligent parents not only provide genetic material but often provide environments for their children that may reflect and promote cognitive development and intellectual activity. Since adoptive families provide only environmental factors and nonadoptive families provide both genetic and environmental factors, it is possible to directly estimate the g–e correlation within a behavior genetic framework given adequate data. Because of data limitations in other traits, only IQ has been subjected to a thorough systematic analysis (Loehlin & DeFries, 1987). Estimates of g–e correlations from existing data bases average about 0.20, a substantial effect. However, a limited analysis from the Colorado Adoption Project (Plomin & DeFries, 1985) yielded a 0.07 passive g–e correlation between infant temperament and environmental factors related to personal growth (Loehlin & DeFries, 1987). Since one focus of current theorizing on the etiology of alcoholism is on early temperament and activity level, this low figure assumes some significance. It would appear that this type of g–e correlation may have much less of an impact on personality development than expected.

2. *Reactive/Evocative.* Individuals react differently to different genotypes. For example, sociable children are responded to differently than shy children, thus creating a g–e correlation (assuming, of course, that sociability has some genetic component). It is possible to measure reactive g–e correlation by assessing the relationship between characteristics of the biological parents with measures of the adoptive home (selective placement effects are assumed to be negligible). Current estimates of reactive g–e correlations in the personality domain are in the 0.15–0.20 range for 7 of 28 correlations found to be significant in the Colorado Adoption Project data (Plomin & Defries, 1985).

3. *Active/Niche-Seeking.* This refers to the notion that individuals will actively seek out environments that complement their genotype. For example, extroverts are likely to engage in sociable activities while introverts are not. To date, no methods of assessing active g–e correlation have been developed. However, this type of g–e correlation can theoretically account for the substantial similarity observed in MZ twins reared apart, including the fact that the most dissimilar pairs were those in which a range of potential environmental influences was not available for one twin.

The importance of g–e correlations is twofold. First, they provide measurement techniques for assessing the combined impact of genetics and environments on phenotypic variance. As long as one does not subscribe to an extreme interactionist position in which genetic and environmental influences are inextricably interwoven, genetic, environmental, and g–e correlated influences can be independently measured and their relative impact assessed.

Second, they fit a general model of development described by Scarr and McCartney (1983). Passive g–e correlation is of major significance during infancy, because parents are the providers of both the infant's genes and a major proportion of its environment. As the child matures, this form of g–e correlation becomes less influential, and reactive and active forms predominate, with active g–e correlations assuming lifelong importance. This model parsimoniously accounts for some intriguing observations from extant data such as:

1. Higher than expected dizygotic (DZ) twin correlations in early childhood.
2. The moderate adoptive sibling correlations in childhood that reduce to zero in late adolescence.
3. The above-mentioned similarity of MZ twins reared apart.

No one to date has considered the implications of g–e correlations for the etiology of alcoholism. There are several ways in which the impact of g–e correlations could be significant.

Passive g–e correlation could have a direct effect through the infant's ingestion of ethanol in the mother's milk. Certain genotypes may be more susceptible than others to the effects of alcohol. Also, an alcoholic mother may provide a hostile intrauterine environment before birth that can result in serious medical complications for the infant, such as fetal alcohol syndrome (FAS). While this could be construed as primarily a congenital effect, particular genotypes may be more vulnerable than others to the effects of alcohol.

If alcohol abuse/dependence is associated with personality traits, and there is some evidence that at least primary alcoholism may be (Cadoret et al., 1984; Tarter et al., 1986), then reactive g–e correlations could have an indirect effect through personality. Impulsive, extroverted children will certainly be reacted to differently than those who are controlled and shy. For example, they are likely to differ on the degree and extent of peer relationships, which may have a substantial influence on early drinking decisions (Kandel, 1984). This notion also applies to the active form of g–e correlation where individuals choose their environments partly as a function of their genetic predispositions.

Some of the g–e correlations associated with alcoholism are likely to be negative, particularly the active form (Cattell, 1982). That is, being exposed to an alcoholic environment may result in an active selection of environments that avoid or preclude alcohol-related properties. In the passive sense, one parent may make special efforts to structure children's environments that emphasize sobriety if the other is an alcoholic. The idea of negative, compensatory g–e correlation has received little research attention in general, and none specific to the development of alcoholism.

These explications of gene × environment interaction and g–e correlation imply that they are quantifiable variance components that can be specified, estimated, and tested in behavior genetic analyses. Naturally, this assumes that these components are, in fact, extricable from the proper data—an assumption that remains controversial despite the increasing sophistication of behavior genetic techniques (Lewontin et al., 1983; Wilson, 1978).

BEHAVIOR GENETIC RESEARCH METHODS: RESULTS FROM SIGNIFICANT STUDIES

Several methods are available for behavior genetic research, each differing in its level of complexity, cost, and yield of appropriate data. The simplest and least costly design is the family or consanguinity study. If genetic factors are important, then the greater the degree of genetic overlap, the stronger the expected relationship. For example, if alcoholism is influenced by genetic factors, then identical twins should be significantly more concordant than DZ twins, who should be as concordant as siblings, who, in turn, should be more concordant than first cousins, and so on. Winokur, Reich, Rimmer, and Pitts (1970) found this relationship in first-degree relatives of male alcoholics but not females. However, in this type of design, genetic and environmental effects are confounded because there is typically a high correlation between the degree of genetic relatedness and the extent of environmental similarity.

The study of half siblings is another method available to behavior genetic researchers. Half sibs of alcoholics share one parent and allow for some interesting comparisons between half sibs who share or do not share an alcoholic biological parent and between half sibs who share or do not share an alcoholic foster parent. To date, the only study that has employed the half sibling methodology found that half sibs who share an alcoholic parent had a higher incidence of alcoholism, regardless of the rearing environment (Schuckit, Goodwin, & Winokur, 1972). That is, there was no increased incidence in half sibs reared by an alcoholic foster parent if they did not have an alcoholic biological parent. Half sibling research presents some serious methodological challenges in separating environmental and genetic effects and has been supplanted by the more methodologically rigorous adoption design. However, this population has been underutilized in behavior genetic analyses of the etiology of alcoholism, especially with regard to investigating nonshared environmental effects.

Twin Studies

Monozygotic (MZ; identical) and dizygotic (DZ; fraternal) twins present a unique opportunity to study individuals who are genetically 100% identical (MZ) compared to those who are, on the average, 50% genetically similar (DZ). This method assumes that both types of twins have equally variable environments. Although this assumption has been questioned (Kamin, 1974; Lewontin et al., 1983), it has been empirically tested and found to be valid (Rowe, 1983; Scarr & Carter-Saltzman, 1979). In any case, even if MZ twins have more similar environments, it must be demonstrated that this would lead to behavioral differences between MZs and DZs. Loehlin and Nichols (1976) examined this question and found that differences in environmental treatment were uncorrelated with personality differences in the two types of twins.

Heritability (h^2) can be directly estimated from twin data as twice the difference between the intraclass correlations of MZ and DZ twins [$h^2 = 2(r_{MZ} - r_{DZ})$] (Falconer, 1960). Although there are other methods available, Falconer's (1960) approach seems to operate well under a wide range of conditions (Plomin, 1986). However, this estimate of h^2 assumes only additive effects and will be biased to the extent that such things as assortative mating (will lead to an underestimate) and dominance (will lead to an overestimate) are operating, as well as the effects of gene × environment interactions and g–e correlations.

Although the methods and assumptions are straightforward, the results across numerous twin studies are not consistent, either in determining the relative contribution of genes and environment or the size of the effects in relation to alcohol use and abuse. Some studies show a substantial genetic effect (Hrubec & Omenn, 1981; Kaij, 1960), some show little effect (Gurling, Clifford, & Murray, 1981; Gurling, Oppenheim, & Murray, 1984), and others are equivocal (Jardine & Martin, 1984). Problems of zygosity determination, reliability of the measures, and young age of most of the twin samples have tended to obscure results with respect to the etiology of alcoholism. More importantly, some of the studies focus on normal social drinking (e.g. Jardine & Martin, 1984) while others look specifically at alcoholism. Since alcoholism and alcohol use may not be on the same continuous dimension and therefore may not share a common genetic mechanism, the results of these studies may have very different implications. Two twin studies (Hrubek & Omenn, 1981; Loehlin & Nichols, 1976) which represent a broad range of age and pathology have been selected for closer attention.

Hrubek and Omenn (1981) examined the medical histories of 15,924 male twin pairs (5,932 MZ pairs, 7,554 DZ pairs, and 2,438 zygosity unknown pairs) in the National Academy of Sciences—National Research Council Twin Registry for alcoholism or alcohol-related diagnoses (e.g., liver cirrhosis). These individuals were identified from a larger cohort of 54,000 multiple births recorded in the United States between 1917 and 1927 as those twin pairs who had served in the United States Armed Forces. This study is noteworthy for several reasons:

1. The size of the sample.
2. The substantial effort made to accurately determine zygosity.
3. The relatively objective information obtained (VA medical records).
4. Most importantly, the age range of the sample was 51–61 years at the time of the study so that the majority would have passed through the highest lifetime risk period for alcohol problems.

Heritability for alcoholism in this study was estimated by the Falconer (1960) method as 0.57. When adjusted for ascertainment (50%), this rose to 0.72. This is one of the highest heritabilities obtained in a sample unselected for alcoholism. However, Murray et al. (1983) point out that this figure may be inflated by a higher ascertainment for MZ than for DZ twin pairs.

Loehlin and Nichols (1976) studied twins who were U.S. high school students participating in the National Merit Scholarship Qualifying Test (NMSQT) in 1962. Of 596,241 students who took the test, 1,507 same-sex twin pairs were identified and asked to participate in the study. A total of 850 pairs completed an extensive test battery, including the California Psychological Inventory (CPI) and a 324-item objective behavior inventory (OBI), among other instruments. The final sample consisted of 514 MZ pairs (217 male, 297 female) and 336 DZ pairs (137 male, 199 female). While the sample sizes are impressive, this study is significant for the inclusion of the intraclass correlation coefficients, means, and standard deviations for each of the *items,* as well as the derived scales from the various instruments. Several items on the OBI and the CPI relate to the use or consequences of use of alcohol. Loehlin (1972) had previously presented an analysis of these items, but he reported them for the combined male and female sample rather than by sex. Since males appear to have a significantly greater risk for alcoholism, it would seem appropriate to analyze the sample accordingly. Table 1.1 presents this analysis, as well as the combined sample heritabilities obtained by Loehlin (1972). All values are derived using Falconer's (1960) formula.

As can be seen by inspection of Table 1.1, there are substantial item-by-item differences in the computed heritabilities for males and females

TABLE 1.1 Heritability Estimates from the NMSQT Twin Data

Item	Loehlin's M & F	Males	Females
Had a hangover	(.62)[b]	(.68)	.46
I have never done any heavy drinking[a]	(.54)	.34	(.70)
I have used alcohol excessively[a]	(.36)	(.52)	−.20
Went on the wagon (swore off drinking)	(.36)	(.44)	.24
Had a drink before breakfast or instead of breakfast	(.36)	.30	.04
Became intoxicated	.16	.30	.18
Mixed a cocktail consisting of three or more ingredients	.34	(.62)	.08
Drank in a bar	.20	.18	.14
Drank wine	.18	.30	.08
Drank beer	.10	.06	.20
Drank whisky, gin, or other hard liquor	−.02	−.02	−.02
I would disapprove of anyone's drinking to the point of intoxication at a party[a]	−.04	−.20	.14
Women should not be allowed to drink in cocktail bars[a]	−.36	−.36	−.32

[a]CPI items.
[b]Numbers in parentheses represent estimates that are greater than the intraclass correlation coefficient for MZ twins

which are masked by combining the samples. Heritability estimates in parentheses are those which are greater than the intraclass correlation for MZ twins. This means that the additive model assumed by the Falconer (1960) formula is inadequate. However, the inflated estimates could result from either a more similar shared environment for MZs relative to DZs or nonadditive genetic variance; these data cannot distinguish between the two.

While all of the items mention alcohol, not all of them are implicative of alcoholism or alcohol abuse. In fact, only the first six relate specifically to the construct of alcohol abuse by indicating either excessive consumption or serious consequences of drinking. The next five items relate to normal drinking behavior; and the last two items may be interpreted in several different ways that have little if anything to do with alcoholism. As can be seen in Table 1.2, these groups of items exhibit differential mean heritability estimates that support a genetic component to alcohol abuse and, to a lesser extent, normal drinking behavior, but not the ambiguous items. Both alcohol abuse and normal drinking heritability estimates are substantially greater for males than females, which is consistent with current theoretical and empirical developments (Goodwin, 1985). However, it should be emphasized that this is a sample of teenagers who have yet to pass through the

TABLE 1.2 Mean Heritability Estimates by Relation to Alcohol Abuse

Grouping	M & F	Males	Females
Indicative of problem drinking or alcohol abuse (1–6)	.40	.43	.24
Indicative of normal drinking (7–11)	.16	.23	.09
Not readily interpretable as alcohol items (12–13)	−.20	−.28	−.09

greatest lifetime risk period for alcoholism. Further, adolescent alcohol use may not be predictive of later adult abuse (Temple & Fillmore, 1986).

Both the Hrubek and Omenn (1981) study and the Loehlin and Nichols (1976) data support a model of alcoholism and alcohol abuse that is substantially influenced by genetic factors. Although these two studies focus on two disparate points in drinking careers, they converge on a common result. Nonetheless, the subject selectivity, cohort, and age differences make direct comparisons problematic. A new study using a panel of Vietnam veteran twins has just begun that will investigate both environmental and genetic influences on alcohol and drug abuse (A. T. McLellan, personal communication, September, 1987). The technical and statistical sophistication of the proposed design is impressive and will potentially yield definitive and undoubtedly provocative results.[5]

However, the twin method still does not completely disentangle genetic from environmental effects. It is possible that the inflated heritability estimates presented above are caused *only* by more similar environments experienced by MZ twins. Because of this ambiguity, twin studies have been regarded as suggestive and supportive of a genetic basis for alcoholism, but not confirmatory.

The Adoption Method

The adoption method conceptually permits the assessment of genetic and environmental factors independently. By comparing the relationships of adopted siblings, nonadopted siblings, biological parents, and adoptive parents, the separate effects can be estimated. Genetically dissimilar individuals reared in the same home yield a direct estimate of shared environmental factors, while genetically related individuals reared in uncorrelated environments provide an appraisal of genetic influences. The adoption design theoretically yields the most powerful and convincing evidence of genetic and environmental contributions to any trait or behavior under study. Due to the time and expense of this type of research, there have only been a few studies reported that relate directly to the etiology of alcoholism.

Two groups of researchers have had a profound impact, and the results of their several studies will now be considered in some detail (Cloninger et al., 1981; Goodwin, Schulsinger, Hermansen, Guze, & Winokur, 1973). These studies were all conducted in Scandinavia (Goodwin et al., 1973, in Denmark and Cloninger et al., 1981, in Sweden), because of the availability of extensive centralized medical, criminal, and personal records kept on the entire population. Therefore, these researchers had considerable data on both the biological and adoptive relatives of adoptees. For example, in Sweden all instances of insobriety resulting in legal, family, medical, or personal difficulties are recorded by a Temperance Board. Data of this type are not available in the United States except retrospectively, and, for the most part, by self-report.

Danish Studies

Goodwin et al. (1973) studied 55 sons of individuals hospitalized for alcoholism (85% fathers) and 78 sons of nonalcoholics who were adopted by nonfamily members within the first six weeks of life. At the time of the study, they ranged in age from 23 to 45 years (mean = 30) and differed on only one sociodemographic variable—the rate of divorce of the probands was three times higher than in the controls. Goodwin et al. (1973) found that the probands had a significantly higher rate of psychiatric treatment, psychiatric hospitalization, and symptoms associated with alcohol abuse (hallucinations, loss of control, morning drinking). Most importantly, the rate of alcoholism was almost four times higher in the probands than in the controls (18% vs. 5%). Goodwin et al. (1974) reported that the 55 probands had 30 brothers who were reared by the alcoholic natural parent. The rate of alcoholism in these biological sons of alcoholics reared by the biological parents was virtually the same as the probands. These results were taken to strongly support a genetic basis for alcoholism. In a related study, there was no difference in the rate of alcoholism in adopted out daughters of alcoholics compared to controls or their nonadopted sisters (Goodwin, Schulsinger, Knop, Mednick, & Guze, 1977); also, the incidence of alcoholism in the females was considerably less than in the males.

The studies by Goodwin and his associates suggest *only* a genetic influence in the etiology of alcoholism. They found that even longtime environmental exposure (over 14 years) to an alcoholic parent did not increase the risk of becoming an alcoholic; in fact, there were *no* identifiable home environmental factors that led to an increased or decreased risk for alcoholism. The results of these studies are problematic for sociological theories of alcoholism that might emphasize family structure and dynamics or social learning influences as causal factors in the development of alcoholism.

It should come as no surprise that the studies by Goodwin and his colleagues were responsible for reviving the nature/nurture question with respect to the etiology of alcoholism. However, it is surprising that there has been so little critical comment regarding the methodology and rather startling results. Tolor and Tamerin (1973) voiced some concerns about the original study including a possible genetic bias on the part of the investigators. Goodwin (in Tolor & Tamerin, 1973) responded and suggested a possible antigenetic bias on the part of Tolor and Tamerin (1973). Only one other critical comment could be located which addressed issues other than the small sample size.[6]

Murray et al. (1983) critically examined a large body of evidence that supports a genetic contribution to alcoholism, including the studies conducted by the Goodwin group. Their main concern was the noncontinuity of the genetic influence along a drinking continuum from abstainer to alcoholic. That is, the fourfold increased risk was found only among those diagnosed as alcoholic; the categories of heavy drinking and problem drinking did not exhibit any genetic loading. In fact, those in the control group were classified more often in these two categories than were the probands. Goodwin and his colleagues have also highlighted this finding, as an unusual and possibly significant discovery. This peculiar finding has yet to be replicated. Murray et al. (1983) suggest that the finding may be more artifactual than real. They also point out that the diagnostic criteria for alcoholism may have been overly broad, and if the categories of problem drinker and alcoholic are combined, the genetic effect disappears. Problems in the diagnostic criteria are also evident in the Swedish studies discussed below. There are other problems with the Danish studies:

Nature of the control group. Initially, Goodwin et al. (1973) selected two control groups: individuals who had a biological parent with a psychiatric hospitalization for something other than alcoholism ($n = 28$), and individuals whose biological parents had no record of any psychiatric hospitalization ($n = 50$). However, in the reported analyses these groups were combined in one group ($n = 78$). The comparison between the probands and the controls without any natural parent psychopathology has never been reported.

High rates of foster parent psychopathology. In both the probands and controls, there was an unusually high proportion of foster parent psychopathology: 42% for the probands and 50% for the controls. These unspecified psychopathological problems may have had differential effects on the development of alcoholism in the two groups and cast doubt on the representativeness of the samples.

High proband divorce rate. The rate of divorce among the index cases was three times higher than the controls. Goodwin et al. (1973) suggested that divorce and alcoholism may both be the result of a genetic predisposition. Tolor and Tamerin (1973) pointed out that the multifactorial nature of causes of divorce make this proposition unlikely. In any case, the direction of the effect is not clear. If for some reason other than alcoholism divorce was more likely in the proband group, then the effects of a broken marriage could quite plausibly lead to excessive drinking and alcoholism.

Prenatal environment. While 85% of the alcoholic biological parents were fathers, it could be that those probands who became alcoholic were those with an alcoholic mother and were subject to a hostile intrauterine environment which *congenitally* influenced their later alcoholism. The proportion of the probands who had alcoholic mothers has never been reported.

An earlier adoption study by Roe and Burks (1945) reported that children of alcoholics did not show an increased risk of alcoholism compared to controls. This study has been criticized by Goodwin et al. (1973) and others for inaccurate parental diagnosis, unspecified subject selection methods, and the questionable comparability of the control group. The concerns outlined above for the Goodwin studies seem equally problematic for drawing unequivocal conclusions about the relative influences of genetic and environmental factors.

An interesting alternative explanation for the similar rate of alcoholism in adopted-away males and their nonadopted brothers suggests that it could be the result of a negative g–e correlation. In the passive form, the nonalcoholic spouse may have structured the environment in such a way as to discourage alcohol use and abuse by the child. In the active sense, the individual himself may have selected environments that discouraged or precluded abusing alcohol in response to the alcoholism of his parent. Either one of these scenerios would result in a suppression of the rate of alcoholism in the nonadopted brothers.[7]

Finally, although a follow-up to this highly influential study would seem appropriate, no such report has been published. It would be particularly important since the mean age of the males in the initial study was too young to assess a lifetime risk for alcoholism.

Swedish Studies

The most analytically sophisticated adoption study thus far has been reported by Cloninger and his colleagues (Bohman, Sigvardsson, & Cloninger, 1981; Cloninger et al., 1981) from data gathered in Sweden on 862 men and 913 women adopted at an early age by nonrelatives. Again, a study such as this is feasible only when extensive records have been maintained on everyone in the population in question. The records available to these researchers were even more complete than those in the Danish studies by Goodwin and associates; and the sample size was considerably larger.

Cloninger et al. (1981) employed a cross-fostering analysis which involved classifying the background of both the biological and adoptive parents by discriminant function analysis as either positively or negatively associated with mild, moderate, severe, or no alcohol abuse in the male adoptees. They identified two distinct types of alcohol abuse which they labeled milieu-limited (Type 1) and male-limited (Type 2). Type 1 was associated with both mild and severe abuse; both a genetic predisposition and postnatal environmental factors were found to influence this type, which was prevalent in 76% of the abusers. Type 2, which was much less prevalent (24%), was associated only with severe alcohol abuse and extensive treatment in the biological fathers, as well as severe criminality in the biological fathers. Heritability of Type 2 abuse was estimated at .90, and relative risks were estimated at 9 for Type 2 and 2 for Type 1.

Bohman et al. (1981) applied the same kind of complex analyses to the sample of 913 female adoptees. Results indicated that daughters of mothers with any alcohol abuse but no paternal alcohol abuse and daughters of mothers with any alcohol abuse and fathers with mild abuse were three times more likely to be alcohol abusers themselves. There was no increased risk associated with a severely abusing father or postnatal environment.

These studies have had a significant impact because they demonstrated several important factors related to the etiology of alcoholism and do so with an adequate sample size:

1. There are multiple pathways to alcohol abuse.
2. Men and women do not exhibit the same patterns of abuse. Daughters of alcoholic mothers are particularly susceptible regardless of the presence of abuse in the fathers.
3. At least one form of alcohol abuse is highly heritable and is found exclusively in males.
4. Environmental factors are significantly associated with the most common type of alcohol abuse.
5. As mentioned earlier, a significant gene × environment interaction is manifest in the Type 1 alcohol abuse for men.

The acceptance of the results of these studies with virtually no critical examination has been remarkable. This may be due to the complex and perhaps intimidating statistical analyses performed on the data. Subsequent publications and reviews, then, usually report only the positive results without reference to methodological and theoretical concerns. While this practice is not restricted to the genetics of alcoholism, this area seems to be a particularly good example of it. The value of these studies may lie more in the methodology proposed (cross-fostering analysis) than in the substantive interpretation of the results.

Close examination of these studies reveals several methodological problems that require an adequate response before the results can be accepted.

1. The prevalence of alcoholism in the United States is estimated at 5% for men and less than 1% for women (Goodwin, 1985). In this sample, 35% of the biological fathers and 6% of the biological mothers were classified as alcohol abusers. Several explanations of this disparity are possible:

a. The prevalence of alcoholism is seven times higher in Sweden than it is in the United States.
b. This particular sample is unrepresentative of the general population in that those willing to adopt out their children may differ in many important aspects, including the rate of alcohol abuse.
c. It may be a function of the loose criteria for alcohol abuse (see 8 below). There is no way to determine this, since the frequencies of mild, moderate, and severe alcohol abusers are only presented for the adoptees and not their parents. However, it is noteworthy that the prevalence among the adoptees for severe abuse is given as 5.9%.

2. The data, while objective in nature, reflect only obvious and reportable instances of the consequences of insobriety. There are no measures of quantity or frequency of drinking or the social and personal consequences of private or unreported drunkenness.

3. There was no nonadopted control group to test for possible idiosyncratic effects of being an adopted child. That is, economic, professional, and a variety of other factors of the natural parents may not be equivalent in shape of distribution, mean, or variability to the general population, which may limit the generalizability of the results. It would be particularly important to control for the effects of differential prenatal environments. This is a problem for most adoption studies but has been taken into account in the Colorado Adoption Project (Plomin & DeFries, 1985).

4. An example of a possible difference in this group as opposed to the general population is the finding of no age effects with regard to risk of alcohol abuse. The sample ranged in age from 23 to 43 years, yet there was no increase in risk as a function of age. This is certainly contrary to epidemiological studies and is particularly noteworthy in view of the identification of a highly heritable type of alcohol abuse found in men. Previous research indicates that this type of alcohol abuse is associated with early onset and severe symptomatology, which is not the case for the Swedish sample. This could mean that the sample is atypical, the data are inadequate, or both. Since the linear relationship between age and diagnosis of alcoholism and the early onset/severe symptoms form of alcoholism is highly reliable, this anomaly in the Swedish study must be addressed.

5. In a sample this large, it is likely that there are unrelated individuals in the same family who vary with respect to their biological history. This type of comparison is one of the main advantages of the adoption study method but was not employed by the Cloninger group. Comparing related

and unrelated individuals in the same family provides a direct estimate of the influence of a shared family environment. Since these researchers have made a point of emphasizing the importance of an environmental contribution, this type of analysis would be of considerable value, especially in further exploring the more common milieu-limited form of alcohol abuse.

6. There is a peculiar ambiguity in the transfer of the results across the male and female samples. The first report (Cloninger et al., 1981) which establishes the two forms of abuse focuses exclusively on the male adoptees. However, in the introduction to the report on the females (Bohman, Sigvardsson, & Cloninger, 1981), the authors state:

> In a recent study of the inheritance of alcoholism in adopted Swedish men, we have identified two types of susceptibility that have distinct genetic and environmental causes. One type affects *both men and women* but is expressed only in particular postnatal environments. The other type of susceptibility is highly heritable from father to son, but mothers of alcoholic sons are seldom alcoholics themselves., (p. 965, emphasis added)

Although the "men and women" mentioned presumably refers to the biological parents of the adoptees, the reference is ambiguous and could be easily interpreted as a reference to the adoptees themselves, in which case the statement is not empirically supportable.

7. The effects of the intrauterine environment are understated, especially for women adoptees. Daughters of alcohol abusing mothers have a threefold increase in risk for alcohol abuse regardless of the abuse status of the biological father, which is consistent with a congenital interpretation. While prenatal effects are acknowledged by Bohman et al. (1981), the results are interpreted in the following manner:

> We have shown that susceptibility to alcoholism in adopted daughters may be inherited from either biological parent but is more often inherited from the mother than from the father. Our findings about adopted women confirm our previous results about adopted men, that there are genetically different types of susceptibility to alcoholism. One type affects both men and women and is usually associated with mild alcohol abuse and minimal criminality. Expression of the other type is limited predominantly to fathers and their sons and is associated with extensive treatment for combined alcohol abuse and criminality. (p. 968)

Also, it should be noted that the association "with extensive treatment for combined alcohol abuse and criminality" is true only for the *fathers* and not the sons. In fact, in this type, alcohol abuse is classified as moderate in the sons and is not associated with criminality in the sons.

8. The most serious problem in the interpretation of the results of these studies is the result of a nonstandard classification or diagnostic system.

The adoptees were classified by the number of times they had been registered with the Temperance Board for insobriety and whether they had ever been in treatment (recommended by the Temperance Board). Those classified as mild abusers had a single registration for abuse and had *never* been treated for alcoholism; moderate abusers had two or three registrations and *no treatment;* and severe abusers had four or more registrations, compulsory treatment for alcoholism, or psychiatric hospitalization with a diagnosis of alcoholism. It is conceptually and empirically difficult to associate abuse with three or less incidents of drunkenness.[8] While it is unlikely that alcoholics are not heavy drinkers, the vast majority of heavy drinkers do not become alcoholics who require treatment. This is even more important when viewed in light of the finding of no age effects. It is quite likely that the obtained results are an artifact of the criteria for abuse. It would be helpful to reanalyze the data with the mild and moderate groups combined. Further, it might be more appropriate to examine only the severe abusers, redefining severity within this subsample. With respect to the female sample, the cross-fostering analysis and conclusions are based on 31 women (3.4% of the sample) who exhibited *any* alcohol abuse, with no specification of severity. It would be of interest to see if there is an equal distribution across the levels of abuse severity for females.

9. However, the combining of the mild and moderate abuse categories would be problematic for these studies, due to the peculiar nature of the obtained types. Type 1 (milieu-limited) categorizes *both* mild and severe abusers, while Type 2 (male-limited) captures the moderate abusers. This unusual classification scheme supports an artifactual interpretation better than a genetic mechanism that would underlie both relatively normal drinking in some cases (mild) and treated alcoholism in others (severe), but not heavy drinking (moderate). In fact, there is no genetic mechanism known that would explain this interpretation of the data.

An alternative method of displaying the data for the 151 adoptees (17.5%) that were classified as alcohol abusers is presented in Table 1.3. This table shows that almost half of the adoptees who were classified as abusers had *neither* a genetic predisposition nor an environmental releasor. Cloninger et al. (1981) investigated an extremely limited set of environmental influences, none of which was directly related to alcohol abuse. Therefore, the causes of alcohol abuse in these cases can probably be found in the environment since there appears to be no genetic linkage. Further, these sporadic cases (i.e., unknown causes) are twice as likely to occur than either genetic or "environmentally" influenced cases, indicating the importance of unidentified environmental influences. Collapsing across the four categories suggests that the main effect of genetics (37.7) is not substantially greater than the main effect of the environment (30.4) despite the narrow scope of the environmental influences described in this study; and

TABLE 1.3 Re-presentation of the Swedish Data For Male Adoptees

Influences		% with any abuse	Mild & moderate	Severe
Genetic	Environmental			
1. N	N	45.0	31.1	13.9
2. N	Y	17.2	13.3	4.0
3. Y	N	24.5	13.3	11.3
4. Y	Y	13.2	8.6	4.6
	Environmental	2. + 4. = 30.4		
	Genetic	3. + 4. = 37.7		

those environmental effects that remain unidentified exert a more powerful influence than either genetic predisposition or the identified environmental variables. It also shows that abuse is least likely if *both* a genetic predisposition and "environmental" factors are operating. Finally, if the mild and moderate categories are combined, the proportion of abusers with genetic and identified environmental influences is identical (13.3). Taken as a whole, this table suggests that environmental pressures, particularly ones that have not been identified, are substantially more important in determining alcohol abuse than are genetic factors.

The limitations of the Swedish studies should preclude premature closure on the genetic and environmental causes of alcoholism. In addition, the "discovery" of two predictable types of alcoholism should be considered, at best, preliminary and, at worst, unfounded. At the very least, these data should be reanalyzed with stricter criteria for abuse.

Other Adoption Studies

Two other adoption studies should be mentioned. Cadoret and his associates have reported on their work at the University of Iowa (Cadoret, Cain, & Grove, 1980; Cadoret & Gath, 1978; Cadoret et al., 1985; Cadoret, Troughton, & O'Gorman, 1987). It should be noted that the Iowa data are not comparable to the Scandinavian data with respect to completeness or accuracy. With limited information on the biological parents, which is typical of adoption studies in the United States, Cadoret's group has found evidence for a genetic factor and an environmental factor, but there was no gene × environment interaction.[9] Unfortunately, Cadoret and his associates rely almost exclusively on odds ratios, which may be misleading for at least two reasons:

1. Very large and impressive sounding odds ratios may not accurately reflect the magnitude of the effect in question. There is no method currently available for assessing effect size associated with odds ratios.

2. Odds ratios represent categorical variables and thus may oversimplify complex processes or overlook subtle, but important, differences. Zucker and Lisansky-Gomberg's (1986) reanalysis of Vaillant's (1983) data emphasizes the masking effect of categorical coding schemes.

Clogg & Eliason (1987) discuss several other general difficulties with log-linear analysis that may be pertinent to the Cadoret studies. Also, Cadoret et al. (1985) present, without explanation, results that indicate that women adoptees with alcoholic first-degree relatives are at greater risk for alcoholism than male adoptees with first-degree alcoholic relatives. This finding is contrary to an entire body of research and is probably an artifact of having only four women identified as definite alcohol abusers. While Cadoret's results are suggestive, they cannot be considered conclusive due to the limitations on the data (e.g., extremely limited secondhand information on the biological father, very high subject attrition, and overly broad diagnostic criteria—see Murray et al., 1983, for a comprehensive critique of the Iowa Adoption Study). In addition, the restrictions of the analytic techniques, as well as several other problems similar to those specified for the Danish and Swedish studies (e.g., no adequate control group, high incidence of psychopathology in the adoptive parents), make unambiguous interpretation of the results problematic.

Perhaps the most ambitious and well-designed adoption study is the Colorado Adoption Project, begun in 1975 (Plomin & DeFries, 1985). Extensive information from behavioral, cognitive, and personality domains is collected from the biological parents, adoptive parents, *and* nonadoptive control parents, as well as the foster home environment. Data are collected on the adoptees, their adoptive families, and the control families at several points in development. Although the initial reports are provocative with respect to cognitive and personality development, the adoptees and controls are still too young for data on alcohol use and/or abuse to be of significance. One interesting finding of a general nature has been that in the cognitive and personality spheres with infants, no evidence of significant g–e correlations have been found. Assuming the study is continuously funded, CAP may eventually provide the most methodologically rigorous test of the genetic and environmental contributions to the etiology of alcoholism.

FAMILY HISTORY AND THE RISK FOR DEVELOPING ALCOHOLISM

An area of considerable recent research interest concerns the identification of individuals with a family history of alcohol abuse or dependence (FH+), but who are not yet alcoholic themselves. They are matched with individuals with no family history of alcohol problems (FH−), but who have similar demographic backgrounds and nonproblematic drinking experience. Both the high risk individuals (FH+) and the controls (FH−) are then subjected to a variety of behavioral, physiological, and psychological tests in the search for presymptomatic trait markers of alcohol abuse. Although these studies are not technically considered behavior genetic in nature since they cannot separate genetic and environmental effects, they are classified as part of the general body of research investigating the genetics of alcoholism. As such, they are included in this review. This domain can be divided into four substantive areas by marker type: biological, neuropsychological, electrophysiological, and psychological.

Biological Markers

Schuckit (1984, 1987; Schuckit & Rayses, 1979) reported that FH+ young men had a significantly elevated level of acetaldehyde in the blood following ethanol ingestion compared to a matched FH− group. However, no differences in blood acetaldehyde concentration were found in a small sample of FH+ and FH− boys (mean age = 12.3 years) with minimal prior exposure to alcohol who had been administered ethanol (Behar, et al., 1983). Results of a number of studies of other potential biochemical markers that attempt to differentiate diagnosed alcoholics and controls have been equivocal and found to be methodologically or practically problematic (Ryback, et al., 1986). No single biological marker has emerged that can reliably differentiate presymptomatic high risk individuals from controls or alcoholics from controls. There is some evidence that a multivariate approach can successfully distinguish alcoholics from controls with a high degree of accuracy, but this strategy has yet to be employed in the high risk design (Ryback et al., 1986).

There appear to be no differences between FH+ and FH− groups on absorption or clearance rates of ethanol, time to peak blood alcohol concentration (BAC), or maximum BAC (Nagoshi & Wilson, 1987; Schuckit, 1981). Although there are demonstrable ethnic differences in biochemical sensitivity and reactions to alcohol (e.g., facial flushing in Orientals: Harada, Agarwal, Goedde, Takagi, & Ishikawa, 1982; Wolff, 1972), no metabolic markers have been shown to distinguish FH+ from FH− groups. Since the most obvious and intuitive genetic mechanism in the transmission of vulnerability to alcoholism would be predictable variation in metabolism of ethanol between FH+ and FH− individuals, the failure to find differences is problematic.

Neuropsychological and Cognitive Markers

Several investigators have reported neuropsychological deficits such as lowered verbal IQ and increased category error scores in offspring of alcoholics compared to controls (Alterman, Bridges, & Tarter, 1985; Drejer,

Thielgaard, Teasdale, Schulsinger, & Goodwin, 1985; Gabrielle & Mednick, 1983; Parsons & Farr, 1981; Tarter, Hegedus, Goldstein, Shelly, & Alterman, 1984). Nagoshi and Wilson (1987) report that FH+ subjects were significantly impaired on two of six cognitive paper and pencil tests compared to controls prior to ethanol dosing. However, the two groups did not differ on these measures following ingestion of alcohol. Workman-Daniels and Hesselbrock (1987) found no differences between FH+ and FH− groups on several neuropsychological tests including Trails A and Trails B, Category Test, Rhythm Test, Tactual Performance Test, and the Wechsler Adult Intelligence Scale from the Halstead battery, as well as the Benton Visual Retention Test and the Wechsler Memory Test. In addition, they found no group differences in the number of childhood hyperkinetic-minimal brain dysfunction symptoms (Hk-MBD), which has been hypothesized as potentially important in the etiology of alcoholism (Tarter, et al., 1985).

None of the research cited above controlled for current level of alcohol consumption, which is positively correlated with category error scores in alcohol abusers. When this and other confounding factors (e.g., age and IQ) are controlled for, the neurocognitive differences between FH+ and FH− groups disappear (Hesselbrock, Stabenau, & Hesselbrock, 1985). Thus, although several studies have reliably identified neuropsychological and cognitive deficits in diagnosed alcoholics, these performance decrements may be a consequence of heavy and prolonged alcohol use rather than a precursor. There is the further complication that neurocognitive deficits in alcoholics may be a function of poor nutrition and/or the increased likelihood of closed-head trauma as a result of falls, physical altercations, and vehicular accidents (Alterman & Tarter, 1985).

Static ataxia (body sway) has been identified as a possible neuropsychological marker for alcoholism, however there have been conflicting reports in the literature as to the extent (yes/no) and under what conditions (eyes open/eyes closed, before alcohol dosing/after dosing) the effect can be demonstrated. Lipscomb, Carpenter, and Nathan (1979), Hegedus, Tarter, Hill, Jacob, and Winsten (1984), Hill, Armstrong, Steinhauer, Baughman, and Zubin (1987), and Lester and Carpenter (1985, cited in Hill et al., 1987) have found in varying degrees an increased body sway in offspring of alcoholics compared to controls. Schuckit (1985) reported no baseline differences between groups, but a significant effect was observed following alcohol ingestion; however, the FH+ group exhibited *less* sway than the FH− group. Nagoshi and Wilson (1987) reported no differences between high and low risk groups at baseline or post-ethanol ingestion for either the eyes open or eyes closed condition. The substantial differences in the results of studies on static ataxia are difficult to reconcile, although disparate subject characteristics (e.g. males vs. females, selection criteria) are a likely contributor (Schuckit, 1985).[10]

Finally, any evaluation of neuropsychological deficits in offspring of alcoholics must consider that these children are six times more likely to suffer physical abuse from their father than offspring of nonalcoholics and seven times more likely to have suffered loss of consciousness at least once as a result of a traumatic head injury (Tarter et al., 1984). Early and repeated blows to the head may have serious neuropsychological consequences associated with being the child of an alcoholic that are independent of any genetic mechanism.

Psychological Markers

The search for presymptomatic personality indicators of alcohol abuse has yielded a voluminous literature but equivocal results. Barnes (1979) reviewed the extant literature and concluded that "past reviewers of an alcoholic personality concept have been correct in noting that the evidence in support of a prealcoholic personality pattern is fairly limited" (p. 623).

Longitudinal studies by Jones (1968, 1971, 1981) found themes of undercontrol and impulsivity in the junior high school ratings of men who eventually became alcoholic; and, although a similar pattern emerged for adolescent females, it was not statistically significant. Most recently, Vaillant (1983) also reported similar but less consequential premorbid personality characteristics for three separate samples of men followed from 10 to 30 years. However, Zucker and Lisansky-Gomberg (1986) reanalyzed Vaillant's data and found that the effects of personality factors and childhood influences were understated by Vaillant, especially with regard to antisocial behavioral tendencies.

High risk studies have found few robust and theoretically meaningful differences between offspring of alcoholics and controls. Tarter et al. (1984) reported that children with alcoholic fathers were significantly more elevated on the neurotic triad (Hysteria, Hypochondriasis, and Depression scales) of the Minnesota Multiphasic Inventory (MMPI), but that both groups scored within the normal range. Schulsinger, Knop, Goodwin, Teasdale, and Mikkelsen (1986) reported that high risk young men were more impulsive, extroverted, and aggressive than matched controls. However, Schuckit (1982, 1983; Morrison & Schuckit, 1983) found no group differences in personality across a number of dimensions including locus of control, trait anxiety, extroversion, and neuroticism. In addition, he found no differences on the clinical scales of the MMPI, but high risk young men scored significantly higher than controls on the MacAndrew Alcoholism Scale, although both groups were in the normal range (Saunders, & Schuckit, 1981).

Schuckit (1985, 1987) has recently emphasized that sons of alcoholics may differ from sons of nonalcoholics in their intensity of subjective reaction to ethanol. Although both groups had similar expectations prior to alcohol dosing, the FH+ group reported feeling significantly less intoxicated than the FH− group following ingestion of a moderate dose of alcohol, even though the groups did not differ on their BAC's; he found the same trend in the data for a higher dose but the differences were not statistically significant. Nagoshi and Wilson (1987), however, found that FH+ subjects were rated as and reported being *more* intoxicated than FH− subjects following a dose similar to Schuckit's high dose. Like Schuckit's subjects, there were no significant differences between groups on the expected level of intoxication prior to receiving alcohol. Although contradictory, the results of the two studies may be reconciled by considering that, while sample sizes were about the same (Nagoshi & Wilson = 35/group; Schuckit = 34/group), Nagoshi and Wilson (1987) used both males and females (16 males and 19 females) and Schuckit (1987) employed only males. Nagoshi and Wilson (1987), however, report that there were no significant sex by family history interactions for any of the intoxication rating measures. Thus, Schuckit's (1987) theory that FH+ individuals have a decreased intensity of reaction to ethanol requires further confirmation.

Electrophysiological Markers

Perhaps the most intriguing and at the same time least understood findings in the high risk literature are the differences between FH+ and FH− groups on certain brain wave patterns. Begleiter, Porjesz, Bihari, and Kissin (1984) have reported that preadolescent sons of alcoholics exhibit a decrease of the P300 wave following presentation of a visual signal. Gabrielli, et al. (1982) reported that sons of alcoholic fathers had electroencephalograms (EEGs) with significantly more relative beta wave activity than did a control group, although this finding was not replicated in another study (Pollock, et al, 1984). In addition, FH+ subjects have been shown to exhibit a decreased P300 wave and slow alpha wave activity subsequent to a small dose of alcohol (Elmasian, Neville, Woods, Schuckit, & Bloom, 1982; Volavka, Pollock, Gabrielli, & Mednick, 1985).

Several competing hypotheses have been proposed to link these results to etiological considerations of alcoholism. Begleiter et al. (1984) suggest that the reduced P300 amplitude could indicate some form of memory impairment which in turn would presumably interfere with an individual's current assessment of behavior. Volavka et al. (1985) hypothesize that the EEG data may conform to a tension reduction theory of alcoholism, while Schuckit (1987) suggests that there may be an association between a decreased ethanol reaction in high risk individuals and brain wave patterns. At this point the data are too tenuous to discriminate between theories of proposed etiological mechanisms or to assess the significance of the findings.

It should be clear from the above discussion that this research approach has not produced consistent empirical findings nor a unified theoretical foundation. Specific study differences such as nonuniform diagnostic criteria (e.g., father alcoholic or any first degree relative alcoholic) and heterogeneity of subjects on such critical variables as age, sex, and socioeconomic background probably contribute substantially to the confusion. The real potential of high risk studies will be realized when subjects in the several longitudinal studies currently underway progress through the age of risk for alcohol problems, and it is determined which set of variables distinguishes those high risk individuals who abuse alcohol from those who remain free of alcohol problems. At this time, there is no articulated link between vulnerability and development of alcoholism. However, data gathered from these studies cannot, in principle, address questions about the causes of alcoholism because genetic and environmental influences are perfectly confounded. High risk studies may be most important in delineating those factors which protect vulnerable individuals from progressing to alcoholism.

DIRECTIONS FOR FUTURE RESEARCH

Although the focus of this chapter is on the genetic transmission of vulnerability to alcoholism, the nature of the critique suggests that environmental influences may have been underemphasized as significant factors in the etiology of alcoholism. Unfortunately, methodologically rigorous studies of environmental influences in the pathogenesis of alcohol abuse have been rare, with longitudinal studies even rarer. Kumpfer and DeMarsh (1986) have suggested several familial factors that may increase a child's risk for alcohol and/or drug abuse such as degree of family conflict, degree of overt modeling of abuse, social isolation, severity of parental neglect, etc. While these factors could have a significant impact on the psychological and emotional development of the child, there are no studies that have systematically linked nongenetic familial influences to adult alcohol abuse despite the intuitive appeal of these social constructs. In fact, those factors that are associated with adolescent problem drinking are uncorrelated with adult drinking status (Temple & Fillmore, 1986), and degree of adolescent alcohol use is not predictive of adult abuse (Donovan, Jessor, & Jessor, 1983).

This suggests several independent but complementary hypotheses that implicitly call for a greater emphasis on individual differences:

1. Genetic influences may have differential developmental (i.e., age related) significance (Plomin, 1986). There are two important ideas embedded in this statement. First, genetic influences can change over

the life course. Second, different genes may control different aspects of the same behavior. For example, social drinking may be under much less or qualitatively different genetic control than alcohol abuse.

2. Unique environmental factors play a major etiologic role (Plomin & Daniels, 1987).
3. G–e correlations (particularly the active sort) are important.
4. Alcohol abuse is the result of some complex function incorporating all of these functions.

This individual difference perspective could provide a more profound understanding of the pathogenesis of alcohol abuse. Future research, then, should recognize not just the relative importance of individuals and environments but also the dynamic aspects of both. Explicit recognition of the importance of the nonstatic nature of the person–environment relationship will necessitate specific methodological improvements and conceptual reformulations, such as:

1. *More refined environmental measurement.* What is termed "environment" in most studies is usually not the complex, multifaceted construct that the word implies. It often is simply what is left after genetic factors are removed, or it reflects overly broad influences of crudely measured variables. For example, in the Swedish adoption studies, four environmental variables were associated with alcohol abuse in the adoptees: reared by biologic mother for more than six months, greater age at time of placement, extent of hospital care prior to placement, and occupational status of the adoptive father. Only the occupational status of the foster father is related to the adoptive home environment. The environmental influences described by Cadoret et al. (1985) have already been discussed. Environments need to be assessed with much greater specificity and precision than is presently being accomplished. The goal of more fine-grained analysis of the environment is to be able to accurately differentiate subtle gene × environment interactions and g–e correlations.

2. *Systematic study of nonshared environmental influences.* Recently, behavior geneticists have begun to stress environmental variables as important factors in cognitive and personality development (see Plomin & Daniels, 1987, for a review of relevant studies). However, this environmental emphasis, for the most part, has not been in the customary sense of regarding home and family as significant socialization agents. In a seminal paper, Rowe & Plomin (1981) discussed two sources of environmental influences. The first, called shared or between-family environment (E_2), acts to make individuals in the same family alike and is most similar to traditional conceptualizations of environment such as common child rearing practices. The second, called nonshared or within-family environment (E_1), acts in such a way as to make family members different from each other and re-

flects those forces that are unique to individual family members. With behavior genetic methods it is possible to estimate the relative influence of these two sources of environmental variance. For example, the correlation of adoptive and nonadoptive children in the same family milieu is a direct estimate of E_2; while 1 minus the intraclass correlation coefficient between MZ twins raised together is an estimate (although an underestimate for nontwins) of sources of variance that make them different from one another (E_1).

Data from both twin and adoption studies suggest that for dimensions of personality the between-family environmental influence is essentially zero (Goldsmith, 1983; Rowe & Plomin, 1981). That is, personality as currently conceptualized and measured appears to be a function of genetic predispositions and nonshared environmental factors. Empirical support for this position is surprisingly compelling. Goldsmith (1983) presents estimates of heritability (h^2), E_1 and E_2 for ten different twin studies of personality. The means across all the studies for all scales are $h^2 = 0.40$, E_2 (shared) = 0.07, E_1 (nonshared) = 0.54. He also reviewed two well-known adoption studies. The mean adoptive sibling correlation for several personality variables was 0.09, which indicates that shared environment has a minimal impact. Studies of infant and childhood temperament, thought to be developmentally related to adult personality (Buss & Plomin, 1984), show a similar pattern. From these data Goldsmith (1983) concludes " . . . common familial environment is not a potent source of similarity in a wide range of personality traits" (p. 341). Rowe and Plomin (1981), after their review of this area, stated: "In other words, whatever environmental variables influence personality—and they are substantial, accounting for half the variance of personality—they are not shared by siblings" (p. 522). Since both temperament and personality factors have been implicated in the etiology of some types of alcoholism, the significance of nonshared environmental influences could be substantial.

It should be noted that inappropriate conceptualization of environmental processes as well as inadequate measurement techniques may account for at least part of the failure to find significant familial environmental influences in the personality domain (Wachs, 1983). Also, direct measurement of nonshared environment has been rare. In most behavior genetic studies to date, E_1 is a residual term that also includes error variance.

3. *Sibling studies.* Because of the potential importance of E_1, multiple members of the same family should be included in future studies. Daniels and Plomin (1985) have developed the Sibling Inventory of Differential Experience (SIDE) to assess nonshared environmental effects. Preliminary reports suggest that the SIDE is environmentally mediated and is sensitive to sibling differences in personality that are a function of E_1 (Daniels, 1986). The inclusion of siblings in high risk studies may be particularly important. Also, with the decreasing availability of adoptees for study as a

result of legal abortion and accessible birth control, half- and step-siblings could be utilized. Although this would require a significant increase over current methodological precision, the improvement in the generalizability of the results may offset the difficulties in solving problems such as variable exposure to environments and degree of genetic overlap.

4. *Long-term prospective longitudinal studies of "at risk" children.* Research that incorporates all the above suggestions, with adequate measurement techniques, and that samples a wide array of factors from the personality, social, and environmental domains would be especially important. Perhaps the most ambitious and significant of the longitudinal studies currently on-going is the Michigan State University Longitudinal Study (Zucker, 1987; Zucker & Noll, 1987). This project identifies and recruits families with very young children (ages 3–6 years) of men convicted of drunk driving in Michigan. Control subjects are recruited from the same neighborhoods as the "high risk" subjects controlling for age, family size, ethnic background, and other important matching variables. An enormous amount of behavioral, psychological, and environmental data is being collected at specified time points throughout the project. The eventual results of this study should provide the best data yet on what factors predict both susceptibility for and vulnerability against developing eventual alcohol problems.

The objective of this selective review is to stimulate even better and more methodologically rigorous studies that focus on the pathogenesis of alcoholism problems. Regardless of their origin, alcohol-related difficulties have a substantial economic impact (Vaillant, 1983), as well as an inestimable social and emotional cost. The early identification of potential alcohol abusers and the eventual amelioration of the deleterious effects of alcoholism may be the result of research in this area.

NOTES

1. While three reviews (four including this one) may seem more like many than few, the nature and content domains of the extant reviews are quite varied. Lester (1988) contributed a somewhat polemical, molecular analysis (and occasional reanalysis) of much of the twin and adoption data, pointing out many significant statistical and computational errors. Murray, Clifford, and Gurling (1983) presented the first substantive published critique of the designs and results of twin and adoption data. Both Lester (1988) and Murray et al. (1983) are chapters in edited volumes; Lester considers his chapter an extension of "the critiques of Cabaniss (1979) and Murray et al. (1983)" (p. 5). Cabaniss (1979) is cited by Lester as an unpublished senior honors thesis from Princeton University. Peele (1986) offered a conceptual critique of genetic models, reevaluat-

ing specific data findings in terms of alternative explanatory paradigms. Searles (1988; this volume) critiqued both the behavior genetic and high risk models and proposed more complex models encompassing gene × environment interactions and gene–environment correlations.

2. The definition offered here is for "broad sense" heritability which includes both additive and nonadditive components. A more restrictive "narrow sense" heritability which includes only additive genetic variance is also computable.

3. Two veterans recently challenged the Veterans Administration policy that alcoholism is a behavioral disorder rather than a medically defined disease. The legal status of the disease concept was thought to be the outcome of the decision rendered by the United States Supreme Court. Genetic studies were offered as evidence supporting the plaintiff's claim that alcoholism is a medical complication as opposed to a behavioral problem (Johnson, 1987). However, the Court upheld the VA on the narrow procedural grounds but did not address the broader question of the disease concept of alcoholism (Taylor, 1988). Subsequent legislation enacted by Congress mandates treatment for alcoholism for veterans regardless of etiological considerations.

4. It should be noted that, in a trivial sense, Lewontin et al. (1983) are correct; that is, behavior never occurs outside some context. The term interaction here is meant in a statistical sense whereby phenotypic expression would be a function of genotypic structure at different measurable levels of the type of environment.

5. Perhaps the most well known of recent twin studies is the Minnesota Study of Twins Reared Apart (Bouchard, 1982). Because of the difficulties involved in identification of potential participants, the sample sizes are relatively small and publication of results from this unique data source has been slow. Media accounts (e.g., *NBC Nightly News* with Tom Brokaw, November 2, 1987) have indicated that strong genetic influences pervade the personality and cognitive domains. Recently, in their first scientific report, this group reported a substantial contribution of genetic factors to personality based on the reared apart twin data (Tellegen et al., 1988; but see Peele, 1983, for a general critique of the methodology of this study). We await reports on alcohol use and abuse.

6. Actually, significant differences found in small samples must be relatively large and robust for them to be detected, since power is an increasing function of sample size. Criticism based on sample size is only appropriate when differences are *not* found.

7. I am indebted to an anonymous reviewer who suggested this intriguing possibility.

8. The Temperance Boards (one for each county) have no American counterpart which makes evaluation of the data difficult. Apparently, instances of alcohol abuse (e.g., family violence, traffic offenses), not just public intoxication, are recorded by the boards. However, the reporting of abuse to the board is not restricted to law enforcement or health professionals. Apparently, an individual's relatives and friends can also report instances of abuse to the board. Since

these persons are likely to have widely varying definitions of alcohol abuse, the situation becomes even more confusing.

9. In this study the null finding of a gene × environment interaction may be due to the small sample size (Cadoret et al., 1985). In a cross-classification analysis, only two subjects could be classified simultaneously as alcoholic with both biologic and adoptive parent alcohol problems.

10. The positive report by Hill et al. (1987) and the negative report by Nagoshi & Wilson (1987) were published in the same issue of the same journal.

REFERENCES

Akiskal, H. S., Hirschfeld, R. M. A., & Yerevanian, B. I. (1983). The relationship of personality to affective disorders. *Archives of General Psychiatry, 40,* 801–810.

Alterman, A. I., Bridges, K. R., & Tarter, R. E. (1985). The influence of both drinking and familial risk statuses on cognitive functioning of social drinkers. *Alcoholism: Clinical and Experimental Research, 10,* 448–451.

Alterman, A. I., & Tarter, R. E. (1985). Assessing the influence of counfounding subject variables in neuropsychological research in alcoholism and related disorders. *International Journal of Neuroscience, 26,* 75–84.

Barnes, G. E. (1979). The alcoholic personality: A reanalysis of the literature. *Journal of Studies on Alcohol, 5,* 41–60.

Begleiter, H., Porjesz, B., Bihari, B., & Kissin, B. (1984). Event-related brain potentials in boys at risk for alcoholism. *Science, 225,* 1493–1496.

Behar, D., Berg, C. J., Rapoport, J. L., Nelson, W., Linnoila, M., Cohen, M., Bozevich, C., & Marshall, T. Behavioral and physiological effects of ethanol in high-risk and control children: A pilot study. *Alcoholism: Clinical and Experimental Research, 7,* 404–410.

Bergeman, C. S., Plomin, R., McClearn, G. E., Pedersen, N. L., & Friberg, L. (1988). Genotype-environment interaction in personality development: Identical twins reared apart. *Psychology and Aging, 3,* 399–406.

Bohman, M., Sigvardsson, S., & Cloninger, C. R. (1981). Maternal inheritance of alcohol abuse: Cross fostering analysis of adopted women. *Archives of General Psychiatry, 38,* 965–969.

Bouchard, T. J. Jr. (1982). Twins reared together and apart: What they tell us about human diversity. In S. W. Fox (Ed.), *Individuality and determinism: Chemical and biological bases* (pp. 147–178). New York: Plenum Press.

Buss, A. H., & Plomin, R. (1984). *Temperament: Early developing personality traits.* Hillsdale, NJ: Erlbaum.

Cadoret, R. J., Cain, C. A., & Crowe, R. R. (1983). Evidence for gene–environment interaction in the development of adolescent antisocial behavior. *Behavior Genetics, 13,* 301–310.

Cadoret, R. J., Cain, C. A. & Grove, W. M. (1980). Development of alcoholism in adoptees raised apart from alcoholic biologic relatives. *Archives of General Psychiatry, 37,* 561–563.

Cadoret, R. J., & Gath, A. (1978). Inheritance of alcoholism in adoptees. *British Journal of Psychiatry, 132,* 252–258.

Cadoret, R. J., O'Gorman, T. W., Troughton, E., & Heywood, E. (1985). Alcoholism and antisocial personality: Interrelationships, genetic and environmental factors. *Archives of General Psychiatry, 42,* 161–167.

Cadoret, R. J., Troughton, E., & O'Gorman, T. W. (1987). Genetic and environmental factors in alcohol abuse and antisocial personality. *Journal of Studies on Alcohol, 48,* 1–8.

Cadoret, R., Troughton, E., & Widmer, R. (1984). Clinical differences between antisocial and primary alcoholics. *Comprehensive Psychiatry, 25,* 1–8.

Cattell, R. B. (1982). *The inheritance of personality and ability.* New York: Academic Press.

Clogg, C. C., & Eliason, S. R. (1987). Some common problems in log-linear analysis. *Sociological Methods & Research, 16,* 8–44.

Cloninger, C. R., Bohman, M., & Sigvardsson, S. (1981). Inheritance of alcohol abuse: Cross fostering analysis of adopted men. *Archives of General Psychiatry, 38,* 861–868.

Cooper, R. M., & Zubek, J. P. (1958). Effects of enriched and restricted early environments on the learning ability of bright and dull rats. *Canadian Journal of Psychology, 12,* 159–164.

Daniels, D. (1986). Differential experiences of siblings in the same family as predictors of adolescent sibling personality differences. *Journal of Personality and Social Psychology, 51,* 339–346.

Daniels, D., & Plomin, R. (1985). Differential experience of siblings in the same family. *Developmental Psychology, 21,* 747–760.

Donovan, J. E., Jessor, R., & Jessor, L. (1983). Problem drinking in adolescence and young adulthood: A follow-up study. *Journal of Studies on Alcohol, 44,* 109–137.

Drejer, K., Theilgaard, A., Teasdale, T. W., Schulsinger, F., & Goodwin, D. W. (1985). A prospective study of young men at high risk for alcoholism: Neuropsychological assessment. *Alcoholism: Clinical and Experimental Research, 9,* 498–502.

Elmasian, R., Neville, H., Woods, D., Schuckit, M. A., & Bloom, F. (1982). Event-related brain potentials are different in individuals at risk for developing alcoholism. *Proceedings of the National Academy of Sciences, 79,* 7900–7903.

Falconer, D. S., (1960). *Introduction to quantitative genetics.* New York: Ronald Press.

Fuller, J. L., & Thompson, W. R. (1960). *Behavior genetics.* New York: Wiley.

Fuller, J. L., & Thompson, W. R. (1978). *Foundations of behavior genetics.* St. Louis: Mosby.

Gabrielli, W. F., & Mednick, S. A. (1983). Intellectual performance in children of alcoholics. *Journal of Nervous and Mental Disease, 171,* 444–447.

Gabrielli, W. F., Mednick, S. A., Volavka, J., Pollack, V. E., Schulsinger, F., & Itil, T. M. (1982). Electroencephalograms in children of alcoholic fathers. *Psychophysiology, 19,* 404–407.

Goldsmith, H. H. (1983). Genetic influences on personality from infancy to adulthood. *Child Development, 54,* 331–355.

Goodwin, D. W. (1976). *Is alcoholism hereditary?* New York: Oxford University Press.

Goodwin, D. W. (1979). Alcoholism and heredity. *Archives of General Psychiatry, 36,* 57–61.

Goodwin, D. W. (1985). Genetic determinants of alcoholism. In J. H. Mendelson & N. K. Mello (Eds.), *The diagnosis and treatment of alcoholism* (pp. 65–88). New York: McGraw-Hill.

Goodwin, D. W., Schulsinger, F., Hermansen, L., Guze, S. B., & Winokur, G. (1973). Alcohol problems in adoptees raised apart from biological parents. *Archives of General Psychiatry, 28,* 238–243.

Goodwin, D. W., Schulsinger, F., Moller, N., Hermansen, L., Winokur, G., & Guze, S. B. (1974). Drinking problems in adopted and nonadopted sons of alcoholics. *Archives of General Psychiatry, 31,* 164–169.

Goodwin, D. W., Schulsinger, F., Knop, J., Mednick, S., and Guze, S. B. (1977). Alcoholism and depression in adopted out daughters of alcoholics. *Archives of General Psychiatry, 34,* 751–755.

Gurling, H. M. D., Clifford, C. A., & Murray, R. M. (1981). Genetic contributions to alcohol dependence and its effect on brain function. In L. Gedda, P. Parisi, & W. A. Nance (Eds.), *Twin Research, Vol. 3* (pp. 77–87). New York: Alan R. Liss.

Gurling, H. M. D., Oppenheim, B. E., & Murray, R. M. (1984). Depression, criminality and psychopathology associated with alcoholism: Evidence from a twin study. *Acta Geneticae Medicae et Gemellologiae, 33,* 333–339.

Harada, S., Agarwal, D., Goedde, H., Takagi, S., & Ishikawa, B. (1982). Possible protective role against alcoholism for aldehyde dehydrogenase isozyme deficiency in Japan. *Lancet, ii,* 827.

Hearnshaw, L. S. (1979). *Cyril Burt, psychologist.* Ithaca, NY: Cornell University Press.

Hegedus, A. M., Tarter, R. E., Hill, S. Y., Jacob, T., & Winsten, N. E. (1984). Static ataxia: A possible marker for alcoholism. *Alcoholism: Clinical and Experimental Research, 8,* 580–582.

Henderson, N. D. (1972). Relative effects of early rearing environment on discrimination learning in housemice. *Journal of Comparative and Physiological Psychology, 79,* 243–253.

Hesselbrock, V. M., Stabenau, J. R., & Hesselbrock, M. N. (1985). Minimal brain dysfunction and neuropsychological test performance in offspring of alcoholics. In M. Galanter (Ed.), *Recent developments in alcoholism, Vol. 3* (pp. 65–82). New York: Plenum Press.

Hill, S. Y., Armstrong, J., Steinhauer, S. R., Baughman, T., & Zubin, J. (1987). Static ataxia as a psychobiological marker for alcoholism. *Alcoholism: Clinical and Experimental Research, 11,* 345–348.

Hrubec, Z., & Omenn, G. S. (1981). Evidence of genetic predisposition to alcoholic cirrhosis and psychosis: Twin concordance for alcoholism and its biological endpoints by zygosity among male veterans. *Alcoholism: Clinical and Experimental Research, 5,* 207–215.

Jardine, R., & Martin, N. G. (1984). Causes of variation in drinking habits in a large twin sample. *Acta Geneticae Medicae et Gemellologiae, 33,* 435–450.

Jensen, A. R. (1976). The problem of genotype-environment correlation in the estimation of heritability from monozygotic and dizygotic twins. *Acta Geneticae Medicae et Gemellologiae, 25,* 86–99.

Jinks, J. L., & Fulker, D. W. (1970). Comparison of the biometrical genetical, MAVA, and classical approaches to the analysis of human behavior. *Psychological Bulletin, 73,* 311–349.

Johnson, D. (1987, October 25). High court faces alcoholism issue. *The New York Times*, p. 1.

Jones, M. C. (1968). Personality antecedents and correlates of drinking patterns in adult males. *Journal of Consulting and Clinical Psychology, 32,* 2–12.

Jones, M. C. (1971). Personality antecedents and correlates of drinking patterns in women. *Journal of Consulting and Clinical Psychology, 36,* 61–69.

Jones, M. C. (1981). Midlife drinking patterns: Correlates and antecedents. In D. Eichorn, J. Clausen, N. Haan, M. Honzik, & P. Mussen (Eds.), *Present and past in middle life* (pp. 223–242.) New York: Academic Press.

Kaij, L. (1960). *Alcoholism in twins.* Stockholm: Almqvist and Wiksell.

Kamin, L. J. (1974). *The science and politics of IQ.* Potomac, MD: Erlbaum.

Kandel, D. B. (1984). Family and peer processes in adolescent drug use. In S. A. Mednick, M. Harway, & K. M. Finello (Eds.), *Handbook of longitudinal research* (pp. 18–33). New York: Praeger.

Kumpfer, K. L., & DeMarsh, J. (1986). Family environmental and genetic influences on children's future chemical-dependency. In S. Griswold-Ezekoye, K. L. Kumpfer, & W. J. Bukoski (Eds.), *Childhood and chemical abuse: Prevention and intervention* (pp. 49–91). New York: The Haworth Press.

Lester, D. (1988). Genetic theory: An assessment of the heritability of alcoholism. In C. D. Chaudron & D. A. Wilkinson (Eds.), *Theories on alcoholism* (pp. 1–28). Toronto: Addiction Research Foundation.

Lewontin, R. C., Kamin, L. J., & Rose, S. (1983). *Not in our genes.* New York: Pantheon.

Lipscomb, T. R., Carpenter, J. A., & Nathan, P. E. (1979). Static ataxia: a predictor of alcoholism? *British Journal of Addictions, 74,* 289–294.

Loehlin, J. C. (1972). An analysis of alcohol related questionnaire items from the National Merit Twin Study. *Annals of the New York Academy of Sciences, 197,* 117–120.

Loehlin, J. C., & Nichols, R. C. (1976). *Heredity, environment, and personality.* Austin: University of Texas Press.

Loehlin, J. C., & DeFries, J. C. (1987). Genotype–environment correlation and IQ. *Behavior Genetics, 17,* 263–277.

Morrison, C., & Schuckit, M. A. (1983). Locus of control in young men with alcoholic relatives and controls. *Journal of Clinical Psychiatry, 44,* 306–307.

Murray, R. M., Clifford, C. A., & Gurling, H. M. D. (1983). Twin and adoption studies: How good is the evidence for a genetic role? In M. Galanter (Ed.), *Recent developments in alcoholism, Vol. 1* (pp. 25–48). New York: Plenum Press.

Nagoshi, C. T., & Wilson, J. R. (1987). Influence of family alcoholism history on alcohol metabolism, sensitivity, and tolerance. *Alcoholism: Clinical and Experimental Research, 11,* 392–398.

Parsons, O. A., & Farr, S. P. (1981). The neuropsychology of alcohol and drug use. In S. B. Filskov & T. J. Boll (Eds.), *Handbook of clinical neuropsychology* (pp. 320–365). New York: Wiley.

Peele, S. (1983). *A direction for psychology.* Lexington, MA: Lexington Books.

Peele, S. (1986). The implications and limitations of genetic models of alcoholism and other addictions. *Journal of Studies on Alcohol, 47,* 63–71.

Peele, S. (1987). Denial—of reality and freedom—in addiction research and treatment. *Bulletin of the Society of Psychologists in Addictive Behaviors, 5,* 149–166.

Petrakis, P. L. (1985). *Alcoholism: An inherited disease*. Washington, DC: National Institute on Alcohol Abuse and Alcoholism.

Plomin, R. (1986). *Development, genetics, and psychology*. Hillsdale, NJ: Erlbaum.

Plomin, R., & Daniels, D. (1987). Why are children in the same family so different from one another? *Behavioral and Brain Sciences, 10*, 1–60.

Plomin, R., & Defries, J. C. (1985). *Origins of individual differences in infancy: The Colorado Adoption Project*. Orlando: Academic Press.

Plomin, R., DeFries, J. C., & Loehlin, J. C. (1977). Genotype-environment interaction and correlation in the analysis of human behavior. *Psychological Bulletin, 84*, 309–322.

Plomin, R., DeFries, J. C., & McClearn, G. E. (1980). *Behavioral genetics: A primer*. San Francisco: W. H. Freeman.

Pollock, V. E., Volavka, J., Mednick, S. A., Goodwin, D. W., Knop, J., & Schulsinger, F. (1984). A prospective study of alcoholism: Electroencephalographic findings. In D. W. Goodwin, K. T. Van Dusen, & S. A. Mednick (Eds.), *Longitudinal research in alcoholism* (pp. 125–145). Boston: Kluwer-Nijhoff.

Roe, A., & Burks, B. (1945). *Adult adjustment of foster children of alcoholic and psychotic parentage and the influence of the foster home*. No. 3. Memoirs of the Section on Alcohol Studies. New Haven, CT: Yale University Press.

Roizen, R. (1987). The great controlled drinking controversy. In M. Galanter (Ed.), *Recent developments in alcoholism, Vol 5*. New York: Plenum Press.

Rowe, D. C. (1983). A biometrical analysis of family environment: A study of twin and singleton sibling kinships. *Child Development, 54*, 416–423.

Rowe, D. C., & Plomin, R. (1981). The importance of non-shared (E_1) environmental influences in behavioral development. *Developmental Psychology, 17*, 517–531.

Ryback, R. S., Rawlings, R. R., Negron, G. L., Correa-Coronas, R., Cirelli, D., & Chobanian, S. (1986). The effectiveness of biological markers to diagnose alcoholism. *Journal of Drug Issues*, Fall, 1986.

Saunders, G. R., & Schuckit, M. Q. (1981). MMPI scores in young men with alcoholic relatives and controls. *Journal of Nervous and Mental Diseases, 169*, 456–458.

Scarr, S., & Carter-Saltzman, L. (1979). Twin method: Defense of a critical assumption. *Behavior Genetics, 9*, 527–542.

Scarr, S., & McCartney, K. (1983). How people make their own environments: A theory of genotype-environment effects. *Child Development, 54*, 424–435.

Schuckit, M. A. (1973). Alcoholism and sociopathy—diagnostic confusion. *Quarterly Journal of Studies on Alcohol, 34*, 157–164.

Schuckit, M. A. 91981). Peak blood alcohol levels in men at high risk for the future development of alcoholism. *Alcoholism: Clinical and Experimental Research, 5*, 64–66.

Schuckit, M. A. (1982). Anxiety and assertiveness in sons of alcoholics and controls. *Journal of Clinical Psychiatry, 43*, 238–239.

Schuckit, M. A. (1983). Extroversion and neuroticism in young men at higher and lower risk for alcoholism. *American Journal of Psychiatry, 140*, 1223–1224.

Schuckit, M. A. (1984). Prospective markers for alcoholism. In D. W. Goodwin, K. T. Van Dusen, & S. A. Mednick (Eds.) *Longitudinal research in alcoholism* (pp. 147–169). Boston: Kluwer-Nijhoff.

Schuckit, M. A. (1985). Ethanol-induced changes in body sway in men at high alcoholism risk. *Archives of General Psychiatry, 42,* 375–379.

Schuckit, M. A. (1987). Biological vulnerability to alcoholism. *Journal of Consulting and Clinical Psychology, 55,* 301–309.

Schuckit, M. A., Goodwin, D. W., & Winokur, G. (1972). A study of alcoholism in half siblings. *American Journal of Psychiatry, 128,* 1132–1135.

Schuckit, M. A., & Rayses, V. (1979). Ethanol ingestion: Differences in blood acetaldehyde concentrations in relatives of alcoholics and controls. *Science, 203,* 54–55.

Schulsinger, F., Knop, J., Goodwin, D. W., Teasdale, T. W., & Mikkelsen, U. (1986). A prospective study of young men at risk for alcoholism: Social and psychological characteristics. *Archives of General Psychiatry, 43,* 755–760.

Searles, J. S. (1988). The role of genetics in the pathogenesis of alcoholism. *Journal of Abnormal Psychology, 97,* 153–167.

Tarter, R. E., Alterman, A. I., & Edwards, K. L. (1985). Vulnerability to alcoholism in men: A behavior genetic perspective. *Journal of Studies on Alcohol, 46,* 329–356.

Tarter, R. E., Hegedus, A. M., Goldstein, G., Shelly, C., & Alterman, A. I. (1984). Adolescent sons of alcoholics: Neuropsychological and personality characteristics. *Alcoholism: Clinical and Experimental Research, 8,* 216–222.

Taylor, S. Jr. (1988, April 21). VA's denial of benefits upheld. *The New York Times,* p. 27.

Tellegen, A., Lykken, D. T., Bouchard, T. J., Wilcox, K. J., Segal, N., & Rich, S. (1988). Personality similarity in twins reared apart and together. *Journal of Personality and Social Psychology, 54,* 1031–1039.

Temple, M. T., & Fillmore, K. M. (1986). The variability of drinking patterns and problems among young men, age 16–31: A longitudinal study. *The International Journal of the Addictions, 20,* 1585–1620.

Tolor, A., & Tamerin, J. S. (1973). The question of a genetic basis for alcoholism: Comment on the study by Goodwin et al., and a response. *Quarterly Journal of Studies on Alcohol, 34,* 1341–1347.

Vaillant, G. E. (1983). *The natural history of alcoholism.* Cambridge: MA: Harvard University Press.

Volavka, J., Pollock, V., Gabrielli, W. F., & Mednick, S. A. (1985). The EEG in persons at risk for alcoholism. In M. Galanter (Ed.), *Recent developments in alcoholism, Vol. 3* (pp. 21–36). New York: Plenum Press.

Wachs, T. D., (1983). The use and abuse of environment in behavior genetic research. *Child Development, 54,* 416–423.

Weissman, M. M., Merikangas, K. R., John, K., Wickramaratne, P., Prussoff, B. A., & Kidd, K. K. (1986). Family-genetic studies of psychiatric disorders: Developing technologies. *Archives of General Psychiatry, 43,* 1104–1116.

Wilson, E. O. (1978). The attempt to suppress human behavioral genetics. *The Journal of General Education, 29,* 277–287.

Winokur, G., Reich, T., Rimmer, J., & Pitts, F. N. (1970). Alcoholism III: Diagnosis and family psychiatric illness. *Archives of General Psychiatry, 23,* 104–111.

Wolff, P. H. (1972). Ethnic differences in alcohol sensitivity. *Science, 175,* 449–450.

Workman-Daniels, K. L., & Hesselbrock, V. M. (1987). Childhood problem behavior and neuropsychological functioning in persons at risk for alcoholism. *Jour-*

nal of Studies on Alcohol, 48, 187–193.

Zucker, R. A. (1987). The four alcoholisms: A developmental account of the etiologic process. In P. C. Rivers (Ed.), *Alcohol and addictive behaviors* (pp. 27–84). Lincoln, NE: University of Nebraska Press.

Zucker, R. A., & Lisansky-Gomberg, E. S. (1986). Etiology of alcoholism reconsidered: The case for a biopsychosocial process. *American Psychologist, 41,* 783–793.

Zucker, R. A., & Noll, R. B. (1987). The interaction of child and environment in the early development of drug involvement: A far ranging review and a planned early intervention. *Drugs and Society, 2,* 57–97.

2

Genetics of Alcoholism

REMI J. CADORET

Alcohol abuse or dependence is a very common condition, as evidenced by current population surveys which show lifetime rates for the population to be about 14% (Helzer & Prysbeck, 1988). Conditions that are common frequently turn out to be heterogeneous with regard to etiology and course, as exemplified by depression, which is one of the most prevalent psychiatric conditions and which has been shown to be divisible into bipolar and unipolar types, each with different course and etiology. A similar theme of heterogeneity runs through the study of alcoholism and its etiology. There is clinical evidence of heterogeneity from studies of alcoholic populations, as demonstrated by the numerous typologies of drinking behaviors (Babor & Lauerman, 1986), as well as the association of alcoholism with other psychopathology (Alterman & Tartar, 1986). Psychiatric diagnoses other than alcoholism contribute significantly to the clinical heterogeneity of alcoholism. The most common codiagnosis is antisocial personality, followed by abuse of other substances (Helzer & Pryzbeck, 1988). Genetic models of alcoholism should account for these clinical findings.

Evidence for a genetic factor in alcoholism has come from a variety of sources: family studies, twin studies, separation studies involving adoptees or halfsibs, and, finally, the most direct evidence for genetic factor, studies of genetic linkage. These are the classical approaches, but more recent studies have also investigated physiological and biochemical processes hypothesized to be relevant to alcoholism and which have genetic bases. Both twins and adoptees have been studied to estimate the genetic involvement, but because of subject availability more studies involving physiological or biochemical measures have been done with so-called "high risk" subjects—those in whom a genetic factor is highly suspect because of alcoholic parentage, or with pure-bred animal strains. Biochemical and physiological findings in high risk subjects are usually contrasted with low risk subjects matched on appropriate variables such as age, sex, diet, etc. One assumes in such studies that the variables being measured have important genetic components (e.g., presence of an enzyme) though in many cases exposure to alcohol or other environmental factors can significantly alter the variable; for example, liver enzyme changes with exposure to alcohol.

This chapter will outline the current state of research in alcoholism in the classical areas of family studies, separation studies, twin studies, and linkage studies. Because of known genetic factors involved in alcohol metabolism—effect of alcohol on the body and on personality and temperament—these areas will also be briefly reviewed, if only to demonstrate the multiplicity of factors that must be considered in the genetic etiology of clinical alcoholism in humans.

FAMILY STUDIES

Alcoholism clearly runs in families. A summary of family studies of alcoholism by Cotton (1979) demonstrates that alcoholism is higher in relatives of alcoholics when compared to a variety of controls. The familial transmission of alcoholism is not disputed, but the mode of transmission—whether genetic, environmental, or by some gene–environment interaction—is not specified by a family study since genetic and environmental factors are confounded when dealing with families where children are reared with their biologic parents. Twin and separation studies such as half-sib and adoption designs can theoretically distinguish genetic from environmental factors.

However, the family study can be used to uncover factors associated with development of alcoholism even though it may not be possible to assign a genetic or environmental cause to the factors identified in this way. Such factors can be followed up in twin or adoption studies, or their roots further investigated by physiological or biochemical studies. One recent example of this type of family study is a follow-up by McCord of men born of alcoholic fathers compared to men whose fathers were not alcoholic (McCord, 1988). The results, as with most family studies, showed that rates of alcoholism were greater in subjects having alcoholic fathers, but that in addition mothers who held the alcoholic fathers in high esteem, who exercised little parental control, or covertly accepted alcoholism also increased the rates of their sons' alcoholism.

A recent development in family studies of alcoholics has been the recognition of the importance of other psychiatric conditions in the etiology of alcoholism, with antisocial personality the most important of these conditions. It has been known for years that antisocial personality is associated with adult alcoholism (Robins, 1966), and its diagnosis has been investigated increasingly in clinical and family studies of alcoholism. The presence of antisocial personality diagnosis is associated with an earlier age of onset of drinking, earlier age of regular drinking, and earlier age of onset of problem drinking (Hesselbrock, Hesselbrock, & Stabenau, 1985). Family studies suggest that alcoholism and antisocial personality are separately and independently inherited (Lewis, Rice, & Helzer, 1983; Vaillant, 1983)—a finding that has been confirmed in the Iowa adoption study of alcoholism (see below) where adoptee adult antisocial personality was predicted by antisocial biologic parental behavior.

Family studies have given rise to the categorization of alcoholism as familial or nonfamilial (Goodwin, 1984). Familial alcoholism, identified with a genetic influence, is supposedly characterized by earlier onset of alcoholism, more severe symptoms at an earlier age, and a worse prognosis than nonfamilial (Goodwin, 1984; Latcham, 1985). However, some studies suggest that some of these differences might be due to the inclusion in the family history positive group of individuals with antisocial background and behavior (Cook & Winokur, 1985; Latcham, 1985). A recent study (Alterman, 1988) questions the value of dichotomizing families by presence or absence of alcoholism in relatives in view of the fact that in their study an antisocial diagnosis or other characterologic disorder was more apparent with increased familial alcoholism. This finding suggests a character spectrum hypothesis disorder of alcoholism or an independent genetic transmission of the characterologic diathesis.

There is a large literature which examines the psychosocial functioning of children of alcoholics (Johnson, 1987; Russell, Henderson, & Blume, 1984). These studies typically involve a comparison of alcoholics' offspring with an appropriate control—usually a child from a family without alcoholism. Some representative recent studies have found: high risk offspring report more family disruptions and are characterized by poor verbal ability and impulsive behavior (Schulsinger, Knop, Goodwin, Teasdale, & Mikkelson, 1986) as well as a more interrupted school career (Knop, 1985; Knop, Teasdale, Schulsinger, & Goodwin, 1985); higher dependent drinking in high risk children, especially if from a low social status occupation (Parker & Harford, 1987); increased rate of divorce in high risk sons and daughters and increased depression in daughters (Parker & Harford, 1988); increased self-reported alcohol, drug, and eating problems in high risk college-age children (Clayton, 1987); increased avoidant coping behaviors such as drinking, eating, and smoking in high risk young adults (Clair & Genest, 1987).

These more recent family studies have focused upon the children of alcoholics, their adjustment and behaviors, and to some extent their social environment. The findings suggest potential behaviors or traits for use in marker studies. They further suggest other psychopathology of importance in predicting alcoholism, such as conduct disorder or hyperactivity. The studies also take into account other conditions such as antisocial personality, which not only colors the clinical appearance of alcoholism but could well be an additional familial or genetic factor in alcoholism.

SEPARATION OR ADOPTION STUDIES

Although alcoholism's familial transmission has been known for years it was only recently that a separation study demonstrated that alcoholism might have genetic roots. In a separation design children are generally reared by adoptive parents. The power of separation studies lies in their ability to separate genetic from environmental factors and to measure gene–environment interaction. The adoption model is the most powerful for these purposes (Cadoret, 1986).

In 1945, Roe published an adoption study of inheritance of alcoholism, with negative findings for a genetic etiology. She followed up as adults 61 foster children, 36 of whom came from alcoholic parentage. At the time of follow-up, the adoptees ranged in age from 22 to 40 years. Approximately 7% of the adult adoptees of alcoholic parents drank "regularly," as opposed to 9% of the controls. There were no alcoholics in either group. It was further noted that, as adolescents, 2 of the 21 boys in the alcohol parent group had been in trouble for drinking too much, while 1 of 11 boys in the normal parent group had had a similar adolescent drinking problem. Again the difference is nonsignificant. There is no obvious explanation for this result.

The first separation study to suggest a genetic etiology to alcoholism was a half-sib design reported by Schuckit, Goodwin, and Winokur (1972). They followed up children of alcoholic probands, including comparisons of full and half-sibling offspring, and found that risk for alcoholism was increased by having an alcoholic biologic parent but *not* by having an alcoholic parenting figure (usually stepfather) in the home. This finding stimulated further adoption studies of alcoholism. Three such studies have appeared since the half-sib study of Schuckit et al. and will be reviewed here in detail.

THE DANISH ADOPTION STUDIES

Goodwin and collaborators (Goodwin, Schulsinger, Hermansen, Guze, & Winokur, 1973) have gathered data on adopted away sons and daughters of alcoholics, using information from centralized Danish registers for adoption, for law enforcement, and for psychiatric hospitalization. The sample was a pool of 5,483 adoptions (by nonrelatives) in Copenhagen city and county from 1924 through 1947. In the study of male adoptees, probands were selected whose biologic parent had been hospitalized for alcoholism. These adoptees had been separated within six weeks of birth from biologic parents and were matched by age and sex with two control groups: in one group none of the controls had a biologic parent with a record of psychiatric hospitalization; in the second control group one biologic parent had

TABLE 2.1. Alcohol Abuse in Adoptees Separated by Study Site, Sex of Adoptee, and Biologic Background

Study site	Parent abuser		Parent nonabuser		Odds ratio diff.
	N	No./% abuse	N	No./% abuse	
		Male adoptee			
Denmark	55	10/18%	78	4/5%	4.1[a]
Stockholm	291	67/23%	571	84/14.7%	1.7[b]
Iowa					
ICFS	6	4/67%	127	27/21%	7.4[b]
LSS	16	10/63%	92	21/23%	5.6[b]
Total Iowa	22	14/64%	219	48/22%	6.2[b]
		Female adoptee			
Denmark	49	2/4%	47	2/4%	0.96NS
Stockholm	336	15/4.5%	577	16/2.8	1.6NS
Iowa					
ICFS	7	1/14%	112	5/4%	3.6NS
LSS	11	4/36%	72	4/6%	9.7[b]
Total Iowa	18	5/28%	184	9/5%	7.5[b]

[a] 5% level significance probands vs. control adoptees.
[b] 1% level significance probands vs. control adoptees.

been hospitalized for a psychiatric condition other than alcoholism, such as depression or character disorder. The probands were personally interviewed by a psychiatrist who had no knowledge of their biologic background. The two control groups were pooled for the analysis. Alcoholism was defined as heavy drinking plus the presence of three of the following four groups of symptoms: (1) trouble with friends or family, (2) job or legal trouble, (3) physical symptoms due to alcohol, and (4) loss of control.

Results for the males, shown in Table 2.1, demonstrate a significant increase in alcoholism between the proband group and the two pooled control groups. Foster home experience, such as psychiatric conditions and socioeconomic levels of the adoptive parents, were similar in the proband and control groups. Heavy drinking by itself in adoptees did not correlate with alcoholic biologic parents, only the presence of clinically defined alcoholism.

Environmental Factors and Alcohol Abuse

In the study cited above, foster home experience was similar for both proband and control adoptees. This included the presence of possible or definite alcoholism in adoptive fathers (13% of probands' fathers vs. 22%

of control). A further study by Goodwin et al. (1974) was designed to detect any environmental effect. Twenty adoptees with an alcoholic background (from the sample described above), separated at birth, had 30 biologic brothers who were reared by the biologic parents. Each brother thus had in common an alcoholic parent, but one had been separated early in life from the biologic home. Both adoptee groups had similar rates of alcoholism: 25% in the adopted away group versus 17% in the nonadopted brothers—a nonsignificant difference. The authors concluded that "environmental factors contributed little, if anything, to the development of alcoholism in sons of severe alcoholics, in this sample" (p. 164). No analyses were published with regard to gene–environment interaction in the etiology of alcohol abuse.

Relationship of Alcohol Abuse to Other Psychopathology

In the first study cited of 55 probands and 78 controls (Goodwin, Schulsinger, Hermansen, Guze, & Winokur, 1975) the incidence of depression and sociopathy, drug abuse, and anxiety neurosis were similar in the two adoptee groups. One later study of retrospectively obtained information from the adoptees indicated an increase in childhood hyperactivity symptoms in those adoptees who as adults were diagnosed alcoholic (Goodwin et al., 1975).

Alcohol Abuse in Females

Adopted away daughters of alcoholics (Goodwin, Schulsinger, Knop, Mednick, & Guze, 1977) were compared to adopted away daughters of controls but no differences were found in alcoholism or problem drinking (see Table 2.1). In a further study Goodwin and collaborators studied nonadopted daughters of alcoholics and found similar rates of alcoholism in the nonadopted daughters, which led to the conclusion that exposure to alcoholism in the environment did not increase the rate of alcoholism (Goodwin, Schulsinger, Knop, Mednick, & Guze, 1979).

With regard to associated psychopathology, however, these investigators noted that the nonadopted daughters of alcoholics had higher rates of depression than the control daughters (27% vs. 7%; $p < .02$).

The Danish studies were the first to show a genetic factor in adult alcoholism. Their failure to find a correlation with heavy drinking (Goodwin et al., 1973) has been interpreted by some to mean that only pathological alcohol intake is inherited, but this conclusion is not warranted in view of the rather small sample of adoptees (and the possibility of missing a true difference) and the fact that more recent studies of twins (see below) have shown evidence for genetic factors in control of drinking behavior in general and not just extremes of such behavior.

THE STOCKHOLM ADOPTION STUDY

This adoption study has been widely reported. The main sources of data for the following discussion are Cloninger, Bohman, and Sigvardsson (1981), Bohman, Sigvardsson, and Cloninger (1981), and Cloninger, Bohman, Sigvardsson, and von Knorring (1985).

The population for this study consisted of 2,324 persons born out of wedlock in Stockholm, Sweden from 1930 to 1949. Subjects were excluded if adopted by relatives (109), if placement in permanent adoptive home occurred after 3 years of age (105), or if the biologic father was unidentified (335), leaving 862 adopted men and 913 adopted women in the final pool. The adoptees ranged in age from 23 to 43 years of age at the time of data collection. Data about alcohol abuse, criminality, social and medical history were obtained for adoptees and their biologic and adoptive parents from the Swedish Temperance Boards, Criminal Boards, and the National Health Insurance Board. Diagnosis of alcohol abuse was based upon hospital records when available but mainly on registration with Temperance Boards.

Most of the adoptees (88%) were separated from biologic parents at birth or before six months of age, and were placed in permanent adoptive homes which represented a restricted range of environments; for example, only 3.3% of adoptive parents were alcoholic in contrast to 16% at risk in the general population and 35% in the biologic parents.

Genetic Factors Predisposing to Alcohol Abuse

The group of adopted away sons of alcoholics had a significantly increased number of alcohol abusers compared to sons of nonalcoholics (Table 2.1). Daughters of alcoholics showed a nonsignificant increase in alcohol abuse when compared to controls (Table 2.1) but daughters of alcoholic mothers included significantly higher numbers of alcohol abusers than controls (9.8% vs. 2.8%). These findings led the investigators to analyze separately families in which only men develop alcoholism and families wherein alcohol abuse occurred in both sexes (see next section).

Gene–Environment Interaction

Low occupational status was a risk factor for alcohol abuse in both sons and daughters. Other environmental variables were found to relate to alcohol abuse only in association with certain genetic backgrounds, and will be discussed below.

The investigators used a novel approach in the detection and analysis of gene–environment interaction. They subdivided the adult adoptee alcohol abusers into three different categories of severity according to number of

Temperance Board registrations and whether the individual had been treated or not. A discriminant analysis was then performed to determine if the groups of adoptees divided by abuse severity had distinctive predictive genetic factors, environmental factors, or a combination of genetic with environmental factors. The investigators' interpretation of the results of this analysis for genetic factors suggested that mild and severe adoptee alcohol abuse had similar biologic backgrounds in contrast to those exhibiting moderate abuse patterns (Table 1 in Cloninger et al., 1981). A similar analysis of a limited set of postnatal environmental factors also found significant differences in predictors of the degree of severity of alcohol abuse. On the bases of these analyses of genetic and environmental factors further analyses were undertaken in an attempt to demonstrate a gene–environment interaction.

Genetic backgrounds (determined from the discriminant analysis) characteristic of each severity group were combined with the environmental factors for that group and tested for their ability to predict alcohol abuse of that grade of severity. Results are shown in Table 2.2 for both mild and severe abusers. The similarity of these two patterns of abuse, with marked increase occurring only in the situation where environmental variables were present with genetic background, led the investigators to hypothesize that mild and severe alcohol abuse represented one type of alcoholism mediated by genetic *and* environmental factors. This is in contrast to the findings in Table 2.3 for moderate abuse where genetic factors alone accounted for the outcome. The difference in patterns shown in Tables 2.2 and 2.3 led the investigators to hypothesize two types of alcohol abuse: Type I (represented in Table 2.2) called milieu limited because both congenital diathesis and postnatal provocation were necessary for expression; and Type II (represented in Table 2.3), male limited, wherein alcohol abuse was increased by the presence of a genetic diathesis regardless of postnatal environment. This type of alcohol abuse was almost entirely confined to the males, hence its name.

TABLE 2.2. Stockholm Adoption Study. Gene–Environment Interaction Found in Type I Alcoholism

Genetic background	Environmental background	% Adoptees with	
		Mild abuse	Severe abuse
Mild	Mild	6.7	4.3
Mild	Severe	5.6	4.2
Severe	Mild	6.5	6.7
Severe	Severe	15.4[a]	11.5[b]

[a] Significantly different from other 3 categories at 1% level.
[b] Significantly different from other 3 categories at 1% level.

TABLE 2.3. Stockholm Adoption Study. Gene–Environment Interaction for Type II Alcoholism

Genetic background moderate	Environmental background moderate	% Adoptees with moderate abuse
No	No	1.9
No	No	4.1
Yes	No	16.9[a]
Yes	Yes	17.9[a]

[a] Significantly different from first two categories at 1% level.

Further characteristics distinguishing these two types was the finding of an excess of daughters in Type II families with somatoform disorders, and differences between the Type I and Type II families in the kinds of environmental factors associated with increased alcohol abuse. These environmental factor differences are shown in Table 2.4.

The investigators also investigated the effect of having an alcoholic adoptive parent and found that the presence of this factor did not increase the risk of adoptee alcohol abuse of any severity.

Relationship of Alcohol Abuse to Other Conditions

Criminality is often associated with alcohol abuse, and the Stockholm Adoption Study showed a high correlation between severity of abuse in adoptees and increased risk of criminality ($r = .61$, $p < .001$). However, criminality only in the biologic parents tended to increase risk of adopted away sons' criminality but *not* to increase their risk for alcohol abuse (Bohman et al., 1982). On the other hand, alcohol abuse only in the biologic parents significantly increased the risk in sons of alcohol abuse only but *not* criminality. Biologic parents with both criminality and alcohol abuse had sons with a significant increase in rate of alcohol abuse but only a nonsig-

TABLE 2.4. Environmental Factors Associated with Increase in Types of Alcohol Abuse

Type I		Type II
Mild	Severe	Moderate
Increased incidence of rearing by biologic mother— longer than 6 months	Increased extent of hospital care prior to adoptive placement	Higher age at final placement
Lower age of final placement	Lower occupational Status of adoptive father	Decreased extent of hospital care prior to adoptive placement

nificant increase in criminality rate. These findings suggested that predisposition to alcohol abuse and criminality were independently inherited.

Depression did not appear to be increased in biologic parents of alcoholics versus controls, nor did substance abuse appear to be higher in biologic parents of adoptees who had depression. Correlation of depression with alcohol abuse in adoptees was not reported.

Alcohol Abuse in Females

As shown in Table 2.1, overall correlation of alcohol abuse in women adoptees with biologic parent alcohol abuse was positive but not quite significant. Women are hypothesized to be affected by a form of abuse occurring in *both* men and women and characterized by mild alcohol abuse and minimal criminality (Type I, see Table 2.2). However, the pattern of Type I gene–environment interaction shown in Table 2.2 was not found in the females.

FURTHER CLINICAL STUDIES TO CONFIRM THE EXISTENCE OF TWO TYPES OF ALCOHOLISM

One of the limitations of the Stockholm data is the fact that the rather complex analyses described above were done on the entire data set. There were no independent adoption data by which to confirm the finding of two distinct types of alcoholism. However, the investigators have continued to look for other types of independent confirmation of the main finding of two types of alcoholism. One approach has involved selecting alcoholic probands, determining their "type" by clinical history (e.g., Type II earlier onset alcohol abuse and more social complications) and then finding evidence of further heterogeneity such as a biochemical finding of different platelet serotonin levels (von Knorring, Bohman, von Knorring, & Oreland, 1985) or personality trait differences (von Knorring, von Knorring, & Smigan, 1987). Another approach has been to study families of alcoholics and show that Type I and II alcoholics exhibit different patterns of inheritance (Gilligan, Reich, & Cloninger, 1987). Whether these biochemical, personality trait, and family differences can be independently confirmed remains to be seen. Most recently the Swedish investigators have suggested that Type II alcoholism is similar to antisocial alcoholism (von Knorring et al., 1987).

THE IOWA ADOPTION STUDIES

Beginning in 1974 and continuing to the present, Cadoret and collaborators have conducted adoption studies which have followed up, as adults, adoptees who were separated at birth from their biologic parents. These studies started by examining adoption agency records and selecting proband adoptees from biologic backgrounds of varying psychopathology ranging from alcohol problems to depression and criminality. Control adoptees without evidence of biologic parent psychopathology were selected from the same adoption agencies and matched to the probands by age, sex, and age of biologic mother. Adult adoptees (18 years or older) were assessed using a personally administered structured psychiatric interview. Adoptive parents were also personally interviewed to determine adoptee development, adoptee school performance, and aspects of the adoptive home environment. To date, data from two private Iowa statewide adoption agencies, Iowa Children's and Family Services (ICFS) and Lutheran Social Services (LSS), have been collected and analyzed for genetic and environmental factors relevant to the development of alcoholism as well as associated psychopathology such as depression and antisocial personality (Cadoret, O'Gorman, Troughton, & Heywood, 1985; Cadoret, Troughton, & O'Gorman, 1987). Interviews of adoptees and adoptive parents were carried out by individuals blind to the biologic parent background.

Proband adoptees were selected on the basis of evidence of psychopathology in biologic parents found in adoption agency records. Definite alcohol problems in biologic parents were defined as heavy drinking plus one or more social, police, employment, or medical problems due to drinking, including hospitalization for detoxification and treatment of alcoholism. Possible alcohol problems in parents usually meant the individual was described as a heavy drinker or drinking too much for his or her own good. Antisocial behavior in a biologic parent was defined as one or more behaviors such as truancy, running away from home, incorrigibility, vandalism, juvenile court record, police trouble, training school record, conviction as a felon, etc.

Information on environmental factors was based on adoption agency records and a personal interview of the adoptive parents. Environmental factors were categorized by type: (1) alcohol problem in an adoptive family member, (2) antisocial problem in family member, (3) other psychiatric problems in family member, (4) physical health problems in adoptive parents, (5) adoptive home broken by divorce, separation, or death, (6) socioeconomic level of adoptive home, (7) rural or urban home, (8) age of final placement in adoptive home, and (9) prenatal, birth, and postnatal medical problems potentially affecting adoptee, for example, precipitous delivery, low birth weight, drinking by mother during pregnancy.

Results for genetic analyses of alcohol problems in males are shown in Table 2.1 and demonstrate a significant increase in rates of alcohol abuse between the proband group and the comparison group (individuals with no psychopathology in their biologic background or a psychiatric condition other than alcohol drinking problem such as mental retardation). Results are similar from both adoption agencies, ICFS and LSS, as can be seen in Table 2.1.

Early analyses of data from ICFS in 1977 and 1980 revealed the following: primary alcoholism (alcohol abuse only without accompanying psychopathology such as antisocial personality, depression) was predicted by biologic parent alcohol problems (Cadoret & Gath, 1977); and adult adoptee alcohol abuse/dependence was predicted in a log-linear analysis by three independent factors. These three factors were: (1) having any first-degree biologic relative with alcohol problem, (2) having any second-degree biologic relative with an alcohol problem, and (3) adoptee diagnosis of conduct disorder as an adolescent (Cadoret, Cain, & Grove, 1980).

The completion in the early 1980s of an independent adoption study with a second private adoption agency (LSS) provided the opportunity to analyze new data using a multivariate method that would simultaneously take into account genetic and environmental factors as well as clinical outcomes of importance such as conduct disorder and its adult counterpart, antisocial personality.

Relationship of Alcohol Abuse to Environmental Factors and Other Psychopathology

The data from LSS were analyzed using a multivariate approach. Genetic and environmental factors and adoptee clinical outcome were analyzed together using log-linear modeling. This technique correlates all of the variables with each other. The result is a model showing which factors are predictive of outcome while at the same time controlling for other relevant factors. For example, by starting with a model containing both genetic variables and outcome variables it is possible to determine which environmental factors add additional significant prediction of the clinical outcome while controlling for genetic factors.

In the LSS data set it was found that clinical outcome was largely represented by alcohol abuse (29% of male adoptees) and antisocial personality (16% of male adoptees) with a rather significant overlap (12% of all adoptees were both alcohol abusers and antisocial). Accordingly these two conditions were included as outcomes in a model, and a variety of genetic backgrounds were tested for inclusion as predictors. The best-fitting model for males showed that a biologic parent alcohol problem was correlated with adoptee alcohol abuse and biologic parent antisocial behavior was correlated with adoptee antisocial personality diagnosis. To this model that considers genetic factors, environmental factors were tested for their ability to increase prediction of outcome as well as improve the goodness of fit. The final best-fitting model for males is shown in Figure 2.1 and includes a number of significant predictors of alcohol abuse. First, then, is a strong

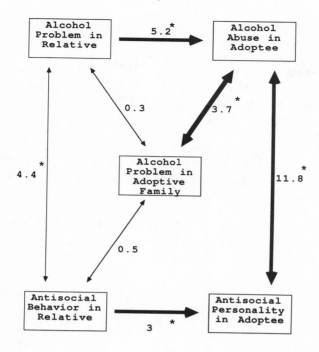

FIGURE 2.1. Interaction diagram for male sample (LSS) between adoptee alcohol abuse and antisocial outcome and genetic and environmental factors. *Heavy arrows* indicate relationships found in log-linear analysis. *Number* adjacent to arrow is odds ratio of relationship. Odds ratios which are significantly different (5% level or less) from 1.0 (no relationship) are marked by an asterisk. Odds ratios shown are "corrected" for the presence of other relationships shown in the model. *Light arrows* are relationships which are forced into the model in order to control for such factors as selective placement. *One-headed arrows* are used to show putative direction of causality. *Double-headed arrows* indicate direction of causality is uncertain.

relationship between antisocial personality and alcohol abuse (odds ratio = 11.8, p < .001). Second, the genetic factor of an alcohol problem in the biologic parent predicts increased adoptee alcohol abuse (odds ratio = 5.2, p = .004). Finally, the environmental factor of an alcohol problem in the adoptive family predicts increased adoptee alcohol abuse (odds ratio = 3.7, p = .008). Thus the results show not only a significant genetic effect, but also a significant environmental effect. In addition there is a specificity of type of inheritance shown by the analysis, with genetic antisocial background predicting antisocial personality and biologic alcohol problems predicting alcohol abuse in the adoptee. The model also demonstrates the importance of antisocial personality disorder in alcohol abuse. No gene–environment interactions predicted alcohol abuse. In the computer program used for log-linear analyses, higher order interactions were generated and tested, but none was found to be significant in these data. Although no significant interactions were found the following caveats are in order: the sample size is small and the log-linear model makes it more difficult to detect nonadditive interaction because of the change in scale introduced by logarithms.

The model presented in Figure 2.1 was also found to be the best-fitting model for the earlier and independently collected ICFS data on male adoptees (Cadoret et al., 1987). Similar relationships between genetic factors and outcomes were found with similar magnitudes of odds ratios. The only additional feature was the discovery of several environmental variables whose presence significantly increased adoptee antisocial personality. However these latter findings did not occur in the LSS data set and so require confirmation in another independently collected sample.

Relationship of Alcohol Abuse to Other Psychopathology

In addition to the relationship between alcohol abuse and antisocial personality found in the two studies described above, a correlation emerged between alcohol abuse and major depression (Cadoret, O'Gorman, Heywood, & Troughton, 1985). This result is shown in Figure 2.2 for the male and female sample. Depression is increased in alcohol abusers of both sexes, and depression is also increased in male adoptees exposed to adoptive families where another individual has an alcohol drinking problem, but to different environmental factors for female adoptees. The possible etiologic role of depression in alcohol abuse will be developed below.

By combining data from the ICFS and LSS studies it was possible to study drug abuse and its relationship to alcohol abuse, as well as other factors (Cadoret, Troughton, O'Gorman, & Heywood, 1986). In adoptees drug abuse was found to be highly correlated with alcohol abuse (odds ratio = 9.1, $p < .001$). However, when antisocial personality diagnosis was added to a log-linear model the correlation between alcohol and drug abuse dropped to nonsignificant value because of the extremely high correlations between antisocial diagnosis and alcohol abuse (odds ratio = 14.9, $p < .0001$) and drug abuse (odds ratio = 18.8, $p < .0001$). Further log-linear modeling showed that drug abuse increased under two conditions: in *non*antisocial adoptees by having a biologic parent with an alcohol problem; and by exposure to an adoptive home where another individual had disturbed behavior. The results suggested that drug abuse has both genetic and environmental roots. The results are shown in the interaction diagram in Figure 2.3.

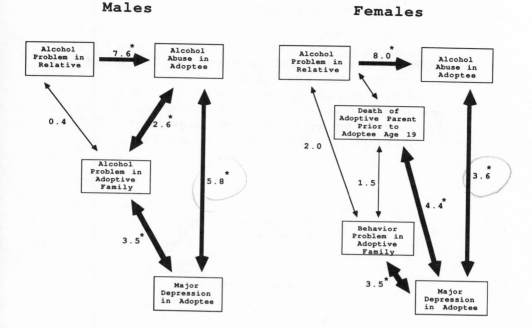

FIGURE 2.2. Interaction diagram for male and female sample (LSS and ICFS) between adoptee alcohol abuse and major depression and genetic and environmental factors. See Figure 2.1 caption for key.

Alcohol Abuse and Comorbidity in Females

In the ICFS data set, alcohol abuse was positively but not significantly correlated with a biologic background of alcohol drinking problem in females (Table 2.1). However, in the LSS data set there is a significant correlation of alcohol abuse in females with having a biologic parent with a drinking problem. The LSS data for females were fitted in a log-linear model similar to the male one and results are shown in Figure 2.4. The odds ratios for relationships are very similar to those shown by the males and suggest that the mode of inheritance in females may not be much different from that of males.

Alcohol abusing female adoptees, like the males, show significant comorbidity with antisocial personality. Females also show significant comorbidity with major depression, as well as showing that environmental factors, different from those in the males, increase the chance of depression (Cadoret, O'Gorman, Troughton, & Heywood, 1985).

The Role of Depression in Alcohol Abuse in Males

Depressive symptoms showed a significant positive correlation with alcohol abuse in male adoptees (see Figure 2.2). Depressive symptoms were also found to be increased in male adult adoptees who as infants were placed in permanent adoptive homes later than five months of age, an action likely associated with more social disruption (Cadoret, Troughton, Moreno, & Whitters, in press). It was found in further analyses (Cadoret & Troughton, 1988) that the number of alcohol abuse symptoms in adult adoptees was also significantly increased by adoptive placement at age five months or

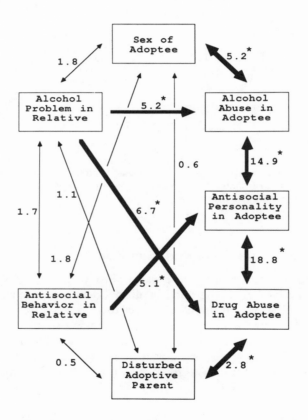

FIGURE 2.3. Interaction diagram for male and female sample (LSS and ICFS) between adoptee drug, alcohol abuse, and antisocial personality and genetic and environmental factors. Note: Sex of adoptee–alcohol abuse relationship holds only when sex is male. Alcohol problem in relative-drug abuse in adoptee relationship holds only when antisocial personality not present in adoptee. See Figure 2.1 caption for key.

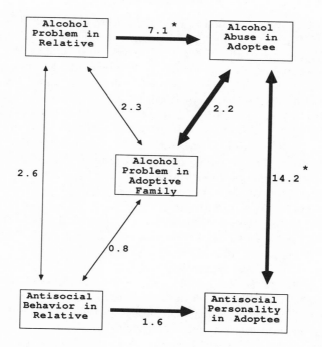

FIGURE 2.4. Interaction diagram for female sample (LSS) between adoptee alcohol abuse and antisocial personality and genetic and environmental factors. See Figure 2.1 caption for key.

later. These results suggest that, in addition to the pathway described through antisocial personality (see above), early life environmental factors that predispose to depressive symptoms might also predispose to adult alcohol abuse.

OVERVIEW AND CRITIQUE OF ADOPTION STUDIES

The adoption studies reported here from Danish, Swedish, and American (Iowa) sources have all demonstrated a significant genetic factor in alcohol abuse in men. Findings in women have been less definitive, with one study (Iowa) of the three showing significant increase of alcohol abuse in daughters of alcoholic biologic background, although the Swedish adoption study also reported a genetic effect in one subset of their female sample. Each of the studies reported a different percentage of alcohol abuse in their adoptee samples. In part this reflects differences in ascertainment. The Stockholm study, which relied on records of hospitalization and registration with the Temperance Board, reported lower percentages than the Iowa studies, which interviewed adoptees either in person or by telephone. The Denmark study shows the lowest percentages of alcoholism even though adoptees were personally interviewed. In large part the low rate appears to be definitional since their criteria for alcoholism were quite stringent and individuals they called "problem drinkers" would likely have been called abusers by the criteria used in the Iowa study, or could have had enough alcohol-related social problems to be registered with the Temperance Board in Sweden. Thus it is difficult to compare rates between studies, but comparison of the studies presented in Table 1, and use of the odds ratios to assess strength of relationship show that, at least for the males, odds ratios for the correlation of alcohol abuse with biologic parent background appear to be similar in magnitude across studies.

Two of the three studies (Sweden and Iowa) address specifically the question of heterogeneity of genetic factors in alcohol abuse. This is a very relevant question since there is much clinical data indicating that alcohol abusers are a heterogeneous group (Helzer & Pryzbeck, 1988; Hesselbrock, Hesselbrock, & Stabe, 1985; Jaffe, Babor, & Fishbein, 1988; Lewis, Robins, and Rice, 1985). The most commonly reported heterogeneity is the distinction between primary alcoholics (no clinical condition present other than alcoholism) and antisocial alcoholics. The Iowa studies address the heterogeneity of primary alcoholics versus antisocial alcoholics by diagnosing both conditions in adoptees and relating both conditions to each other as well as to the background genetic and environmental factors using log-linear modeling. These analyses reveal a specific and independent inheritance of antisocial behavior and alcohol abuse, a result that has been found in family studies (Lewis et al., 1983; Vaillant, 1983) and in the Stockholm adoption study (Bohman et al., 1982). According to the model of alcohol abuse suggested by the Iowa data, there are several independent pathways to alcohol abuse: (1) from a biologic parent with a drinking problem; (2) by having a biologic parent with antisocial behavior, and becoming alcoholic through behavior associated with antisocial personality; and (3) being exposed to an environment where a family member has a drinking problem.

The Stockholm study approaches the problem of heterogeneity by looking for different patterns of inheritance including gene–environment interactions. Two types of inheritance have been reported: Type I (milieu limited), with late clinical onset, which appeared to require environmental factors to allow expression of the genetic diathesis; and Type II (male limited), with early clinical onset and genetic diathesis, which expressed itself, despite environmental factors, almost entirely in males. Swedish investigators have pursued these differences in clinical studies (von Knorring et al., 1985, 1987) and found that onset of alcohol abuse and social complications of drinking could distinguish the two groups of alcoholics, and in their recent publications indicate that Type II alcoholism is similar to the antisocial alcoholism described in the literature (von Knorring et al., 1987). It has not been possible to confirm directly the association of alcohol abuse with antisocial personality in the Stockholm study since the adoptees were not psychiatrically interviewed. With regard to heterogeneity in the Danish data, although the presence of antisocial and other personality diagnoses was assessed in the adoptees, there is no information provided for their relation to diagnosed alcoholism or heavy drinking.

Considerations of alcoholic heterogeneity are not limited to antisocial personality. Other conditions have been implicated such as depression, with evidence that in some individuals depression precedes the onset of alcoholism (Winokur, Rimmer, & Reich, 1971). The Iowa study addresses this question and shows a significant relationship in both male and female alcohol abusers with major depression. Unfortunately, because of the retrospective nature of the psychiatric information the time course of alcohol use and abuse and depressive symptoms could not be sorted out. However, in analyzing genetic and environmental factors predicting adult depressive symptoms it was found that final adoptive placement at a late age (over five months of age) was associated with both increased adult depressive symptoms and increased number of alcohol abuse symptoms as adults (Cadoret & Troughton, 1989). This finding, and the correlation of alcohol abuse with major depression, raises the possibility that depression is an etiologic factor in alcohol abuse, or that alcohol abuse and depression are a manifestation of one underlying diathesis in some individuals.

Various methodologic and interpretive criticisms have been leveled at the Danish, Swedish, and Iowa adoption studies (Searles, 1988). The Swedish studies have been faulted for the interpretation that both mild and severe alcohol abuse are due to one genetic background and moderate alcohol abuse to a second genetic background (Searles, 1988). This interpretation is counterintuitive to the usual association of increased severity with increased genetic loading. Obviously such an interpretation must be independently confirmed by other evidence which conceivably could be found in extant family studies or further adoption data. The other major criticism by Searles of the Swedish study is the limitation of generalizability imposed by the use of Temperance Board data.

The Iowa studies have been faulted for their small numbers and especially for their reliance upon adoption agency records for the diagnosis of psychopathology in biologic parents (Murray, Clifford, & Gurling, 1983). The reliance on agency records undoubtedly diminishes the detection of conditions such as depression which might appear later in life (the typical biologic parent is usually in the teens or early twenties). Also, the quality of the records usually does not permit the use of modern diagnostic criteria for biologic parents. Nevertheless the results show that biologic parents with some evidence of a drinking problem, however meager, appear to have offspring with an increased chance for alcohol abuse.

The adoption designs allow environmental factors to be tested for their effect upon alcoholism. The three adoption studies from Denmark, Sweden, and the United States have examined specifically the effect of placement in an adoptive home with an alcohol problem in a parent. Only the Iowa study has reported such an environmental effect, but it was found in two independent data sets from that study. A further feature of the Iowa finding is that having an *adoptive* relative, such as an aunt or grandparent who did not live in the home, with an alcohol problem increased adoptee alcohol abuse as much as having an adoptive parent with an alcohol problem. This suggests that the adoptive family alcohol problem may be a type of marker for an environmental effect such as attitude toward alcohol, or increased exposure to alcohol, rather than purely imitative behavior. No explanation is apparent for the failure to find a similar environmental factor in the Scandinavian studies. However, adoptive family alcoholism in the Scandinavian studies was defined by parental alcoholism only and did not include alcoholism in sibs, aunts, uncles, or grandparents.

EVIDENCE OF GENETIC FACTORS IN ALCOHOLISM AND DRINKING BEHAVIOR FROM TWIN STUDIES

The rationale of the twin study method to assess genetic factors harkens back to Sir Francis Galton (Pearson, 1914–1930). The basis of the approach is the genetic fact that monozygotic (MZ) twins have in common all of their genes, but dizygotic (DZ) twins share on the average only 50% of their genes. If the environments of MZ and DZ twins are the same then excess concordance (presence of similar clinical condition in both members) shown by MZ twin pairs over DZ twin pairs is assigned to genetic factors. Twin pairs are *pairwise concordant* if both members are ill or both are not ill. Proband concordance is computed somewhat differently in that if two twins both independently become probands that pair is counted once for each proband. Smith (1974) has shown that proband concordance for a dichotomous character (e.g., alcoholic vs. not alcoholic) is equal to the intraclass correlation (r) for that character. Further, the quantity $2(r_{MZ}-r_{DZ})$ estimates the heritability (h^2) of the character.

Results of twin studies are generally expressed as concordance rates, heritability (h^2), or, when more elaborate genetic models are fit, estimates of different types of environmental factors are included in addition to the estimates of genetic heritability.

Interpretation of studies of twins must be tempered by assessing the biases and errors which can shape the conclusions from a study. Determination of twin zygosity, sample bias, especially that involving sample selection, diagnosis of alcoholism in the sample, and other factors must be considered in evaluating twin studies. It is usually possible to fault a twin study in some methodologic detail. However, it is useful to keep in mind the larger interpretative picture by weighing the number of positive studies against the negative. In this type of meta-analysis it is likely that the individual errors in each study would balance out, since studies often present different weaknesses when compared to each other.

In order to gain an overview of the twin studies relevant to alcoholism and drinking behavior consider Table 2.5, which presents information extracted from 13 published twin studies; the reader can see the variation in sample source, size, selection, and determination of alcoholism or drinking behavior in the twins. The studies are displayed in order of publication of the results. Notable is the increase in number of studies as well as the development of large samples of twins in the last decade. The Scandinavian countries of Sweden and Finland are renowned for their centralized public records of births, hospitalization, temperance boards, and other records of behavior, which allow representative samples to be selected and objective assessments of outcome to be made, such as hospitalization for alcoholism. Studies numbered 1, 3, 6, 9, and 13 from these countries made use of these registers. Other studies used samples ranging from volunteers recruited in a variety of ways (5, 10, 11) or town registries (2). (See study description columns.) Ascertainment of drinking habits and/or alcoholism varies from use of hospital and Temperance Board registration to questionnaires and personal interviews. (See determination of alcohol behavior column.) In some studies questionnaires were given twin pairs, and rates of return of these questionnaires must be considered in assessing the results (e.g., studies 4 and 6); in others twins were interviewed (e.g., studies 1, 3, 8), while still others utilized centralized medical records (e.g., 1 and 7). Some were concerned with drinking behaviors in general (e.g., 2, 3, 12, 13), while others concentrated on abnormal, or excessive, drinking behavior (e.g., 1, 4, 5, 6, 7, 8).

The results represent a number of aspects of drinking behavior, including excessive drinking and alcoholism, which demonstrate MZ–DZ differences consistent with a genetic factor. Studies of drinking behavior in general (consisting of drinking practices ranging from teetotaling through social drinking to chronic alcoholism) have shown more concordance in MZ than in DZ for the amount of alcohol consumed (studies 2, 3, 13, 12, 9, 10). One of these studies (Pederson et al., 1984) shows that MZ twins reared apart are more concordant for alcohol consumed than DZ reared together. The Hayakawa study (1987), which recorded only the occurrence of daily drinking in a Japanese sample, shows a nonsignificant preponderance of MZ concordance, but separation of the twins early in life appears to have little effect on the MZ–DZ difference. Abnormal drinking behavior is addressed by the following studies: 1, 3, 4, 7, 6, 8, 9, and 10. Heavy drinking appears to show more MZ concordance (studies 10, 6, 1, 4); however, one study of twins separated early in life (Pedersen et al., 1984) fails to

TABLE 2.5 Twin Studies in Alcoholism

Investigators (date)	Study description	Source of information about alcohol behavior	Behavior measures and results
1. Kaij (1960)	Twins born since 1840 who were reported to Temperance Boards in Sweden. In 1953 records researched. $N = 214$ pairs	Structured interview and Temperance Board records	Concordance rate MZ $N = 59$ / DZ $N = 146$ Heavy drinking and chronic alcoholism: 63.0% / 26.7% Chronic alcoholism alone: 71.4% / 32.3%
2. Conterio & Chiarelli (1962)	Twin registry of three Italian towns (Parma, Pavia, and Florence)	Adults contacted and questioned about drinking habits, smoking and coffee consumption (median daily wine consumption ¼ to ½ liter/day)	Quantity of alcohol consumed MZ ($N = 34$) 65% concordant DZ ($N = 43$) 44% concordant
3. Partanen, Bruun, & Markkanen (1966)	Male same-sexed twin pairs living in Finland in 1958. $N = 902$.	Interview instrument items factored to characterize drinking pattern. Five factors extracted. Two presented here: amount drunk and loss of control	MZ / DZ Drinking behavior Amount drunk: .38[a] / .11 Loss of control: .35 / .27
4. Jonsson and Nilsson (1968)	$N = 1500$ twin pairs in Sweden	Questionnaires mailed to 7500 twin pairs with 20% return rate	Frequent consumption of large amounts of alcohol Pairwise concordance MZ 43% / DZ 35%
5. Lochlin (1972)	$N = 850$ pairs of adolescent twins in USA taking Nat'l Merit Scholarship Test	Mailed questionnaire. 12 items mentioned drinking.	Answer to one item: "I have never used alcohol excessively" MZ .36[a] / DZ .24

6. Cederlof, Friberg and Lundeman (1977)	Swedish like-sexed pairs born 1886–1925 and 1926–1967 from twin registers	Mailed questionnaires. Response rate 58–91%. Other medical topics covered.	Excessive drinking (½ bottle of spirits or 1 of wine at sitting)

			Male coincidence ratio[b]	1.50
			Female coincidence ratio	2.14

7. Hrubec and Omenn (1981)	Male twin pairs from NAS-NRC Twin Registry 15,924 twins born 1917–1927 who have served in Armed Forces	Medical records from veterans service records	Alcoholism (at least one in twin pair affected)

MZ (N = 271) 26.3% concordant
DZ (N = 444) 11.9% concordant

8. Gurling, Oppenheim, & Murray (1984)	Consecutive admission to Maudsley Hospital (psychiatric). Subsample of twins with ICD diagnosis of alcohol addiction, psychosis, or habitual excessive use (males and females)	SADS-L interview	Alcoholism

MZ (N = 28) 21% pairwise concordant
DZ (N = 28) 25% pairwise concordant

1987 Report Gurling & Murray showed in discordant twins that ventricular enlargement related amount of alcohol

9. Pederson, Friberg, Floderus-Myrrhed, McClearn, & Plomin (1984)	Subsample of Swedish Twin Registry of those separated early in life (961 pairs) matched to twins living together	Not specified				
				MZ (A)	MZ (T)	DZ (A)	DZ (T)

	MZ (A)	MZ (T)	DZ (A)	DZ (T)
Young cohort				
Total alcohol	.42[b]	.60	.17	.28
Old cohort				
Total alcohol	.71	.64	.47[c]	.27
Heavy consump.	.14	.50	.13	.08

10. Gabrielli & Plomin (1985)	Colorado Adoptee and Twin Registry Analysis used: MZ, DZ, nontwin sib pairs, and pairs of unrelated adoptees living together N = 346 total	Colorado Alcohol Behavior Questionnaire	Intraclass correlations of alcohol drinking variables

	MZ	DZ	Non-twin sibs	Adoptee pairs
Av. month amount	.47	−.01	−.08	.15
Heavy drinking	.33	.17	−.12	−.09

(cont.)

TABLE 2.5 Twin Studies in Alcoholism (cont.)

Investigators (date)	Study description	Source of information about alcohol behavior	Behavior measures and results
11. Hayakawa (1987)	Japanese twins (like sex) weak determination of zygosity (based on one question regarding alikeness)	Mailed questionnaires on drinking, smoking, and health habits	Daily drinking MZ (N = 220) 59.5% concordant DZ (N = 85) 49.4% concordant Separation appeared to have little effect on concordance rates
12. Martin (1987) (Jardine & Martin) (1984)	5,967 adult pairs enrolled on Australian Twin Register	Questionnaires sent to adult twin pairs 64% pairwise response rate	Alcohol consumption sources of variance analysis (see table below)
13. Kaprio et al (1987)	Finnish Adoption Registry. Twins born prior to 1958 and alive in 1967	Mailed questionnaire on frequency and quantity drunk. 88.5% return	(see table below)

Study 12 — Alcohol consumption, sources of variance analysis:

	Females		Males	
age	≤30	>30	≤30	>30
Individual environment	42%	45%	34%	49%
Shared environment	—	—	21%	—
Genetic	58%	55%	45%	51%

Study 13:

	MZ	DZ
Quantity drunk	.37[a]	.19[d]
Frequency of beer	.41	.22
Frequency of spirits	.32	.13

[a]Intraclass correlations.
[b]Coincidence ratio = MZ coincidence rate/DZ coincidence rate
  Coincidence rate = pairs concordant for behavior
      discordant pairs + pairs free of behavior
Ratio >1 consistent with genetic transmission.
[c]Twins differ significantly from twins reared together.
A = Twins reared apart.   T = Twins raised together.
[d]Amount of social contact between twins and their ages did not materially alter estimates of alcohol use.

show a MZ–DZ difference, but does show a difference with nonseparated twins. Diagnosed alcoholism shows more MZ concordance than DZ in studies 7 and 1 but not in study 8. As with quantity of alcohol drunk, abnormal drinking including alcoholism appears to show more MZ than DZ concordance in the majority of studies.

These results, considered as a whole, suggest a genetic factor in regulating alcohol consumption. The finding that separated twins show similar results (studies 13, 11, 9) with regard to total alcohol consumed lends more weight to the genetic interpretation since one alternate hypothesis explaining increased MZ concordance is possible increased environmental similarity for MZ twins, for example, dressed alike, treated more alike, which could lead to greater twin similarity of behavior.

Excessive or heavy drinking (studies 6, 1, 4, 10) appears to have greater MZ than DZ concordance, but one study (Pedersen et al., 1984) of separated twins fails to find such a difference. However, the twins from this study who were brought up together do show a MZ–DZ difference. Of the three studies that look at extreme drinking behavior such as alcoholism (studies 7, 8, 1) two show evidence for a genetic factor while one (Gurling, Oppenheim, & Murray, 1984) does not. In addition, Partanen, Bruun, and Markkanen (1966) suggest that loss of control, a behavior generally associated with alcoholism, may have a genetic component.

Thus, the twin studies are consistent with a genetic factor operating not only in the regulation of "normal" alcohol consumption, but also affecting those more extreme behaviors labeled alcoholism. Heritability measures in most of the twin studies indicate a significant amount of variability even in MZ twin samples. While these differences could be a result of variation introduced by methodologic factors, such as measurement error, this finding suggests that environmental factors play a very important role in determination of alcohol use (or abuse) dependence. Since MZ twins share a common environment, the differences found would have to reflect specific environmental factors affecting only one twin. The possible importance of individual specific or unique environmental factors is shown by the analysis of twins in the Martin study (1987). Their mathematical modeling suggests a rather sizable component of outcome associated with individual environments.

GENETIC MARKERS IN ALCOHOLISM

Genetic markers are certain genetically determined characteristics, such as an enzyme, eye color, a blood group, a tissue protein, which occur more frequently with an illness. If the gene for the genetic marker is located on the same chromosome as a gene responsible for the illness and the physical distance between the two genes is very small, this is known as genetic *link-*

age. In the case of linkage, the illness and the marker characteristic segregate together in families. For a characteristic to be useful as a genetic linkage marker it must demonstrate polymorphism, that is, have two or more distinct and detectable variations such as found, for example, with the ABO blood groups. Thus one could trace the gene for the A blood group protein through a family tree and determine if it were associated with a pathologic condition such as alcoholism. The marker gene need have no etiologic connection to alcoholism. It serves merely as a convenient signpost. Studies of genetic linkage and disease are best described as "fishing expeditions" since investigators generally have no preconceived hypothesis as to linkage and test the association of as many available markers as is practical. Thus it is difficult to "correct" any significant associations for the chance factor and positive findings must be confirmed in independent samples. At present there is no conclusive evidence of a genetic linkage between a blood group system and alcoholism although a recent study by Tanna, Wilson, Winokur, and Elston (1988) reports a possible linkage between alcoholism and esterase-D, a protein associated with red blood cells. Another recent study by Hill, Aston, and Rabin (1988) has reported evidence for genetic linkage between alcoholism and the MNS blood group gene which is located on chromosome 4. As noted above, findings such as those reported by Hill et al. and Tanna et al. must be confirmed in independent studies.

One other possible linkage with alcoholism has been reported. For a number of years Winokur and coworkers (Winokur, 1974, 1982) have hypothesized a condition which they currently call familial depression spectrum disease (FDSD). This condition is defined by the presence in a family pedigree of individuals with major, minor, or intermittent depression, schizoaffective depression, alcoholism, or antisocial personality. Linkage between individuals with FDSD as defined above and a serum protein marker, orosomucoid, have been reported in two separate and independent studies (Hill, Wilson, Elston, & Winokur, in press). Finding evidence for genetic linkage would be the most direct proof of a genetic etiology in alcoholism; hence the importance of this kind of research. Also, the finding of linkage would further localize the gene concerned with alcoholism to a specific chromosome. In turn this could eventually lead to a chemical characterization of the gene and enable carriers of the gene to be identified and counseled as to their genetic liability. Eventually a gene product could be identified and its role in the etiology of alcoholism determined, with the possibility of direct manipulation of the process that leads to alcoholism.

Another type of marker finding which involves a correlation of a genetically determined characteristic with alcoholism is called association. In association it is not necessary that there be linkage between the two genes; instead the presence of a certain allele of the "marker" gene is correlated with alcoholism. Positive association studies have been reported for several genetically determined traits and alcoholism: secretion of ABO blood groups in saliva; taste sensitivity to phenylthiourea (PTC); and various color vision defects (Swinson, 1983). ABO secreter status in blood group A individuals has been associated with alcoholism in two studies (Camps, Dodd, & Lincoln, 1969; Swinson & Madden, 1973). Two studies have reported an excess of nontasters of PTC in alcoholics but one has found no such increase (Swinson, 1983). The loss of taste could be a consequence of alcohol abuse itself. In 1964 Cruz-Coke reported an increase in color vision defects among male and female patients with liver cirrhosis (Cruz-Coke, 1964), and similar results were found in later studies (Cruz-Coke & Varela, 1966). Criticism of these associations has included concern that the color vision defects are acquired and do not represent a genetic etiology (Swinson, 1983).

Association studies are important because they could represent genetic characteristics that predispose to alcoholism. Recent research has concentrated on biologic "markers" for alcoholism. Most of these "markers" are not proven to be genetically determined but are hypothesized to be because they often involve biochemical or physiologic processes. Some of these processes are behavioral, for example, body sway when sober or intoxicated, while others are physiological processes such as secretion of hormones, or brain wave activity. Twin studies have contributed to information about the genetic etiology of some of these physiological processes such as motor coordination (Martin et al., 1985) and EEG (Propping, 1977). Because the biologic marker studies are so numerous and potentially important they will be discussed separately in the next section.

BIOLOGIC MARKERS IN ALCOHOLISM

As developed over the past decade, biologic markers in alcoholism represent a variant of the genetic markers discussed above. These studies are potentially important because they try to delineate biologic processes which are present prior in time to alcoholism and which could serve to identify individuals at high risk for the development of alcoholism in the future (Radouco-Thomas et al., 1984). To detect markers, studies are usually made of high risk populations such as children of alcoholics who are then contrasted with suitable low risk controls (children of nonalcoholics). Using alcoholics themselves as a demonstrated high risk group leaves the interpretation of differences obscured by the fact that heavy drinking itself could produce any observed effect. Using very young children of alcoholics is another approach, but this strategy may not detect a marker that does not manifest itself until puberty or later. Hypothesized biologic markers have ranged from behavioral traits to hormonal secretion, to electrophysiological events in the brain. A number of recent studies involving biologic markers are shown in Table 2.6. This list is not meant to be exhaustive but merely to reflect the range and variety of biologic marker studies. As

TABLE 2.6. Representative Biologic Marker Studies

	Investigators (date)	Study sample	Study design	Results
1.	Schuckit (1980)	Young men (not alcoholic) with (FHP) and without (FHN) family history of alcoholism	Alcohol challenge. Self-ratings of intoxication by questionnaire	FHP subjects rated self less intoxicated than FHN group though blood alcohol concentration similar in both groups.
2.	Schuckit, Gold & Risch (1987a)	Similar to (1)	Alcohol challenge. Change in plasma cortisol level due to alcohol measured	FHP subjects demonstrated lower cortisol levels after drinking.
3.	Radouco-Thomas et al. (1984)	Patients with alcoholism and controls without illness	Thyroid releasing hormone (TRH) administered all subjects and output of subjects' thyroid stimulating hormone (TSH) measured	Alcoholic subjects showed lower (blunted) TSH response. (Blunted response also noted in non-alcoholic sons of sons of alcoholics but difference not significant)
4.	Swartz, Drews & Cadoret (1987)	Adoptees of both sexes from biologic parents with alcohol problems and control parents	Stress-induced by alcohol ingestion and by playing competitive game	Both types of stress in adoptees from alcohol background resulted in less epinephrine release than in control adoptees.
5.	Schmidt & Neville (1985)	Similar to (1)	EEG event-related potentials (ERP) recorded during letter rhyming task	Amplitude of ERP ($N - 450$) smaller in FHP subjects
6.	Schuckit, Gold & Risch (1987b)	Similar to (1)	Alcohol challenge. Circulating prolactin measured	FHP sons had lower prolactin levels than controls in response to higher dose ethanol challenge

	Study	Sample	Measure	Results
7.	Moss, Guthrie & Linnoila (1986)	Similar to (1) but sample of both sexes matched for age, sex and past alcohol exposure	Basal and protirelin stimulated T_3, prolactin, growth hormone, and thyrotropin measured	FMP sons had higher basal and stimulated thyrotropin levels. FHP daughters showed no differences in thyrotropin
8.	Pollock et al. (1984)	Similar to (1). Sample from Denmark perinatal birth cohort FHP matched to controls (FHN) on age, sex, social status. Age 19–21	Resting EEG and EEG change following alcohol administration	Suggestive increases in fast EEG activity in certain brain areas in resting EEG. Following alcohol FHP subjects showed greater increases of slow alpha energy and decrease in mean alpha frequency
9.	Schuckit (1985)	Similar to (1)	Alcohol challenge. Change in body sway following alcohol	FHP showed less change in body sway than FHN following alcohol despite similar blood alcohol levels
10.	Whipple, Parker, & Noble (1988)	Prepubescent sons of alcoholics (high risk). Control group matched for age, education, sex and father's income (low risk)	EEG event related potentials measured during complex visual task and visual perceptive performance tests	High risk showed reduction in amplitude of late positive complex of event related potential and lower visual perceptual performance on tests. Lower test scores correlated with change in late positive complex
11.	Begleiter, Porjesz Bihari, & Kissin (1984)	Preadolescent sons of alcoholics FHP and age and sex matched controls	EEG event related potential to stimulus	FHP showed decreased size of P300 component of event related brain potential compared to control

shown in column 2 of the table, a high risk design is very popular and reflects the belief in a transmitted factor which can be detected in offspring. For some behaviors or traits there is evidence of genetic factors (e.g., twin studies of body sway and EEG), although other studies do not show this effect. Many of the studies use an alcohol challenge to elicit differential responses in a trait or behavior (see column 3). How this use of alcohol challenge is relevant to alcoholism is not always clear, though in some cases a rationale is given; for example, less body sway and lower self-ratings of intoxication in high risk subjects (see Table 2.6, studies 1 and 9) suggest high risk subjects might be able or tempted to consume more alcohol per drinking occasion and thus be at higher risk for eventual alcohol abuse. Although positive findings are reported in all of the studies shown in the table, it does not mean that all of the findings are repeatable or have been independently confirmed. For example, Moss, Guthrie, and Linnoila (1986) fail to find the prolactin changes reported by Schuckit, Gold, and Risch (1987b); and though the event-related potential changes described by Begleiter et al. (1984) have generally proven to be repeatable and robust there have been negative studies (Polich, Harer, Buchsbaum, & Bloom, 1988).

However, to date there is no study that has followed up individuals with any of these biologic markers to determine how many of them actually become alcohol abusers. When this is done it is likely that a number of markers will turn out to be irrelevant. Those that are actually predictive of later alcoholism should provide some clues regarding the developmental process of becoming an alcoholic. In view of the relative ease of measuring rather complex physiological and neurophysiological processes with current technology, it is extremely likely that many more so-called biologic marker studies will appear in the future. As yet the findings are too tentative to suggest any one underlying process leading to alcoholism. The wide variety of markers so far described, if uncorrelated with each other, could lead to the conclusion that a large number of independent factors contribute to the development of alcoholism. Another problem left to the future is the question of the genetic etiology of biologic markers and to what extent gene–environment interactions enter into the appearance and detection of a marker trait.

BIOCHEMICAL AND PHYSIOLOGIC FACTORS IN ALCOHOLISM

Many biochemical reactions catalyzed by enzymatic action have long been known to be genetically determined. Alcohol is also known as a substance with profound and widespread effects upon biochemical and physiological processes. It is natural, then, that genetic factors be sought which influence the body's metabolism of ethanol and the body's reaction to ethanol, both in acute and chronic exposure. The body's reaction to alcohol withdrawal following acute or chronic alcohol administration has also been examined for the influence of genetic factors.

The study of alcohol metabolism has been greatly stimulated in recent years by advances in molecular biology which have facilitated recognition of genetic variants of the enzymes involved in the breakdown of alcohol to acetaldehyde (Agerwal & Goedde, 1987). Genetic variations in these enzymes determine the rate of alcohol metabolism, the concentration of breakdown products such as acetaldehyde, and in turn physiological responses to these products. For example, slower acetaldehyde oxidation because of the presence of aldehyde dehydrogenase I isoenzyme usually leads to elevated blood acetaldehyde levels, and this causes physiologic changes marked by skin flushing (especially of the face) and feelings of dysphoria (Agarwal & Goedde, 1987; Li & Bosron, 1986). Low incidences of aldehyde I isoenzyme deficiencies of 2% to 5% have been observed in Japanese alcoholics as contrasted with 40% in a control group (Harada, Agarwal, & Goedde, 1987). This suggests a possible protective role of certain enzymes in alcoholism—in the case above conceivably the unpleasant flushing and dysphoria discourage alcohol intake. Whether such "protective" action extends to other ethnic groups remains to be seen.

Research on animal models of human alcohol behaviors has become increasingly important in the search for genetic factors involved in alcoholism. Results of animal studies show that genes have a strong influence on choice of alcohol and its consumption (Fuller, 1985). Strains of mice have been developed which manifest different behavioral effects following alcohol administration, and these strains have been used to study possible neurophysiological mechanisms responsible for sensitivity to ethanol (Palmer, 1985; Smollen & Collins, 1985). Animal models have been developed for alcohol dependence (Wilson, 1985) and for tolerance (Erwin, 1985; Tabakoff, Cornell, & Hoffman, 1986; Tabakoff & Hoffman, 1987). Evidence suggests that dependence and tolerance are influenced by both genetic and environmental factors.

Thus the burgeoning animal and biochemical studies indicate a genetic influence in many areas relevant to alcoholism in humans, and suggest that a rather wide variety of genetically determined factors could operate independently to produce the varying clinical pictures seen in human alcoholism. What is currently needed in this area is more evidence linking the animal behavioral studies and metabolic studies with clinical alcoholism in humans.

PERSONALITY, TEMPERAMENT, AND ALCOHOLISM

Studies already cited in this chapter show that antisocial personality disorder plays a significant role in some forms of alcoholism, that antisocial alcoholics have a different course of alcoholism, and, further, that antisocial personality is inherited independent of alcoholism. Other types of disorders of personality could be involved as well in alcoholism. This view is supported by a review of earlier family studies (Cadoret, 1976) which found a higher incidence of varied types of personality disorder in families of alcoholics compared to families of controls. There is also evidence from twin (Eysenk, 1982; Loehlin & Nichols, 1976; Plomin, DeFries & McClearn, 1980) and adoption studies (Loehlin, Horn, & Willerman, 1981; Loehlin, Willerman, & Horn; 1982; Scarr, Webber, Weinberg, & Wittig, 1981) that genetic factors play a role in the transmission of temperament and personality traits. However, studies suggest that much of the explanation for personality variation lies in within-family environmental variation or nonadditive genetic factors (e.g., Loehlin, Willerman, & Horn, 1985).

Recently Cloninger (1987a) has proposed a systematic scheme of personality with three bipolar and independent factors, and applied this system to define clinical subgroups of alcoholics (Cloninger, 1987b). The personality schema was applied to a sample of Swedish children (age 11 years) and results correlated with alcohol abuse when the sample was 27 years old. It was found that childhood characteristics of high novelty seeking and low harm avoidance predicted higher rates of early onset alcohol abuse (Cloninger, Sigvardsson, & Bohman, 1988). The temperament–personality perspective on alcoholism has been further developed by Tarter, Alterman, and Edwards (1985).

SUMMARY

Evidence for a genetic basis of alcoholism has increased greatly in the past decade and a half. Twin and separation studies have provided the best indication for a genetic factor, and recent studies using these approaches are focusing more on environmental factors and gene and environmental interaction. The studies also are more concerned with the psychiatric (and presumably etiologic) heterogeneity of alcoholism and seek to divide alcoholics into clinically and etiologically significantly different subgroups, for example, antisocial alcoholics (Alterman & Tarter, 1986). With a genetic explanation (at least in part) for alcoholism and for associated conditions which also influence social adjustment (such as antisocial personality) we have come a long way from the 19th century view of alcohol as a *cause* of heritable disease in offspring and the basis for progressive hereditary degeneration leading to epilepsy, feeblemindedness, etc. (Bynum, 1984; Crowe, 1985)

The preponderance of evidence from marker and biologic studies suggests that many independent biochemical and physiological mechanisms could be involved in the development of alcoholism (Tartar & Hegedus,

1985). The adoption and twin studies do not tell us which of these bio-chemical or physiological processes is relevant to clinical alcoholism. The adoption studies are consistent with genetic (as well as clinical) heterogeneity in alcoholism and have the best potential of all the techniques to separate out genetic from environmental effects.

The adoption studies and studies of clinical alcoholism support the hypothesis of two types of alcoholism, one associated with antisocial personality and the other with "familial" alcoholism (Stabenau, 1985). The studies testify to the importance of environmental factors. If specific environmental factors are responsible for a major portion of variability in the outcome of alcoholism (e.g., see Searles' 1988 reanalysis of Stockholm adoption data; also Martin's 1987 twin study) then a more direct search must be made to identify such factors rather than estimating them by "subtraction" in a mathematical model paradigm. Some recent proposals for such specific environmental factors include parental disciplinary practices (Holmes & Robins, 1988), childhood abuse (Famularo, Stone, Barnum, & Wharton, 1986; Kroll, Stock, & James, 1985) and ethnic differences (Marjoribanks, 1985). General environmental factors will likely prove more important than has been shown to date in the adoption studies. Recent findings pointing to increases in alcohol abuse in more recent birth cohorts suggest a source in the changing sociocultural background of alcohol use and availability (Reich, Cloninger, van Eerdewegh, Rice, & Mullaney, 1988). As Peele (1986) has pointed out all genetic models proposed to account for alcoholism "leave room for the substantial impact of environmental, social and individual factors (including personal values and intentions) so that drinking to excess can only be predicted within a complex, multivariate framework" (p. 63). In the perennial debate over heredity versus environment in the etiology of alcoholism we now know that it is "nature and nurture" interacting together (Omenn, 1987).

REFERENCES

Agarwal, D., & Goedde, H. (1987). Genetic variation in alcohol metabolizing enzymes: implications in alcohol use and abuse. In H. W. Goedde and D. P. Agarwal (Eds.), *Genetics in alcoholism* (pp. 121–139). New York: Alan R. Liss.

Alterman, A. J. (1988). Patterns of familial alcoholism, alcoholism severity and psychopathology. *Journal of Nervous and Mental Disease, 176,* 167–175.

Alterman, A., & Tarter, R. (1986). An examination of selected typologies. Hyperactivity, familial, and antisocial alcoholism. In M. Galnter (Ed.), *Recent Developments in Alcoholism, Vol. 4* (pp. 169–189). New York: Plenum Press.

Babor, T., & Lauerman, R. (1986). Classification and forms of inebriety. Historical antecedents of alcoholic typologies. In M. Galanter (Ed.), *Recent developments in alcoholism, Vol. 4* (pp. 113–144). New York: Plenum.

Begleiter, H., Poryesz, B., Bihari, B., & Kissin, B. (1984). Event-related brain potentials in boys at risk for alcoholism. *Science, 227,* 1493–1496.

Bohman, M., Cloninger, C. R., Sigvardsson, S., & von Knorring, A. L. (1982). Predisposition to petty criminality in Swedish adoptees. I. Genetic and environmental heterogeneity. *Archives of General Psychiatry, 39,* 1233–1241.

Bohman, M., Sigvardsson, S., & Cloninger, C. R. (1981). Maternal inheritance of alcohol abuse. *Archives of General Psychiatry, 38,* 965–969.

Bynum, W. F. (1984). Alcoholism and degeneration in 19th century European medicine and psychiatry. *British Journal of Addiction, 79,* 59–70.

Cadoret, R. J. (1976). Genetic determinants of alcoholism. In R. Tarter and A. Sugerman (Eds.), *Alcoholism: Interdisciplinary approaches to an enduring problem* (pp. 225–256). Reading, MA: Addison-Wesley.

Cadoret, R., Cain, C., & Grove, W. (1980). Development of alcoholism in adoptees raised apart from alcoholic biologic relatives. *Archives of General Psychiatry, 37,* 561–563.

Cadoret, R., & Gath, A. (1978). Inheritance of alcoholism in adoptees. *British Journal of Psychiatry, 132,* 252–258.

Cadoret R. J. (1986). Adoption studies: Historical and methodological critique. *Psychiatric Developments, 1,* 45–64.

Cadoret, R., O'Gorman, T., Troughton, E., & Heywood, E. (1985). Alcoholism and antisocial personality: Interrelationships, genetic and environmental factors, *Archives of General Psychiatry, 42,* 161–167.

Cadoret, R. J., O'Gorman, T., Heywood, E., & Troughton, E. (1985). Genetic and environmental factors in major depression. *Journal of Affective Disorders, 9,* 155–164.

Cadoret, R. J., & Troughton, E. (1989). Genetic and environmental factors in alcohol abuse. In K. Kiianma, B. Tabahoff, & T. Saito (Eds.), *Genetic aspects of alcoholism,* Vol. 37. Helsinki: Foundation for Alcohol Studies.

Cadoret, R. J., Troughton, E., O'Gorman, T., & Heywood, E. (1986). An adoption study of genetic and environmental factors in drug abuse. *Archives of General Psychiatry, 43,* 1131–1136.

Cadoret, R. J., Troughton, E., & O'Gorman, T. (1987). Genetic and environmental factors in alcohol abuse and antisocial personality. *Journal of Studies on Alcohol, 48,* 1–8.

Cadoret, R. J., Troughton, B. A., Moreno, L., & Whitters, A. (in press). Early life psychosocial events and adult affective symptoms. In M. Rutter and L. Robins (Eds.), *Straight and devious pathways from childhood to adulthood,* Chapter 16. London: Cambridge University Press.

Camps, F. E., Dodd, B., & Lincoln, R. (1969). Frequencies of secretors and nonsecretors of ABH substance among 1,000 alcoholic patients. *British Medical Journal, 4,* 457–459.

Cederlof, R., Friberg, L., & Lundman, T. (1977). The interactions of smoking, environment, and heredity and their implications for disease etiology. *Acta Medica Scandinavica Supplement 202, 612,* 1–128.

Clair, D., & Genest, M. (1987). Variables associated with the adjustment of offspring of alcoholic fathers. *Journal on Studies of Alcohol, 48,* 348–355.

Clayton, P. (1987). Self-reported alcohol, drug, and eating disorder problems among male and female collegiate children of alcoholics. *Journal of American College Health, 36,* 111–116.

Cloninger, C. R. (1987a). A systematic method for clinical description and classification of personality variants. A proposal. *Archives of General Psychiatry, 44,* 573–588.

Cloninger, C. R. (1987b). Neurogenetic adoptive mechanisms in alcoholism. *Science, 236,* 410–436.

Cloninger, C. R., Bohman, M. & Sigvardsson, S. (1981). Inheritance of alcohol abuse. *Archives of General Psychiatry, 38,* 861–868.

Cloninger, C. R., Bohman, M., Sigvardsson, S., & von Knorring, A. L. (1985). Psychopathology in adopted-out children of alcoholics. The Stockholm Adoption Study. In M. Galanter (Ed.), *Recent developments in alcoholism, Vol. 3* (pp. 37–51). New York: Plenum.

Cloninger, C. R., Sigvardsson, S., & Bohman, M. (1988). Childhood personality predicts alcohol abuse in young adults. *Alcohol: Experiments in Clinical Research, 12,* 494–505.

Conterio, F., & Chiarelli, B. (1962). Study of the inheritance of some daily life habits. *Heredity, 17,* 347–359.

Cook, B., & Winokur, G. (1985). A family study of familial positive vs. familial negative alcoholics. *Journal of Nervous and Mental Disease, 173,* 175–178.

Cotton, N. S. (1979). The familial incidence of alcoholism: A review. *Journal of Studies on Alcohol, 40,* 89–116.

Crowe, L. (1985). Alcohol and heredity: Theories about the effects of alcohol use on offspring. *Social Biology, 32,* 146–161.

Cruz-Coke, R. (1964). Colour blindness and cirrhosis of the liver. *Lancet, ii,* 1064–1065.

Cruz-Coke, R., & Varela, A. (1966). Inheritance of alcoholism: Its association with colour blindness. *Lancet, ii,* 1282–1284.

Erwin, V. G. (1985). Genetic influences on acquisition of tolerance to alcohol. *Social Biology, 32,* 222–228.

Eysenk, H. J. (1982). *Personality, genetics, and behavior.* New York: Praeger.

Famularo, R., Sone, K., Barnum, R., & Wharton, R. (1986). Alcoholism and severe child maltreatment. *American Journal of Orthopsychiatry, 56(3),* 481–485.

Fuller, J. L. (1985). The genetics of alcohol consumption in animals. *Social Biology, 32,* 210–221.

Gabrielli, W., & Plomin, R. (1985). Drinking behavior in the Colorado adoptee and twin sample. *Journal of Studies on Alcohol, 46,* 24–31.

Gilligan, S. B., Reich, T., & Cloninger, C. R. (1987). Etiologic heterogeneity in alcoholism. *Genetic Epidemiology, 4,* 395–414.

Goodwin, D. (1984). Studies of familial alcoholism: A review. *Journal of Clinical Psychiatry, 45,* 14–17.

Goodwin, D., Schulsinger, F., Hermansen, L., Guze, S., & Winokur, G. (1973). Alcohol problems in adoptees raised apart from alcoholic biologic parents. *Archives of General Psychiatry, 28,* 238–243.

Goodwin, D., Schulsinger, F., Hermansen, L., Guze, S., & Winokur, G. (1975). Alcoholism and the hyperactive child syndrome. *Journal of Nervous and Mental Disorders, 160,* 349–353.

Goodwin, D., Schulsinger, F., Knop, J., Mednick, S., & Guze, S. (1977). Alcoholism and depression in adopted-out daughters of alcoholics. *Archives of General Psychiatry, 34,* 751–755.

Goodwin, D., Schulsinger, F., Moller, N., Hermansen, L., Winokur, G., & Guze, S. (1974). Drinking problems in adopted and nonadopted sons of alcoholics. *Archives of General Psychiatry, 31,* 164–169.

Goodwin, D., Schulsinger, F., Knop, J., Mednick, S., & Guze, S. (1979). Psychopathology in adopted and nonadopted daughters of alcoholics. In D. Goodwin and C. Erickson (Eds.), *Alcoholism and affective disorders. Clinical, genetic and biochemical disorders* (pp. 89–98). New York: Spectrum.

Gurling, H., Oppenheim, B., & Murray, R. (1984). Depression, criminality and psychopathology associated with alcoholism: Evidence from a twin study. *Acta Geneticae Medicae et Gemellologiae, 33,* 333–339.

Harada, S., Agarwal, D., & Goedde, H. (1987). Aldehyde dehydrogenase and glutathione-S-transferase polymorphism: Association between phenotype frequences and alcoholism. In H. Goedde and D. Agarwal (Eds.), *Genetics and alcoholism* (pp. 241–250). New York: Alan R. Liss.

Hayakawa, K. (1987). Smoking and drinking discordance and health condition: Japanese identical twins reared apart and together. *Acta Geneticae Medicae et Gemellologiae, 36,* 493–501.

Helzer, J., & Pryzbeck, T. (1988). The cooccurence of alcoholism with other psychiatric disorders in the general population and its treatment. *Journal of Studies on Alcohol, 49,* 219–224.

Hesselbrock, V. M., Hesselbrock, M. N., & Stabenau, J. R. (1985). Alcoholism in men patients subtyped by family history and antisocial personality. *Journal of Studies on Alcohol, 46,* 59–64.

Hill, E., Wilson, A., Elston, R., & Winokur, G. (1988). Evidence for possible linkage between genetic markers and affective disorders. *Biological Psychiatry, 24,* 903–917.

Hill, S., Aston, C., & Rabin, B. (1988). Suggestive evidence of genetic linkage between alcoholism and the MNS blood group. *Alcoholism: Clinical and Experimental Research, 12,* 811–814.

Holmes, S. J., & Robins, L. N. (1988). The role of parental disciplinary practices in the development of depression and alcoholism. *Psychiatry, 51,* 24–36.

Hrubec, Z., & Omenn, G. (1981). Evidence of genetic predisposition to alcoholic cirrhosis and psychosis: Twin concordance for alcoholism and its biological endpoints by zygosity among male veterans. *Alcoholism: Clinical and Experimental Research, 5,* 207–215.

Jaffe, J., Babor, T., & Fishbein, D. (1988), Alcoholics, aggression and antisocial personality. *Journal of Studies on Alcohol, 49,* 211–218.

Jardine, R., & Martin, N. (1984). Causes of variation in drinking habits in a large turn sample. *Acta Geneticae Medicae et Gemellologiae, 33,* 435–450.

Johnson, J. (1987) Selected references on psychosocial characteristics of children of alcoholics. *Alcohol research utilization system.* Rockville, MD: National Clearinghouse for Alcohol and Drug Information.

Jonsson, E., & Nillson, T. (1968). Alkohol konsumtion hos monozygota och alizygota twilling par. *Nordisk Hygiensk Tidskrift, 49,* 21–25.

Kaij, L. (1960). *Alcoholism in twins: Studies on the etiology and sequels of abuse of alcohol.* Stockholm: Almquist & Weksell.

Kaprio, J., Koshenviro, M., Langenvainio, H., Romanov, K., Sarna, S., & Rose, R. (1987). Genetic influences on use and abuse of alcohol: A study of 5638 adult

Finnish twin brothers. *Alcoholism: Clinical and Experimental Research, 11,* 349–356.

Knop, J. (1985). Premorbid assessment of young men at high risk for alcoholism. In M. Galanter (Ed.), *Recent developments in alcoholism, Vol. 3* (pp. 53–64). New York: Plenum.

Knop, J., Teasdale, T. W. Schulsinger, F., & Goodwin, D. W. (1985). A prospective study of young men at high risk for alcoholism: School behavior and achievement. *Journal of Studies on Alcohol, 46,* 273–278.

Kroll, P., Stock, D., & James, M. (1985). The behavior of adult alcoholic men abused as children. *Journal of Nervous and Mental Disease, 173,* 689–693.

Latcham, R. W. (1985). Familial alcoholism: Evidence from 237 alcoholics. *British Journal of Psychiatry, 147,* 54–57.

Lewis, C., Rice, J., & Helzer, J. (1983). Diagnostic interactions: Alcoholism and antisocial personality. *Journal of Nervous and Mental Disorders, 171,* 105–113.

Lewis, C., Robins, L., & Rice, J. (1985). Association of alcoholism with antisocial personality in men. *Journal of Nervous and Mental Disorders, 173,* 166–174.

Li, T. K., & Bosron, W. F. (1986). Genetic variability of enzymes of alcohol metabolism in human beings. *Annals of Emergency Medicine, 15,* 997–1004.

Loehlin, J. (1972). An analysis of alcohol-related questionnaire items from the national turn merit study. *Annals of the New York Academy of Sciences, 197,* 117–120.

Loehlin, J., Horn, J., & Willerman, L. (1981). Personality resemblance in adoptive families. *Behavioral Genetics, 11,* 309–330.

Loehlin, J. C., & Nichols, R. C. (1976). *Heredity, environment and personality: A study of 850 sets of twins.* Austin: University of Texas Press.

Loehlin, J. C., Willerman, L., & Horn, J. M. (1982). Personality resemblance between unwed mothers and their adopted-away offspring. *Journal of Personality and Social Psychology, 42,* 1089–1099.

Loehlin, J. C., Willerman, L., & Horn, J. M. (1985). Personality resemblances in adoptive families when the children are late-adolescent or adult. *Journal of Personality and Social Psychology, 48,* 376–392.

Marjoribanks, K. (1985). Sibling and environmental correlates of adolescents' perceptions of family environments: Ethnic group differences. *Social Biology, 32,* 71–81.

Martin, N. G. (1987). Genetic differences in drinking habits, alcohol metabolism and sensitivity in unselected samples of twins. In H. Goedde and D. Agarwal (Eds.), *Genetics and alcoholism* (pp. 109–119). New York: Alan R. Liss.

Martin, N. G., Oakeshott, J. G., Gibson, J. B., Starmer, G. A., Perl, J., & Wilks, A. V. (1985). A twin study of psychomotor and physiological responses to an acute dose of alcohol. *Behavioral Genetics, 15,* 305–347.

McCord, J. (1988). Alcoholism: Toward understanding genetic and social factors. *Psychiatry, 51,* 131–141.

Moss, H. B., Guthrie, S., & Linnoila, M. (1986). Enhanced thyrotropin response to thyrotropin releasing hormone in boys at risk for development of alcoholism. *Archives of General Psychiatry, 43,* 1137–1142.

Murray, R., Clifford, C., & Gurling, H. (1983). Twin and adoption studies: How good is the evidence for a genetic role? In M. Galanter (Ed.), *Recent developments in alcoholism, Vol. 1* (pp. 25–48). New York: Plenum.

Omenn, G. (1987). Heredity and environmental interactions. In H. W. Goedde and D. P. Agarwal (Eds.), *Genetics and alcoholism* (pp. 323–325). New York: Alan R. Liss.

Palmer, M. R. (1985). Neurophysiological mechanisms in the genetics of ethanol sensitivity. *Social Biology, 32,* 241–154.

Parker, D. A., & Harford, T. C. (1987). Alcohol-related problems of children of heavy-drinking parents. *Journal of Studies of Alcohol, 48,* 265–268.

Parker, D. A., & Harford, T. C. (1988). Alcohol-related problems, marital disruption, and depressive symptoms among adult children of alcohol abusers in the United States. *Journal of Studies on Alcohol, 49(4),* 306–313.

Partanen, J., Bruun, K., & Markkanen, T. (1966). *Inheritance of drinking behavior, Vol. 14.* Helsinki: Finnish Foundation for Alcohol Studies.

Pearson, K. (1914–1930). *The life, letters, and labours of Francis Galton, vols. I, II, IIIA and IIIB.* Cambridge University Press.

Pedersen, N., Friberg L, Floderus-Myrrhed, B., McClearn, G., & Plomin, R. (1984). Swedish early separated twins: Identification and characterization. *Acta Geneticae Medicae Gemellologiae, 33,* 243–250.

Peele, S. (1986). The implications and limitations of genetic models of alcoholism and other addiction. *Journal of Studies on Alcohol, 47,* 63–73.

Plomin, R., DeFries, J. C., & McClearn, G. E. (1980). *Behavioral genetics: A primer.* San Francisco: Freeman.

Polich, J. Harer, R., Buchsbaum, M., & Bloom, F. (1988). Assessment of young men at risk for alcoholism with P300 from a visual discrimination task. *Journal of Studies on Alcohol, 49,* 186–190.

Pollock, V. E., Volavka, J., Mednick, S. A., Goodwin, D. W., Knop, J., & Schulsinger, F. (1984). A prospective study of alcoholism: Electroencephalographic findings. In D. W. Goodwin, Van Dusen R., and Mednick, S. A. (Eds.), *Longitudinal research in alcoholism* (pp. 125–145). Boston: Kluver Nijhoff.

Propping, P. (1977). Genetic control of ethanol action on central nervous system. *Human genetics, 35,* 309–334.

Radouco-Thomas, S., Garcin, F., Murthy, M., Faure, N., Lemay, A., Forest, J., & Radouco-Thomas, C. (1984). Biological markers in major psychosis and alcoholism: Phenotypic and genotypic markers. *Journal of Psychiatric Research, 18,* 513–539.

Reich, T., Cloninger, C. R., van Eerdewegh, P., Rice, J. P., & Mullaney, J. (1988). Secular trends in the familial transmission of alcoholism. *Alcoholism: Clinical and Experimental Research, 12,* 458–464.

Robins, L. (1966). *Deviant children grown up.* Baltimore: Williams & Wilkins.

Roe, A. (1945). Children of alcoholic parents raised in foster homes. In *Alcohol, science and society* (pp. 378–393). New Haven: Quarterly Journal of Studies on Alcohol.

Russell, M., Henderson, C., & Blume, S. (1984). *Children of alcoholics: A review of the literature.* Buffalo, NY: New York State Division of Alcoholism and Alcohol Abuse, Research Institute on Alcoholism.

Scarr, S., Webber, P. L., Weinberg, R. A., & Wittig, M. A. (1981). Personality resemblance among adolescents and their parents in biologically related and adoptive families. *Journal of Personality and Social Psychology, 40,* 885–898.

Schmidt, A., & Neville, H. (1985). Language processing in men at risk for alcoholism: An event-related potential study. *Alcohol, 2,* 529–533.

Schuckit, M. (1980). Self-rating alcohol intoxication by young men with and without family histories of alcoholism. *Journal of Studies on Alcohol, 41,* 242–249.

Schuckit, M. A. (1985). Ethanol-induced changes in body sway seen at high alcoholism risk. *Archives of General Psychiatry, 42,* 375–379.

Schuckit, M. A., Gold, E. O., & Risch, C. (1987a). Plasma cortisol levels following ethanol in sons of alcoholics and controls. *Archives of General Psychiatry, 44,* 942–945.

Schuckit, M., Gold, E., & Risch, C. (1987b). Serum prolactin levels in sons of alcoholics and control subjects. *American Journal of Psychiatry, 144,* 854–859.

Schuckit, M., Goodwin, D., & Winokur, G. (1972). A study of alcoholism in half siblings. *American Journal of Psychiatry, 128,* 122–216.

Schulsinger, F., Knop, J., Goodwin, D., Teasdale, T., & Mikkelsen, U. (1986). A prospective study of young men at high risk for alcoholism. *Archives of General Psychiatry, 43,* 755–760.

Searles, J. (1988). The role of genetics in the pathogenesis of alcoholism. *Journal of Abnormal Psychology, 97,* 153–167.

Smith, C. (1974). Concordance in twins: Methods and interpretation. *American Journal of Human Genetics, 26,* 434–466.

Smollen, T. N., & Collins, A. C. (1985). Neurochemical mechanisms in the genetics of alcohol phenotypes. *Social Biology, 32,* 255–271.

Stabenau J. R. (1985). Basic research on heredity and alcohol: Implications for clinical application. *Social Biology, 32,* 297–321.

Swartz, C. M., Drews, V., & Cadoret, R. (1987). Decreased epinephrine in familial alcoholism: Initial findings. *Archives of General Psychiatry, 44,* 938–941.

Swinson, R. (1983). Genetic markers and alcoholism. In M. Galanter (Ed.), *Recent advances in alcoholism* (pp. 9–24). New York: Plenum.

Swinson, R., & Madden, J. (1973). ABO blood groups and ABH substance secretion in alcoholics. *Quarterly Journal of Studies on Alcohol, 34,* 64–70.

Tabakoff, B., Cornell, N., & Hoffman, P. L. (1986). Alcohol tolerance. *Annals of Emergency Medicine, 15,* 1005–1012.

Tabakoff, B., & Hoffman, P. (1987). Ethanol tolerance and dependence. In H. Goedde and D. Agerwal (Eds.), *Genetics and alcoholism* (pp. 253–269). New York: Alan R. Liss.

Tanna, V., Wilson, A., Winokur, G., & Elston, R. (1988). Possible linkage between alcoholism and esterase-D. *Journal of Studies on Alcohol, 49,* 472–476.

Tarter, R. E., Alterman, A. J., & Edwards, K. (1985). Vulnerability to alcoholism in men: A behavior-genetic perspective. *Journal of Studies on Alcohol, 46,* 329–356.

Tarter, R. E., & Hegedus, A. M. (1985). Neurological mechanisms underlying inheritance of alcoholism vulnerability. *International Journal of Neuroscience, 28,* 1–10.

Vaillant, G. (1983). *The natural history of alcoholism.* Cambridge, MA: Harvard University Press.

von Knorring, L., von Knorring, A. L., & Smigan, L. (1987). Personality traits in subtypes of alcoholics. *Journal of Studies on Alcohol, 48,* 523–527.

von Knorring, A. L., Bohman, M., von Knorring, L., & Oreland L. (1985). Platelet MAO activity as a biological marker in subgroups of alcoholism. *Acta Psychiatrica Scandinavica, 72,* 51–58.

Whipple, S., Parker, E., & Noble, E. (1988). An atypical neurocognitive profile in alcoholic fathers and their sons. *Journal of Studies on Alcohol, 49,* 240–244.

Wilson, J. R. (1985). Development of an animal model of alcohol dependence. *Social Biology, 32,* 229–240.

Winokur, G. (1974). The division of depressive disease into depression spectrum disease and pure depressive disease. *International Pharmacopsychiatry, 9,* 5–13.

Winokur, G. (1982). The development and validity of familial subtypes in primary unipolar depression. *Pharmacopsychiatria, 15,* 142–146.

Winokur, G., Rimmer, J., & Reich, T. (1971). Alcoholism IV: Is there more than one type of alcoholism? *British Journal of Psychiatry, 118,* 525–531.

3

Biological Markers for Vulnerability to Alcoholism

RALPH E. TARTER, HOWARD MOSS, and SUSAN B. LAIRD

Alcoholism is not randomly distributed in the population. The presence of alcoholism in first-degree family members of alcoholics (Reich, Winokur, & Mullaney, 1975), in the urban demographic populace (Room, 1983), and in those of Northern European ethnic origin (Vaillant, 1983) is, for example, higher than found in the general population. An issue of paramount importance, therefore, for understanding the multifactorial etiology of alcoholism is to document the characteristics of individuals who are susceptible to alcoholism. Once the vulnerability characteristics are known, it will then be possible to devise and implement interventions which are specifically targeted to this high risk population.

Diathesis—stress models of psychopathology afford the opportunity to elucidate the causes of alcoholism. The cardinal assertion is that there is a composite of liabilities (vulnerability) intrinsic to the organism which augment the likelihood (risk) for an adverse outcome. A myriad of factors mediating the pathway between vulnerability and outcome can either exacerbate the risk for an adverse outcome or alternatively attenuate the risk. Figure 1 outlines schematically the dynamic interplay between vulnerability or diathesis and key developmental and environmental parameters which, through idiosyncratic pathways, promotes either a positive or negative outcome. It can be seen that within this conceptual framework there is no single cause of alcoholism or one sufficient condition comprising the etiology. Nor is the outcome topologically homogeneous; indeed the complexity of factors and their interactions intervening between vulnerability and outcome argues against the likelihood of defining one specific diagnostic entity or an alcoholism syndrome.

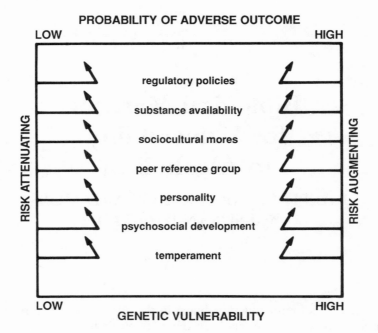

FIGURE 3.1. Interplay between vulnerability and developmental and environmental parameters.

Research directed at elucidating the biobehavioral characteristics associated with alcoholism vulnerability is guided by recognition that there is substantial individual variability in the population with respect to the time of drinking onset, pattern of beverage consumption, rate of ethanol metabolism, and the biomedical consequences of excessive and prolonged alcohol use. The end point, a psychiatric syndrome labeled alcohol abuse or dependence, reflects in very general terms the culmination of genetic predisposition, social learning, and precipitating environmental influences. This chapter reviews the literature pertaining to the putative genetic determinants of alcoholism vulnerability in human subjects. Reviews of research employing animal models have recently been published elsewhere (McClearn, 1988.).

WHAT IS A MARKER?

The term "marker" has been employed in a variety of different contexts. Radouco-Thomas, Garcia, Faure, and Leman et al. (1984) classify markers into several different types. Their interrelationship is depicted in Figure 2.

The most general term, "biological marker," simply denotes a concomitant characteristic of some condition. A "state marker" is a concomitant feature of the active disease. As such, it is sometimes referred to as an episode marker. It is essentially a diagnostic measure of the presence of a disease phenomenon, as for example, low serum albumin levels in liver disease. Substantial research effort has been devoted, for instance, to diagnosing alcoholism based on hepatologic and hematologic laboratory indices subjected to sophisticated statistical techniques. This research has yielded very accurate methods of detection; however, the complexity of the equations derived from combinations of numerous predictor variables mitigates the general applicability of these procedures for clinical practice. Nonetheless, the point to be made is that state markers for diagnosing the disease sequelae of chronic excessive drinking have been revealed which have a better than acceptable level of sensitivity.

In contrast, a "trait marker" is a characteristic of the individual that is present independently of the disease. As such it is present during the lifespan of the individual and may indicate a predisposing factor for the

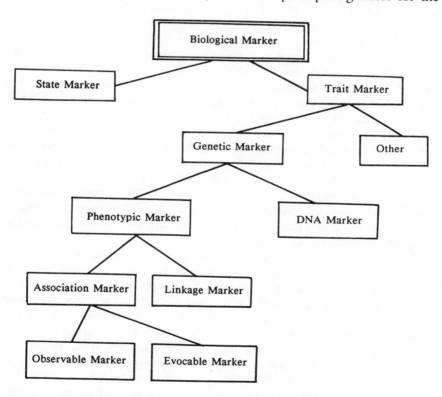

FIGURE 3.2. Interrelationship of markers for alcoholism.

disease. Generally, research in this area has been much less rewarding; however, the preliminary findings suggest that this avenue of investigation may identify persons at risk for alcoholism. It is this program of research that comprises the primary focus of this review.

Genetic markers are one particular type of trait marker. The key requirement of a genetic marker is that it is present in persons affected with the condition; this is referred to as nonindependent assortment or segregation.

There are two subtypes of genetic markers. Phenotypic markers reflect gene expression with respect to morphology, biochemistry, physiology, behavior, or any other observable characteristic. As such, they are indirect indicators of gene activity. However, nonhereditary alterations in phenotype, termed phenocopies (usually produced by environmental factors), may mimic the effects of specific genes. Thus, techniques that employ phenotypic markers may lack specificity. Genotype or DNA markers derive from the analysis of DNA sequences, which is readily accomplished as the result of recent advances in recombinant DNA technology. These newer techniques of molecular biology yield results with superior specificity, but are limited by our current rudimentary knowledge of the DNA sequences comprising the human genome.

Association and linkage markers comprise the two types of phenotypic markers. A linkage marker is a phenotype where the gene is physically proximal on the chromosome to the gene underlying the putative condition. A functional association between the marker gene and disease gene is not implied, but because they are geographically close on the chromosome they are assumed to be inherited together. Research investigating color blindness or blood type in alcoholism attempts to identify markers using the linkage approach. In contrast, an associative marker is related functionally to the putative condition. These markers are integral to either the pathogenesis of the disorder or are reflected as a biological process in the causal chain of events culminating in the disorder. Biochemical, neurophysiologic, and enzymatic characteristics that have yielded encouraging results, vis à vis detection of a marker for alcoholism, fall, for the most part, in the category of associative markers.

Associative markers are either dispositionally observable or evoked (Radouco-Thomas et al., 1984). The former marker is always present dispositionally whereas the latter is revealed only following a biological challenge. Evoking an abnormal or atypical response comprises the basic paradigm of pharmacogenetic research and is a useful procedure for unmasking biological variability in the population or for detecting the mechanisms of vulnerability to the disorder of interest. With respect to alcoholism, the most common practice has been to administer a challenge dose of alcohol (Schuckit, 1987); however, other methods such as infusion of thyrotropin releasing hormone have also been utilized (Moss, Guthrie, & Linnoila, 1986).

Thus, the term marker can denote either a general or specific phenomenon. As will be discussed subsequently, with respect to alcoholism, vulnerability markers have been implicated having either a genetic or nongenetic basis, and in the former context, in paradigms attempting to identify associative (observable and evocable) as well as linkage markers.

ALCOHOLISM VULNERABILITY: ETIOLOGY AND CONSEQUENCES

The fundamental question concerns why a minority of the alcohol consuming population develops an habitual and problematic association with this beverage. This issue bears directly on vulnerability as a predisposing characteristic. A secondary but closely related question concerns whether there is a differential vulnerability in certain individuals to experience the adverse consequences of excessive prolonged drinking. This issue bears on vulnerability to medical disease where alcohol use is itself a risk factor. Two areas of research have attracted wide interest.

Central Nervous System Sensitivity

Heavy drinking, particularly its clinical concomitants, hangovers, loss of control, and drinking pattern, appear to be influenced strongly by genetics (Kaij, 1960; Partanen, Brun, & Markkanen, 1966). These findings indicate that there are differential effects of alcohol on the CNS in the population. It has also been shown that alcohol's effects on EEG activity are largely under genetic control (Propping, 1977). Significantly, nonalcoholics who are at known high risk for alcoholism (Pollock, et al., 1983) exhibit a different EEG response than controls following an ethanol challenge. Prolactin levels (Schuckit, Gold, & Reisch, 1987) discriminate low from high risk individuals following an acute alcohol challenge, suggesting that persons vulnerable to alcoholism may be differentially reactive to alcohol's neuropharmacologic effects.

Other lines of research suggest that high risk individuals may experience a stronger reinforcing effect from alcohol than persons who are at low risk. High risk status, determined on the basis of either the presence of familial alcoholism or antisocial personality characteristics of the subjects, is associated with both stress dampening and concomitant sympathetic nervous system attenuation following acute alcohol administration (Finn & Pihl, 1987; Levenson, Oyama, & Meek, 1987; Schuckit, 1984a; Sher & Levenson, 1982).

With respect to the consequences of alcoholism, a susceptibility to develop clinical neurologic disease may be present in certain individuals who drink excessively and for a prolonged period. For example, strong evidence has been reported indicating that the Wernicke-Korsakoff syndrome is due to an inherited deficit in transketolase activity. This enzyme is required for the absorption and utilization of thiamine (vitamin B_1) (Mukerjee, Svoronos, Ghazanfari, & Martin, 1987). Significantly, in concordance with the diathesis-stress model, the enzyme deficiency is insufficient to induce the Korsakoff syndrome which also requires a history of alcohol abuse for this amnestic disorder to be manifest. The observation that the morphologic brain changes in amnesic alcoholics occur while they are still young and relatively early in their drinking career (Wilkinson & Carlen, 1980) suggests that chronic alcohol consumption may have particularly deleterious effects on CNS integrity for some people. The point to be made, however, is that not all individuals in the alcoholic population share the same liability to suffer neurologic disease from their drinking, and that the Korsakoff syndrome, perhaps the most debilitating neurologic sequela, is associated with a genetic predisposition that may be easily detectable biochemically.

Ethanol Metabolism

The pathogenesis of alcoholism may also be facilitated by genetically determined mechanisms regulating alcohol metabolism. In this regard, the acute actions and effects of alcohol on various organ systems can directly influence the development of physical addiction in addition to predisposing to alcohol-related diseases. Alcohol elimination rate is to a large degree under genetic control. Where the rate is slow it can be expected that because of higher peak blood alcohol concentrations due to longer half-life of alcohol in systemic circulation the ethanol can potentially cause greater injury to all organs and systems.

Alcohol is metabolized in two stages. First, ethanol is oxidized into acetaldehyde which in turn is reduced to acetate. Acetate subsequently enters the general metabolic pathway for sugar and fats to be oxidated into water and carbon dioxide. Of particular interest is alcohol dehydrogenase (ADH) since it is this enzyme which primarily determines the rate of alcohol metabolism. Significantly, there are numerous forms of this enzyme that differ with respect to their catalytic properties (Bosron & Li, 1981). Moreover, because the location of this enzyme is in the liver, where most of the oxidation of alcohol takes place, the functional characteristics of the liver and its susceptibility to injury in persons vulnerable to alcoholism has become a subject of prime interest.

Although it would appear likely that vulnerable persons would be expected to metabolize ethanol differently from nonvulnerable individuals, the results of research to date have not supported this notion. Ethanol metabolism and elimination rates have not been shown to discriminate between individuals at high and low risk for alcoholism (Moss, Yao, Maddock, 1989; Schuckit, 1984b). Similarly, specific forms of ADH have not been shown to segregate among alcoholic individuals (Von-Wartburg & Buhler, 1984), nor does possession of an atypical form of ADH invariably alter the rate of alcohol metabolism (Edwards & Evans, 1967). Although both of these latter kinetic properties are largely under genetic control, it is clear that rates of ethanol metabolism and elimination are not markers for alcoholism.

Acetaldehyde dehydrogenase (ALDH), on the other hand, may be a protective marker and indeed reduce risk for developing alcoholism. For example, an atypical acetaldehyde dehydrogenase genetic trait (Bosron & Li, 1981) is present in about 50% of Orientals and, compared to Caucasians, appears to be responsible for their slower rate of acetaldehyde metabolism. Indeed, Orientals with this trait appear to suffer from alcohol intolerance (Mizoi et al., 1979). The slow metabolism of acetaldehyde due to atypical ALDH activity underlies the facial flushing response which is accompanied by rapid heart rate, nausea, low blood pressure, and, in severe cases, vomiting. This punishing effect of alcohol consumption is thus likely to reduce the probability of voluntary alcohol consumption and hence the development of habitual use. To date, no alcohol metabolizing enzyme has been identified in humans, which appears to augment the risk for alcoholism.

Alcohol is metabolized almost entirely in the liver with minor contribution by the kidneys and other organs. Not surprisingly, the most prevalent biological injury is to the liver, which histopathologically progresses from the stage of fatty liver to hepatitis, and ultimately to cirrhosis. Significantly, most individuals who consume excessive amounts of alcoholic beverages over the long term do not develop cirrhosis. Although estimates vary across studies, the available findings suggest that less than 25% of the alcoholic population develop cirrhosis (Lelbach, 1975). While the pattern of drinking may be more malignant in alcoholics who develop cirrhosis and in whom nutritional deficiency may be more severe, it is becoming increasingly appreciated that there may also be a genetic vulnerability (Hrubec & Omenn, 1981). This end stage sequela of alcoholism is poorly correlated with drinking pattern or duration (Galambos, 1977). Recent research has supported the notion that alcoholic cirrhosis may be an immunologically mediated disease. Increased immunoglobulin levels in alcoholic cirrhosis seems to be related to the severity of disease (Wilson, Onstad, & Williams 1969). Immune markers have also been examined with respect to identifying individuals at risk for alcoholism; however, the results have been generally negative.

Population based research is required to clarify the association between immune markers and hepatic disease. For example, the demonstration of Laennec cirrhosis in a young female with only very modest levels of alcohol beverage consumption suggests that this disease condition is not merely the product of longstanding alcohol abuse (Cueller, Tarter, Hays, & Van

Thiel, 1987). Moreover, females are especially susceptible to developing cirrhosis (Gavaler, 1982). In addition, Arria, Tarter, Williams, and Van Thiel (1988) found that the age of onset of nonalcoholic autoimmune liver disease (and alcoholic cirrhosis) is earlier among individuals who have a family history of alcoholism. Whether this vulnerability reflects a specific genetic predisposition, is the product of general biological and sociocultural factors, or is the combination of both, remains to be elucidated.

As discussed previously, a marker does not necessarily imply that the phenotype is under genetic control. Indeed, the term marker has been widely applied to refer to any characteristic that may presage alcoholism. The use of the concept of a genetic marker for nongenetic phenomena can unfortunately lead one to infer that a genetic mechanism is present. For this reason, it is important to specify the criteria for a genetic marker.

Predictive Validity. The marker must identify individuals at risk for the outcome. With respect to alcoholism etiology, the marker should be present before the onset of drinking as well as before any other comorbid psychopathology. The marker should ideally be specific to the alcoholism and not be merely reflective of any other type of psychopathology. No marker has yet been identified for alcoholism which meets this condition.

Construct Validity. The marker should have a genetic basis. Research on genetic markers has yielded inconclusive results. For example, inherited phenotypes (e.g., blood grouping) which are totally under genetic control have not been found to be associated with the risk for alcoholism. Other characteristics which are largely, but not entirely, under genetic control (e.g., EEG parameters, platelet MAO level) have been shown to be related to alcoholism risk. Indeed, the strongest support to date for the presence of markers for alcoholism has been obtained measuring biological processes having uncertain genetic contribution (e.g., static ataxia, cognitive deficit, P300 of the evoked potential, behavioral deviance). Thus, with respect to the criterion that the marker have a known genetic basis, it should be emphasized that the available evidence is equivocal; virtually all of the findings to date implicate predisposing traits which have significant nongenetic contribution.

Discriminative Validity. The marker should segregate among the population who have alcoholism or among individuals who have a first degree relative with alcoholism. This criterion has also not been met.

Prevalence. The marker should have a low base rate in the population. This criterion has not been met for any putative marker for alcoholism. The markers investigated to date have relatively high population base rates (e.g., blood types).

In summary, none of the criteria required for invoking the presence of a pure genetic marker for alcoholism have been satisfied. Although numerous clues about markers for vulnerability have been hypothesized, spanning all levels of biological organization, the evidence supporting any one of the plethora of traits implicated is, at best, equivocal.

MODELS OF GENETIC TRANSMISSION

Two different genetic models have been applied to research into the heritability of alcoholism. These are the single gene model and the multifactorial genetic model. Four modes of transmission are possible within a single gene or Mendelian model of heredity, these being autosomal dominant, autosomal recessive, sex-linked dominant, and sex-linked recessive. The single gene model receiving the most attention asserts that alcoholism is transmitted via a recessive gene located on the X chromosome. The supporting evidence based on studies of color blindness (Cruz-Coke & Varela, 1966) has been faulted for both methodologic and statistical reasons. Other single gene hypotheses have likewise not received empirical support.

The multifactorial hypothesis of genetic transmission has received stronger empirical support. Significantly, multifactorial models of genetic transmission have the advantage of accommodating nongenetic as well as genetic factors. Alcoholism per se is not hypothesized to be inherited but rather it is the underlying vulnerability to develop alcoholism which is conjectured to be transmitted. Furthermore, the vulnerability is assumed to be normally distributed in the population, which upon surpassing a threshold, culminates in the adverse outcome. The mode of transmission is polygenic; that is, it involves the concurrent action of many genes. Although conceptually appealing and consistent with a diathesis-stress perspective of vulnerability, it should be noted that multifactorial models cannot separate environment from genetic modes of transmission when studying intact families. The strength of the multifactorial model lies in its ability to accommodate assortative mating and for investigating nonintact families.

Research applying the multifactorial model has provided strong evidence for a genetic contribution to alcoholism (Cloninger, Reich, & Wetzel, 1979). Moreover, two general subtypes of alcoholism (Cloninger, Bohman, & Sigvardsson, 1981) have been proposed having varying degree of heritability and a different natural history. Recently, secular changes with respect to age of onset and prevalence of alcoholism have also been documented employing a multifactorial genetic model (Reich, Cloninger, Van Eerdewegh, Rice, & Mullaney, 1988).

Family, adoption, and twin studies generally support a genetic predisposition to alcoholism although it should be noted that the evidence is not entirely consistent (Murray, Clifford, & Gurling, 1983; Searles, 1988). A multifactorial model of genetic transmission nonetheless best fits the available data. The biological pathways or mechanisms of gene expression are, however, unknown. Only recently have the biochemical, physiological, or behavioral expressions of gene activity been investigated. The ensuing discussion summarizes the status of these research findings.

TRAIT MARKERS FOR ALCOHOLISM

Alcoholism is a heterogeneous disorder. Labels such as "alcohol abuse" or "alcohol dependence" characterize diverse individuals with respect to comorbid psychopathology, psychosocial history, and behavioral patterns. Indeed, only a minority of persons who are designated as alcoholic have problems confined only to alcohol consumption or its consequences. Additionally, the natural history, clinical presentation, and familial transmission of alcoholism differs between males and females. For these reasons, it is highly unlikely that one genetic marker will be discovered which characterizes all persons at risk. Furthermore, it is important to reiterate and underscore the point that a marker only serves to characterize persons at risk for alcoholism; that is, it describes a genetically mediated liability expressed at one or more levels of biological organization. The presence of a marker does not imply an invariant or causal relationship to outcome. Depending on familial and extrafamilial factors, acquired social skills and interpersonal interactional patterns, personality and behavioral competencies, the person may surmount a genetic vulnerability and hence not succumb to an alcoholism outcome. The following discussion reviews the literature and current status of the evidence pertaining to markers of alcoholism risk.

Morphologic Markers

Physique is largely genetically determined although it is modifiable by diet, drugs (e.g., anabolic steroids), and exercise. Somatotype has been shown to be related to quantity of alcohol consumption, with mesomorphs having the highest consumption levels (Rees & Eysenck, 1945). It has also been found that boys having both a "gynic" or feminine appearing physique and antisocial propensities are at heightened risk for alcoholism (Monnelly, Hartl, & Elderkin, 1983). Indeed, in this latter study, 85% of a sample could be correctly classified at outcome according to these two variables.

Body morphology has not been systematically studied as a vulnerability trait. Its importance as a vulnerability marker is evident in its role as a social stimulus. As the child disengages from parental authority, and becomes increasingly influenced by peers, acceptance into a particular peer reference group is mediated by dimensions of attractiveness and maturity. Hence, at puberty, when alcohol use is likely to be initiated, the youngster who is sexually and physically mature may be more inclined to drink simply because this behavior is more normative among older adolescents. Similarly, athletically inclined and physically stronger boys may drink more because drinking often accompanies sporting pastimes. At the other extreme, physical unattractiveness may induce drinking because of social withdrawal or loneliness. The point to be made is that for different reasons, physical appearance and body morphology can be a vulnerability factor which, combined with other psychosocial risk factors, can precipitate problem drinking. This issue has not been explored empirically, although it has been found in one prospective study that in females, early pubertal development combined with older group peer affiliation is associated with subsequent antisocial behavior, low academic achievement, and substance abuse by the third decade of life (Magnusson, Stattin, & Allen, 1986). This finding illustrates how social mediational factors interact with a biologically determined vulnerability to produce adverse outcomes.

Biochemical Markers

Genes are expressed biochemically, and a number of biochemical characteristics appear to differentiate high from low risk individuals. The most researched trait has been monoamine oxidase (MAO) level measured in platelet membranes. Low MAO levels have been observed in alcoholics and first degree relatives of alcoholics (Alexopoulos, Lieberman, & Frances, 1983). Moreover, MAO level is particularly low in alcoholics with antisocial propensities (von Knorring, Bohman, von Knorring, & Oreland, 1985). Of particular interest is the finding of an association between low platelet MAO level and behavioral traits reflecting poor self-regulatory capacity. In this regard, it is noteworthy that low platelet MAO level correlates with sensation seeking, impulsivity, and behavioral disinhibition (Zuckerman, 1984). Also, persons selected for these traits have low MAO levels (von Knorring et al., 1985). However, the finding that chronic exposure to alcohol itself lowers platelet MAO activity (Tabakoff, Lee, DeLeon-Jones, & Hoffman, 1985) confounds this area of research.

Biochemical indicators of central neurochemical mechanisms have also been investigated. Low brain serotonin, measured by peripheral metabolites, has also been implicated to underlie alcoholism vulnerability (Boismare et al., 1987). This neurotransmitter is particularly interesting in light of its association with impulsive and violent behavior (Schalling, Asberg, & Edman, 1984); these latter features are commonly associated with antisocial alcoholism. Moss, Yao, Burns, Maddlock, and Tarter (in press) observed that sons of alcoholics had lower plasma gamma-aminobutyric acid (GABA) levels than male offspring of nonalcoholics. This is a major inhibitory amino acid neurotransmitter, and disturbances in this neural system may contribute to the behavioral dysregulation observed in alcoholics.

Neuropeptides have also been the subject of research (Van Ree, 1986). These are hormone fragments which modulate neurotransmitter activity and are particularly integral to brain reward mechanisms and regulation of homeostasis. Numerous pituitary and brain opioid peptides and other pituitary hormones (e.g., ACTH, prolactin, vasopressin, melanophore stimulating hormone) have been implicated on theoretical grounds; however, there is currently no empirical evidence supporting the role of these neuropeptides in alcoholism. Endorphins are endogenous opiates and are intimately involved in regulating reinforcement. Although theoretically plausible, evidence has yet to be provided implicating these transmitters to alcoholism in humans. Moss et al. (1986) observed higher basal thyrotropin levels and an enhanced thyrotropin response which they attribute to a disruption of biogenic mechanisms in persons at risk for alcoholism.

For several reasons, the neurochemical studies have not been very rewarding with respect to elucidating the neurotransmitter systems underlying alcoholism. First, although the observed differences between high and low risk subjects have been reported and may reflect phenotypic characteristics, and although there may be sensitive indicators of alcoholism vulnerability, their specificity and impact on alcoholism outcome remains unknown. Second, the complexity of behavior defining alcoholism in all likelihood is the end point of the synergistic interplay among multiple neurotransmitter systems. Thus, while single mechanism investigations have been informative, the need remains to more fully characterize the neurochemical substrate which may be altered in vulnerable individuals. For example, it has been hypothesized that, at least with respect to antisocial behavior, a disruption of equilibrium between cholinergic and adrenergic neurotransmitter systems occurs (Mawson & Mawson, 1977). It would appear to be important to know how different neural systems combine to characterize the vulnerability to alcoholism so as to fully describe the biochemical vulnerability. To date, research has focused almost entirely on the monoaminergic and peptidergic systems.

Because alcohol is metabolized primarily in the liver, extensive research has been conducted with the aim of clarifying genetic markers of alcoholism which may be expressed phenotypically in liver function. The liver is a major organ of immune regulation and because the gene loci are already known for the human histocompatibility complex, studies have been undertaken to characterize immune processes in alcoholics or high risk persons with the aim of implicating specific chromosomes carrying the alcoholic genes. Most of the effort has focussed on human (leucocytic) antigens (HLA) located on chromosome number six. The results of this line of research, however, have been disappointing. In a study of 27 HLA antigens, Rosler, Bellaire, Hengesch, Giannitsis, and Jarovici (1983), for example, found no evidence for an association with alcoholism.

There also appears to be genetic vulnerability to develop cirrhosis (Hrubec & Omenn, 1981). Hepatic markers for cirrhosis have not, however, been identified. The bulk of research has focused on the HLA complex and has yielded inconclusive results (Watson, Mohs, Eskelson, Sampliner, & Hartman, 1986). Interestingly, individuals with autoimmune cirrhosis develop their disease earlier in life if there is a family history of alcoholism (Arria et al., in press). Thus, the consequences of alcoholism vis à vis cirrhosis may be genetically determined, although the biological mechanisms still remain to be elucidated.

Neurophysiological Markers of Alcoholism

One mode of expression of the vulnerability to alcoholism may be in the form of disturbed physiological functioning of the brain. The waveform frequency on the EEG is to a great extent under genetic control (Propping, 1983). However, it should be pointed out that children of alcoholics are at greater risk of experiencing physical abuse and bouts of unconsciousness (Tarter, Hegedus, Goldstein, Shelly, & Alterman, 1984). Only when the neurologic history is known can inferences about inherited brain abnormality be made.

Two studies have been conducted that measure the EEGs in children of alcoholics. Gabrielli et al. (1982) observed that children of alcoholics had an excess of high frequency activity. Pollock et al. (1983) observed a greater augmentation of alpha energy after an acute alcohol challenge in children of alcoholics. The results of these latter experiments are difficult to interpret but may reflect higher resting organismic activation level and greater sedation after an acute alcohol challenge than occurs in low risk persons. Significantly, Naitoh (1972) has reported that alcohol exerts both a calming and arousing effect in alcoholics, suggesting perhaps that alcohol beverage consumption exerts its reinforcing effects by destabilizing homeostatic states.

Measurement of event related potentials (ERP) enables analysis of neurophysiologic phenomena that are time-locked to sensory stimuli. Following exteroceptive stimulation (e.g., flashes, tones, visual patterns, mild electric shock) it is possible to directly measure processing of the stimulus at various loci in the afferent pathway, and, particularly for the late components of the ERP, detection of the stimulus at the cortical level. This procedure is accomplished by the use of computer averaging in which sensory signals are extrapolated from the background EEG.

Research employing evoked potential methods has elicited much media attention. However, an objective appraisal of the empirical evidence underscores the tentative status of the findings. The initial study by Elmasian, Neville, Woods, Schuckit, and Bloom (1982) investigated a small sample of children of alcoholics who were administered placebo or low dose or high dose of ethanol. The ERP response was recorded in response to a series of tones of which the target tone had a shorter duration. The main finding from this investigation was that subjects with a family history of alcoholism demonstrated a relatively lower amplitude of the P300 component. This late appearing waveform component is generally assumed to constitute a neurophysiologic substrate for attention. Significantly, it was observed that P300 attenuation occurred also when the children of alcoholics were tested in the placebo condition.

Subsequent research has yielded inconsistent results. Schmidt and Neville (1985), controlling for maternal alcohol consumption, found no differences in P300 amplitude between sons of alcoholics and nonalcoholics. It should be noted, however, that the sample was small ($n = 10$) and that the subjects were young adults who were experienced drinkers. Among the children of alcoholics, drinks per occasion was associated with lower amplitude and a longer P300 latency.

The third study, conducted by Begleiter, Porjesz, Bihari, and Kissin (1984), controlled for history of exposure to alcohol. In a sample of young boys, they found that the P300 amplitude was attenuated where there was a family history of alcoholism. Unlike the previous two studies they investigated the visual modality using a task that required the subjects to discriminate target from nontarget stimuli. Subsequent studies have provided partial confirmation of Begleiter et al.'s findings of lower P300 amplitude in children of alcoholics. Investigations by Schuckit (1985), Whipple, Parker, and Noble (1988), O'Connor, Hesselbrock, and Tasman (1986), and Hill, Steinhauer, Zubin, and Baughman (1988) have found P300 differences between sons of alcoholics and nonalcoholics, although the magnitude of effects and specific aspect of the waveform difference (latency or amplitude) is not consistent across studies. In one investigation comparing alcoholics with a positive family history of alcoholism to those without such a family history (Patterson, Williams, McLean, Smith, & Schaeffer, 1987), it was observed that the former subjects had a lower P300 amplitude although latency was indistinguishable between the groups. Polich, Burns, and Bloom (1988), on the other hand, failed to find any differences between children of alcoholics and nonalcoholics. The reasons for these discrepancies among studies are uncertain but may be due to sampling factors. For example, Polich et al. (1988) assessed young adult university students who may represent a less severely impaired group, as indicated by the fact that the subjects have made a successful adjustment by their status as university students. The important point thus needs to be raised that the putative CNS dysfunction may not be present in all individuals predisposed to alcoholism and that its utility as a marker for vulnerability may be limited.

To date, almost all of the ERP research has focused on the P300 waveform component. Evidence for disturbances in the early waveform components of the ERP has not been reported, illustrating that sensory disturbances are not associated with alcoholism vulnerability. One late component, which has been recorded in one study, concerns the N430 waveform. In a pilot study of five cases, Schmidt and Neville (1985) found that the amplitude of the N430 wave was lower in sons of alcoholics. This negative wave appears approximately 400–450 milliseconds after stimulus onset and appears to be associated with the processing of linguistic information.

Taken as a whole, the available evidence implicates a perceptual information processing deficit in persons at risk for alcoholism. The causes of this disturbance are, however, unknown. Also, it should be emphasized that the neurophysiologic deviations are not observed in all high risk persons. Moreover, neither the meaning nor significance of the P300 findings is understood. They may reflect the neurophysiologic substrate of an attention disorder which, as will be noted in the next section, is probably present in a high proportion of boys at known risk for alcoholism. The extent to which this type of cognitive disorder contributes to an adverse outcome, and the manner by which attentional factors interact with other predisposing risk factors (e.g., conduct disorder, impulsivity) remains unknown. Thus, reservations need to be enunciated so as to not uncritically accept the presence of the ERP data to reflect a specific biological marker of alcoholism. Nevertheless, the research using ERP measurements has been very encouraging with respect to identifying a neural coding disturbance, possibly mediated in part in the hippocampus (since this is one generator source for the P300) in individuals at risk for alcoholism.

Psychophysiologic Markers

Numerous motivational theories of alcoholism etiology have been advanced. Among the earliest theories, the one that has received the most empirical confirmation promotes the hypothesis that alcohol consumption for alcoholics is especially tranquilizing. Although it is unlikely that tension reduction is the prime reason for drinking in all alcoholics, three investigations have reported that alcohol exercises a "stress dampening" effect in high risk individuals (Finn & Pihl, 1987; Levenson, Oyama, & Meek, 1987; Sher & Levenson, 1982). The finding that ethanol is more reinforcing in high risk young adults suggests that a dysregulation of sympathetic nervous system reactivity may comprise an important component of alcoholism vulnerability. It is also interesting to note that it has been hypothesized that alcohol has a homeostatic effect on autonomic nervous system regulation in alcoholics. The evidence implicating a disorder of autonomic regulation is buttressed by emerging data indicating that psychopathy, which characterizes *Type II alcoholics*, is featured by a disturbance in arousal regulation. These individuals have an alcoholism onset early in life, exhibiting recurring patterns of alcohol use and multiple treatment involvement as well as paternal history of crimes. It may be that alcohol consumption for such individuals represents an attempt to stabilize an otherwise labile arousal disposition.

Neurologic Markers

Alcoholism vulnerability may be expressed as a neurologic disturbance. Preliminary research suggests that this may occur in at least two ways—as either a clinical neurologic disorder or as an idiosyncratic cortical organization of functional psychological capacities. Familial tremor (Nasarallah, Keelor, & McCalley-Whitters, 1983) and static ataxia (Hegedus, Tarter, Hill, Jacob, & Winsten, 1984; Lester & Carpenter, 1985) have been reported to be more prevalent in first degree relatives of alcoholics, suggesting that an inhibitory motor system disorder may comprise one component of a generalized disinhibitory disturbance. The higher prevalence of left-handedness among alcoholics compared to the normal population (London, Kibbee, & Holt, 1985) indicates that there may be an idiosyncratic neurologic organization of functional capacities in a subset of the population predisposed to alcoholism. These neurologic correlates of alcoholism vulnerability are, however, based on relatively small clinical samples. Furthermore, while these latter features may be sensitive markers of alcoholism vulnerability, it is very unlikely that they specifically characterize persons at risk for only this disorder.

Psychologic Markers

Cognitive Impairment

Findings accrued to date indicate that children of alcoholics perform deficiently on certain cognitive tests (Bennett, Wolin, & Reiss, 1988; Hegedus, Tarter, et al., 1984; Tarter, Hegedus, Goldstein, et al., 1984). Deficits have also been reported on cognitive tests in offspring of alcoholics (Knop, Teasdale, Schulsinger, & Goodwin, 1985). The impairments appear to encompass a variety of cognitive processes involving short-term memory, planning, visuospatial analysis, and attention. Furthermore, it has been demonstrated that children of alcoholics do not progress in school as expeditiously as children of nonalcoholic parents (Knop et al., 1985), and perform less well than other children on standardized tests of educational achievement (Hegedus, Alterman, & Tarter, 1984). These latter findings may reflect the effects of an adverse home environment; however, the possibility exists that the slower educational progress may be due in part to suboptimal cognitive development due to nonenvironmental factors.

Little formal research has been conducted to delineate the severity and pattern of cognitive impairment in children of alcoholics. Where deficits are found they do not merely reflect a generalized cognitive impairment. Rather, the deficits appear to be somewhat circumscribed. Tarter, Alterman, & Edwards (1988), upon reviewing the available literature, concluded that the pattern of cognitive and behavioral impairment is consistent with a disorder of neural systems lying along the frontal–midbrain neuroaxis. It is significant to point out that the anterior cerebrum does not functionally mature until about mid-adolescence (Luria, 1961, 1966; Vygotsky, 1962); thus the cognitive sequelae observed may reflect a functional immaturity of the CNS substrate. Hence, relative to their chronologic age, children of alcoholics may have a neuromaturational retardation.

Behavioral Disturbance

Offspring of alcoholics domiciling with their parents have a higher prevalence of personality and emotional disturbances than their peers (Tarter, Hegedus, Goldstein, et al. 1984). A conduct disorder has also been found to be more frequently present as well (Cloninger & Reich, 1983). Although it is generally recognized that there is no single "alcoholic personality," a review of the literature indicates that certain trait dimensions indicative of a disposition toward behavioral disinhibition is more prevalent among children of alcoholics. Indeed, a syndrome of disinhibitory psychopathology has been conjectured to underlie alcoholism vulnerability, which has as its neural substrate a dysfunctional frontal-septal system and which, at the behavioral level, is reflected in impaired self-regulation (Tarter, Alterman, & Edwards, 1985).

The origins of personality are in temperament. Temperaments are behavioral propensities which have a high heritable contribution and are present and measurable within the first few weeks or months of life (Garrison & Earls, 1987). Although numerous temperament traits have been suggested at one time or another, empirical evidence strongly implicates the presence of only a few such traits. Activity level, emotionality, attention span persistence, and sociability are among the temperaments for which the strongest empirical evidence exists. Significantly, there is emerging evidence documenting extreme manifestation of each of these latter traits in children of alcoholics or in individuals who subsequently became alcoholic (Tarter et al., 1985). How these inherited behavioral propensities are shaped by the social environment to establish habitual styles of behavior or personality disposition is the central research question pertaining to elucidating the psychological basis of alcoholism vulnerability.

In addition, it appears that high behavioral activity level, or hyperactivity, may be a sensitive but nonspecific precursor to alcoholism. Hyperactive children have a higher prevalence of paternal alcoholism than their peers even if reared away from their biologic parents (Cantwell, 1975; Morrison & Stewart, 1971). Children of alcoholics (Tarter, McBride, Buonpane, & Schneider, 1977; Wood, Wender, & Reimherr, 1983) and boys who subsequently develop alcoholism (McCord, McCord, & Gudeman, 1960) have been reported to have a higher prevalence of hyperactivity. This behavioral disturbance is, however, embedded in a conduct disorder and thus may not comprise a pure behavioral trait.

EVOKED TRAIT MARKERS FOR ALCOHOLISM

A substantial literature has developed in the past two decades which attempts to identify abnormalities that may be detectable when the vulnerable person is challenged pharmacologically. Most of this research has involved the administration of alcohol to individuals at known high risk. Several studies have employed the challenge of thyroid-releasing hormone or have examined taste sensitivity to solutions of phenylthioureas. These latter studies will be briefly reviewed before addressing the ethanol challenge literature.

A number of disease states are associated with taste insensitivity. Phenylthiocarbamide, one of a group of phenylthioureas, is a two-phase genetic polymorphism; 70% are tasters and 30% are nontasters. Although encouraging results have been reported in one study (Eckardt, Rawlings, & Martia, 1986), the majority of findings are inconclusive with respect to alcoholics being over- or underrepresented on this phenotype.

The findings with respect to thyrotropin-releasing hormone (TRH) challenge are more encouraging. In a number of studies of recently abstinent and long-term abstinent alcoholic men (Loosen, Prange, & Wilson, 1979), a blunted thyrotropin (TSH) response was observed (Loosen, Wilson, Dew, & Tipermas, 1983). However, enhanced baseline and stimulated TSH responses were found in nine sons of alcoholic fathers (Moss et al., 1986). Interestingly, thyrotropin-releasing hormone appears to antagonize the CNS depressant effects of alcohol and other drugs (Cott, Breese, Cooper, Barlow, & Prange, 1976).

Paradigms employing an ethanol challenge have primarily compared the differences between individuals at high and low risk for alcoholism. The investigations have been directed to a variety of biological and psychological processes. The basic objective of this research is pharmacogenetic; that is, the identification of individual variability in drug response having a genetic basis.

Alcohol Metabolism

Blood alcohol curves of young men who are either positive or negative for familial alcoholism are indistinguishable (Schuckit 1987). Lex, Lucas, Greenwald, & Mendelson (1988) obtained similar results for women following an alcohol challenge. Numerous other investigations have also failed to find a difference between subjects dichotomized according to family history (Lipscomb & Nathan, 1980; O'Malley & Maisto, 1985; Pollock et al., 1983; Schuckit, 1984c; Schuckit, O'Connor, Duby, Vega, & Moss, 1981; Schuckit, Parker, & Rossman, 1983), including one study (Utne, Hansen, Winkler, & Schulsinger, 1977) in which the subjects were adoptees who were not living with their alcoholic biological parents. Alcohol dehydrogenase is the rate determining enzyme for alcohol metabolism, but in view of the similarities in ethanol elimination between high and low risk individuals it is unlikely that this comprises a biochemical vulnerability marker.

There are, however, pronounced differences among various ethnic and racial groups (Agarwal & Goedde, 1987; Del Villano, Miller, Schacter, & Tischfield, 1980) with respect to alcohol metabolism. Because of the finding that there are multiple molecular forms of ADH which fit a genetic model encompassing five gene loci (Bosron & Li, 1981), interest has remained high in this area. The unequal distribution of the ADH variants among different racial or ethnic groupings, which correspond roughly to alcoholism prevalence rates in the population, has been the major reason for the sustaining interest in this topic.

The first product of alcohol metabolism is acetaldehyde caused by the enzymatic actions of ADH. One report (Schuckit & Rayses, 1979) has suggested that offspring of alcoholics have higher acetaldehyde levels after an alcohol challenge compared to children of nonalcoholics. This study has been criticized on methodological grounds, particularly the fact that the assay procedure cannot yield valid measurement due to the facility of aldehyde binding and production of acetaldehyde following acid treatment of the sample. Hence, accurate determinations were not possible given the analytical procedures used. Moreover, other investigators have not been able to replicate the findings of higher acetaldehyde levels (Von Wartburg & Buhler, 1984).

The second stage of alcohol metabolism involves the reduction of aldehyde to acetate by acetaldehyde dehydrogenase. There has been increasing interest in this enzyme because of its reported association with the facial flushing response common in Asians and the production of substances that have opioid properties. Although there is suggestive evidence that ALDH mitochondrial activity may be lower in alcoholics with cirrhosis than nonalcoholics, no studies of high risk populations have yet been conducted.

The final stage in alcohol metabolism involves the conversion of acetate to carbon dioxide and water. This reaction occurs outside of the liver, unlike the first two stages. No research has yet been conducted on this stage of the metabolic process in high risk individuals.

Subjective Effects of Ethanol Metabolism

Schuckit and Rayses (1979) report that sons of alcoholics experience less subjective euphoria from a given dose of alcohol than do low risk subjects. Two other groups have confirmed this diminished perception of intoxication by high risk individuals (O'Malley & Maisto, 1985; Moss et al., in press). This finding cannot be attributed to alcohol metabolism as discussed above. Nor, as Lipscomb and Nathan (1980) have shown, are differences between men having a positive or negative family history of alcoholism distinguishable according to their capacity to estimate blood alcohol concentration. Other investigators have also reported differential mood effects in high and low risk subjects (Ricciardi, Saunders, Williams, & Hopkinson, 1983), which, although important to document, may be related to differential expectancies regarding alcohol's effects.

Biochemical Markers

A number of biochemical mechanisms have been investigated following an alcohol challenge. Schuckit and his colleagues have conducted most of the research in this area and have found no differences between high and low risk subjects with respect to dopamine-B-hydroxylase (Schuckit, 1981), inconsistent results for plasma cortisol level (Schuckit, 1984c), and modest differences in prolactin release (Schuckit et al., 1983). Swartz, Drews, and Cadoret (1987) observed that a stress-induced increase in epinephrine level was greater in subjects having no family history of alcoholism compared to subjects having a positive family history. Significantly, this latter study was conducted on adoptees; thus the stress response cannot be inferred to be affected by living with an alcoholic family member.

Neurophysiologic Markers

Pollock et al. (1983) found that sons of alcoholics exhibited a greater increase in slow alpha energy than controls 30 and 120 minutes after an alcohol challenge. Mean alpha activity also discriminated the offspring of alcoholics and nonalcoholics at 30, 60, and 120 minutes after alcohol consumption.

In a study measuring event related potentials, Elmasian et al. (1982) found a lower amplitude and longer P300 latency in sons of alcoholics compared to controls to target visual stimuli. A group–drug condition interaction was not reported. Schuckit and Rayses (1979) found no consistent differences to an ethanol challenge in young men having either a positive or negative family history of alcoholism.

Neurologic Markers

The only process reflective of CNS functional capacity studied to date is static ataxia. This quantification of the Romberg test is particularly sensitive to a dorsal column or cerebellar injury. In the first study of high risk subjects, Lipscomb, Carpenter, and Nathan (1979) found that upon controlling for predrinking ataxia, no differences in body sway were detected between subjects having either a positive or negative family history of alcoholism. In contrast, Schuckit (1985) found that alcohol induced less body sway in family history positive than negative subjects 125 minutes following an alcohol challenge. Interestingly, differences between family history positive and negative subjects were found for only a low dose challenge but not at a higher dose. The findings obtained to date are thus inconclusive; indeed even the positive results reported by Schuckit are inconsistent and somewhat paradoxical.

Psychophysiologic Markers

Three studies have reported less sympathetic reactivity to stress in young adults who have a family history of alcoholism compared to subjects not having alcoholism in the family (Levenson et al., 1987; Finn & Pihl, 1987; Swartz et al., 1987). The results of these investigations have been interpreted to reflect a differentially greater stress dampening effect among individuals at risk for alcoholism.

SUMMARY

This chapter has reviewed findings associated with the risk for onset of alcoholism as well as its medical sequelae. A cardinal assumption is that outcome, either the behavioral correlate of alcoholism or alcoholic diseases, is multifactorially determined. Markers have not been implicated, having strong empirical support, which reveal the predisposition or diathesis to specifically alcoholism. A diathesis, even if discovered by itself, is not presumed to be sufficient to result in the adverse outcome. A facilitative environment is additionally required. This can consist of numerous factors, including availability of alcohol, deviant peer network, stress, and acute life crisis. The point to be made is that environmental factors have the ability to modify predisposing risk. Nonetheless, the first task is to identify markers of risk, which to date has, unfortunately, not been very rewarding.

This interactive framework, subserved within the diathesis-stress model of psychopathology, provides the basis for delineating multiple pathways to an adverse outcome. From the practical standpoint, the diathesis–stress model emphasizes how risk can be attenuated by altering either organismic or environmental processes. Thus, invariant causal theories of alcoholism etiology will not be forthcoming, nor will any marker be discovered which can identify at birth a person who will invariably experience the outcome. In effect, the risk for alcoholism must be viewed as a complement of increasingly complex processes existing across multiple levels of biologic organization. The adverse outcome depends, in addition to a vulnerability, on exposure to an appropriate environmental opportunity to drink habitually. How vulnerable individuals both seek out as well as react to specific types of environmental circumstance would thus appear to comprise an important agenda for research in charting the pathways linking predisposition to an adverse outcome.

Acknowledgment. Preparation of this chapter was supported by Grant No. 5 R01 AA 066936 from the National Institute on Alcohol Abuse and Alcoholism.

REFERENCES

Agarwal, D. P., & Goedde, H. W. (1987). Human aldehyde dehydrogenase isozymes and alcohol sensitivity. *Isozymes—Current Topics in Biology and Medical Research, 16,* 21–48.

Alexopoulos, G. S., Lieberman, K. W., & Frances, R. J. (1983). Platelet MAO activity in alcoholic patients and their first-degree relatives. *American Journal of Psychiatry, 140*(11), 1501–1504.

Arria, A. M., Tarter, R. E., Williams, R. T., & Van Thiel, D. H. (in press). Early onset of nonalcoholic cirrhosis in patients with familial alcoholism. *Alcoholism: Clinical and Experimental Research.*

Begleiter, H., Porjesz, B., Bihari, B., & Kissin, B. (1984). Event-related brain potentials in boys at risk for alcoholism. *Science, 225*(4669), 1493–1496.

Bennett, L. A., Wolin, S. J., & Reiss, D. (1988). Cognitive, behavioral and emotional problems among school aged children of alcoholic parents. *American Journal of Psychiatry, 145*(2), 185–190.

Boismare, F., Lhuintre, J. P., Daoust, M., Moore, N., Saligaut, C., & Hillemand, B. (1987). Platelet affinity for serotonin is increased in alcoholics and former alcoholics: A biological marker for dependence? *Alcohol and Alcoholism, 22*(2), 155–159.

Bosron, W. F., & Li, T. K. (1981). Genetic determinants of alcohol and aldehyde dehydrogenases and alcohol metabolism. *Seminars in Liver Disease, 1,* 179–188.

Cantwell, D. (1975). Familial-genetic research with hyperactive children. In D. N. Cantwell (Ed.), *The hyperactive child: Diagnosis, management and current research* (pp. 93–105). New York: Halstead Press.

Cloninger, C., Bohman, M., & Sigvardsson, S. (1981). Inheritance of alcohol abuse: Cross-fostering analysis of adopted men. *Archives of General Psychiatry, 38,* 661–668.

Cloninger, C. R., & Reich, T. (1983). Genetic heterogeneity in alcoholism and sociopathy. *Res. Publ. Assoc. Nerv. Ment. Dis., 60,* 145–166.

Cloninger, C. R., Reich, T., & Wetzel, R. (1979). Alcoholism and affective disorders; familial associations and genetic models. In D. W. Goodwin & C. K. Erickson (Eds.), *Alcoholism and affective disorders: Clinical, genetic and biochemical studies* (pp. 57–86). New York: SP Medical & Scientific Books.

Cott, J. M., Breese, G. R., Cooper, B. R., Barlow, T. S., & Prange, Jr., A. J. (1976). Investigation into the mechanism of reduction of ethanol by thyrotropin-releasing hormone (TRH). *Journal of Pharmacological Experiments and Therapeutics, 196,* 594–604.

Cueller, R., Tarter, R., Hays, A., & Van Thiel, D. (1987). The occurrence of alcoholic hepatitis in a patient with bulimia in the absence of alcoholism. *Hepatology, 7,* 878–883.

Cruz-Coke, R., & Varela, A. (1966). Inheritance of alcoholism: Its association with colour-blindness. *Lancet, ii,* 1282–1284.

Del Villano, B. C., Miller, S. I., Schacter, L. P., & Tischfield, J. A. (1980). Elevated superoxide dismutase in black alcoholics. *Science, 207*(4434), 991–992.

Eckhardt, M. J., Rawlings, R. R., & Martin, P. R. (1986). Biological correlates and detection of alcohol abuse and alcoholism. *Progress in Neuropsychopharmacology and Biological Psychiatry, 10,* 135–144.

Edwards, J. A., & Evans, P.D.A. (1967). Ethanol metabolism in subjects possessing typical & atypical liver alcohol dehydrogenase. *Clinical Pharmacology and Therapeutics, 8,* 824.

Elmasian, R., Neville, H., Woods, D., Schuckit, M., & Bloom, F. (1982). Event-related brain potentials are different in individuals at high risk and low risk for developing alcoholism. *Proceedings of the National Academy of Sciences of the USA, 79,* 7900–7903.

Finn, P. R., & Pihl, R. O. (1987). Men at high risk for alcoholism: The effect of alcohol on cardiovascular response to unavoidable shock. *Journal of Abnormal Psychology, 96*(3), 230–236.

Gabrielli, W. F., Mednick, S. A., Volavka, J., Pollock, V. E., Schulsinger, F., & Stil, T. M. (1982). Electroencephalograms in children of alcoholic fathers. *Psychophysiology, 19,* 404–407.

Galambos, J. (1977). Cirrhosis: Epidemiology. In L. Smith (Ed.), *Major problems in internal medicine* (pp. 91–127). Philadelphia: W. B. Saunders.

Garrison, W. T., & Earls, F. J. (1987). *Temperament and child psychopathology, Vol. 12. Developmental clinical psychology and psychiatry,* Newbury Park, CA: Sage Publications.

Gavaler, J. S. (1982). Sex-related differences in ethanol-induced liver disease: Artifactual or real? *Alcoholism: Clinical & Experimental Research, 6*(2), 186–196.

Hegedus, A., Alterman, I., & Tarter, R. E. (1984). Learning achievement in sons of alcoholics. *Alcoholism: Clinical and Experimental Research, 8,* 330–333.

Hegedus, A., Tarter, R., Hill, S., Jacob, T., & Winsten, N. (1984). Static ataxia: A biological marker for alcoholism? *Alcoholism: Clinical and Experimental Research, 8,* 580–582.

Hill, S. Y., Steinhauer, S. R., Zubin, J., & Baughman, T. (1988). Event-related potentials as markers for alcoholism risk in high density families. *Alcoholism: Clinical and Experimental Research,* 545–554.

Hrubec, Z., & Omenn, G. (1981). Evidence of genetic predisposition to alcoholic cirrhosis and psychosis: Twin concordances for alcoholism and its biological end points by zygosity among male veterans. *Alcoholism: Clinical and Experimental Research, 5*(2), 207–215.

Kaij, L. (1960). *Alcoholism in twins. Studies on the etiology and sequels of abuse of alcohol.* Stockholm: Almquist & Wiksell.

Knop, J., Teasdale, T. W., Schulsinger, F., & Goodwin, D. W. (1985). Prospective study of young men at high risk for alcoholism: School behavior and achievement. *Journal of Studies on Alcohol, 46*(4), 273–278.

Lelbach, W. K. (1975). Cirrhosis in the alcoholic and its relation to the volume of alcohol abuse. *Annals of the New York Academy of Science, 252,* 85–105.

Lester, D., & Carpenter, J. A. (1985). Static ataxia in adolescents and their parentage. *Alcoholism: Clinical and Experimental Research, 9*(2), 212.

Levenson, R. W., Oyama, O. M., & Meek, P. S. (1987). Greater reinforcement from alcohol for those at risk: Parental risk, personality risk, and sex. *Journal of Abnormal Psychology, 96*(3), 242–253.

Lex, B. W., Lukas, S. E., Greenwald, N. E., & Mendelson, J. H. (1988). Alcohol-induced changes in body sway in women at risk for alcoholism: A pilot study. *Journal of Studies on Alcohol, 49,* 346–356.

Lipscomb, T. R., Carpenter, J. A., & Nathan, P. E. (1979). Static ataxia: A predictor of alcoholism? *Journal of Addiction, 74,* 289–294.

Lipscomb, T. R., & Nathan, P. E. (1980). Blood alcohol level discrimination: The effects of family history of alcoholism, drinking pattern, and tolerance. *Archives of General Psychiatry, 3,* 571–576.

London, W. P., Kibbee, P., & Holt, L. (1985). Handedness and alcoholism. *Journal of Nervous and Mental Disease, 173*(9), 570–572.

Loosen, P. T., Prange, A. J., & Wilson, I. C. (1979). TRH (protirelin) in depressed alcoholic men. *Archives of General Psychiatry, 36,* 540–547.

Loosen, P. T., Wilson, I. C., Dew, B. W., & Tipermas, A. (1983). Thyrotropin-releasing hormone (TRH) in abstinent alcoholic men. *American Journal of Psychiatry, 140,* 1145–1149.

Luria, A. (1961). *The role of speech in the regulation of normal and abnormal behavior.* London: Pergamon.

Luria, A. (1966). *Higher cortical functions in man.* New York: Basic Books.

Magnusson, D., Stattin, H., & Allen, V. (1986). Differential maturation among girls and its relation to social adjustment: A longitudinal perspective. In P. B. Baltes, D. R. Featherman, & R. M. Learner (Eds.), *Life-span development and behavior.* Hillsdale, NJ: Erlbaum.

Mawson, A., & Mawson, C. (1977). Psychopathy and arousal: A new interpretation of the psychophysiological literature. *Biological Psychiatry, 12,* 49–74.

McClearn, G. E. (1988). Animal models in alcohol research. *Alcoholism: Clinical and Experimental Research, 12*(5), 573–576.

McCord, W., McCord, J., & Gudeman, J. (1960). *Origins of alcoholism.* Stanford, CA: Stanford University Press.

Mizoi, Y., Ijiri, J., Tatsuno, Y., Kijima, T., Fujiwara, S., & Adachi, J. (1979). Relationship between facial flushing and blood acetaldehyde levels after ethanol intake. *Pharmacology, Biochemistry and Behavior, 10,* 303–311.

Monnelly, E. P., Hartl, E. M., & Elderkin, R. (1983). Constitutional factors predictive of alcoholism in a follow-up of delinquent boys. *Journal of Studies on Alcohol, 44,* 530–537.

Morrison, J., & Stewart, M. (1971). A family study of the hyperactive child syndrome. *Biological Psychiatry, 3,* 189–195.

Moss, H. B., Guthrie, S., & Linnoila, M. (1986). Enhanced thyrotropin response to thyrotropin releasing hormone in boys at risk for development of alcoholism. *Archives of General Psychiatry, 43,* 1137–1142.

Moss, H. B., Yao, J. K., Burns, M., Maddock, J., & Tarter, R. E. (in press). Plasma GABA-like activity in response to ethanol challenge in men at high risk for alcoholism. *Biological Psychiatry.*

Moss, H., Yao, J. K., & Maddock, J. M. (1989). Responses by sons of alcoholic fathers to alcoholic and placebo drinks: Perceived mood, intoxication and plasma prolactin. *Alcoholism: Clinical and Experimental Research, 13*(2), 252–257.

Mukherjee, A. B., Svoronos, S., Ghazanfari, A., & Martin, P. R. (1987). Transketolase abnormality in cultured fibroblasts from familial chronic alcoholic men and their male offspring. *Journal of Clinical Investigations, 79*(4), 1039–1043.

Murray, R. M., Clifford, C. A., & Gurling, H. M. (1983). Twin and adoption studies: How good is the evidence for a genetic role? In M. Galanter (Ed.), *Recent developments in alcoholism, Vol. I* (pp. 25–48). New York: Plenum.

Naitoh, P. (1972). The effect of alcohol on the autonomic nervous system of humans: Psychophysiological approach. In B. Kissin & H. Begleiter (Eds.), *The biology of alcoholism, Vol. 2, Physiology and behavior* (pp. 367–425). New York: Plenum.

Nasarallah, H. A., Keelor, D., & McCalley-Whitters, M. (1983). Laterality shift in alcoholic males. *Biological Psychiatry, 18,* 1065–1067.

O'Connor, S., Hesselbrock, V., & Tasman, A. (1986). Correlates of increased risk for alcoholism in young men. *Progress in Neuropsychopharmacology and Biological Psychiatry, 10*(2), 1–218.

O'Malley, S. S., & Maisto, S. A. (1985). Effects of family drinking history and expectancies on response to alcohol in men. *Journal of Studies on Alcohol, 46,* 289–297.

Partanen, J. K., Brun, K., & Markkanen, T. (1966). *Inheritance of drinking behavior. A study on intelligence, personality, and use of alcohol in adult twins.* Finnish Foundation for Alcohol Studies Pub. No. 14. Helsinki: Finnish Foundation for Alcohol Studies.

Patterson, B. W., Williams, H. L., McLean, G. A., Smith, L. T., & Schaeffer, K. W. (1987). Alcoholism and family history of alcoholism: effects on visual and auditory event-related potentials. *Alcohol, 4*(4), 265–274.

Polich, J., Burns, T., & Bloom, F. E. (1988). P300 and the risk for alcoholism: Family history, task difficulty, and gender. *Alcoholism: Clinical and Experimental Research, 12*(2), 248–254.

Pollock, V. W., Volavka, J., Goodwin, D. W., Mednick, S. A., Gabrielli, W. F., Knopp, J., & Schulsinger, F. (1983). The EEG after alcohol administration in men at risk for alcoholism. *Archives of General Psychiatry, 40,* 857–861.

Propping, P. (1977). Genetic control of ethanol action on the central nervous system. *Human Genetics, 35,* 309–334.

Propping, P. (1983). Pharmacogenetics of alcohol's CNS effect: implications for the etiology of alcoholism. *Pharmacology, Biochemistry, and Behavior, 18*(1), 549–553.

Radouco-Thomas, S., Garcin, F., Faure, N., & Lemay, A. et al. (1984). Biological markers in major psychosis and alcoholism: Phenotypic and genotypic markers. *Journal of Psychiatric Research, 18*(4), 513–539.

Rees, L., & Eysenck, H. (1945). A factorial study of some morphological and psychological aspects of human constitution. *Journal of Mental Science, 91,* 8.

Reich, T., Cloninger, R., Van Eerdewegh, P., Rice, J. P., & Mullaney, J. (1988). Secular trends in the familial transmission of alcoholism. *Alcoholism: Clinical and Experimental Research, 12*(4), 458–464.

Reich, T., Winokur, G., & Mullaney, J. (1975). The transmission of alcoholism. In R. Fieve, D. Rosenthal, & H. Brill, (Eds.), *Genetic research in psychiatry* (pp. 259–271). Baltimore: John Hopkins University Press.

Ricciardi, B. R., Saunders, J. B., Williams, R., & Hopkinson, D. A. (1983). Hepatic ADH & ALDH isoenzymes in different racial groups and in chronic alcoholism. *Pharmacology, Biochemistry, and Behavior, 18*(1), 61–65.

Room, R. (1983). Region and urbanization as factors in drinking practices and problems. In B. Kissin & H. Begleiter (Eds.), *The Biology of Alcoholism, Vol. 7, The pathogenesis of alcoholism: Psychosocial factors* (pp. 555–604). New York: Plenum.

Rosler, M., Bellaire, W., Hengesch, G., Giannitsis, D., & Jarovici, A. (1983). Genetic markers in alcoholism: no association with HLA. *Archiv fur Psychiatrie und Nervenkrankheiten, 233*(4), 327–331.

Schalling, D., Asberg, M., & Edman, G. (1984). *Personality and CSF monamine metabolites.* Unpublished manuscript. Department of Psychiatry and Psychology, Karolinski Hospital, Department of Psychology, University of Stockholm, Stockholm, Sweden.

Schmidt, A. L., & Neville, H. J. (1985). Language processing in men at risk for alcoholism: An event-related potential study. *Alcohol, 2*(3), 529–533.

Schuckit, M. A. (1984a). Differences in plasma cortisol after ingestion of ethanol in relatives of alcoholics and controls: preliminary results. *Journal of Clinical Psychiatry, 45*, 374–376.

Schuckit, M. A. (1984b). Subjective responses to alcohol in sons of alcoholics and control subjects. *Archives of General Psychiatry, 41*(9), 879–884.

Schuckit, M. (1984c). Biochemical markers of a predisposition to alcoholism. In S. B. Rosalki (Ed.), *Clinical biochemistry of alcoholism* (pp. 20–55). Edinburgh: Churchill Livingstone.

Schuckit, M. A. (1985). Behavioral effects of alcohol in sons of alcoholics. *Recent Developments in Alcoholism, 3*, 11–19.

Schuckit, M. A. (1987). Biological vulnerability to alcoholism. *Journal of Consulting and Clinical Psychology, 55*(3), 301–309.

Schuckit, M. A., & Gold, E. O. (1988). A simultaneous evaluation of multiple markers of ethanol/placebo challenges in sons of alcoholics and controls. *Archives of General Psychiatry, 45*(3), 211–216.

Schuckit, M. A., Gold, E., & Reisch, C. (1987). Serum prolactin levels in sons of alcoholics and control subjects. *American Journal of Psychiatry, 144*(7), 854–859.

Schuckit, M. A., O'Connor, D. T., Duby, J., Vega, R., & Moss, M. (1981). Dopamine-B-hydroxylase activity levels in men at high risk for alcoholism and controls. *Biological Psychiatry, 16*, 1067–1075.

Schuckit, M. A., Parker, D. C., & Rossman, L. R. (1983). Ethanol-related prolactin responses and risk for alcoholism. *Biological Psychiatry, 18*, 1153–1159.

Schuckit, M. A., & Rayses, V. (1979). Ethanol ingestion: Differences in blood acetaldehyde concentrations in relatives of alcoholics and controls. *Science, 203*(4375), 54–55.

Schuckit, M. A., Shaskan, E., Duby, J., & Moss, M. (1982). Platelet monoamine oxidase activity in relatives of alcoholics: Preliminary study with matched control subjects. *Archives of General Psychiatry, 39*, 137–140.

Searles, J. (1988). The role of genetics in the pathogenesis of alcoholism. *Journal of Abnormal Psychology, 97*(2), 153–167.

Sher, K., & Levenson, R. (1982). Risk for alcoholism and individual differences in the stress-response-dampening effect of alcohol. *Journal of Abnormal Psychology, 91*, 350–367.

Swartz, C. M., Drews, V., & Cadoret, R. (1987). Decreased epinephrine in familial alcoholism: Initial findings. *Archives of General Psychiatry, 44*, 938–941.

Tabakoff, B., Lee, J. M., DeLeon-Jones, F., & Hoffman, P. (1985). Ethanol inhibits the activity of the B form of monoamine oxidase in human platelet brain tissue. *Psychopharmacology, 87*, 152–156.

Tarter, R., Alterman, A., & Edwards, K. (1985). Vulnerability to alcoholism in men. A behavior-genetic perspective. *Journal of Studies on Alcohol, 46*, 329–256.

Tarter, R., Alterman, A., & Edwards, K. (1988). Neurobehavioral theory of alcoholism etiology. In C. Chaudron & D. Wilkinson (Eds.), *Theories of alcoholism* (pp. 73–93). Toronto: Addiction Research Foundation.

Tarter, R. E., Hegedus, A., Goldstein, G., Shelly, C., & Alterman, A. (1984). Adolescent sons of alcoholics: Neuropsychological & personality characteristics. *Alcoholism: Clinical and Experimental Research, 8*, 216–222.

Tarter, R., Hegedus, A., Winsten, N., & Alterman, A. (1984). Neuropsychological, personality and familial characteristics of physically abused juvenile delinquents. *Journal of Academy of Child Psychiatry, 23*, 668–674.

Tarter, R. E., McBride, H., Buonpane, N., & Schneider, D. U. (1977). Differentiation of alcoholics. *Archives of General Psychiatry, 34*, 761–768.

Utne, H. E., Hansen, F. V., Winkler, K., & Schulsinger, F. (1977). Alcohol elimination rates in adoptees with and without alcoholic parents. *Journal of Studies on Alcohol, 38*(7), 1977.

Vaillant, G. E. (1983). *The natural history of alcoholism*. Cambridge, MA: Harvard University Press.

Van Ree, J. M. (1986). Role of pituitary and related neuropeptides in alcoholism and pharmacodependence. *Progress in Neuro-Psychopharmacology and Biological Psychiatry, 10*, 219–228.

von Knorring, A. L., Bohman, M., von Knorring, L., & Oreland, L. (1985). Platelet MAO activity as a biological marker in subgroups of alcoholism. *Acta Psychiatrica Scandinavica, 72*(1), 51–58.

Von-Wartburg, J. P., & Buhler, R. (1984). Alcoholism and aldehydes: New biomedical concepts. *Laboratory Investigation, 50*, 5–15.

Vygotsky, L. (1962). *Thought and language*. Cambridge, MA: M.I.T. Press.

Watson, R. R., Mohs, M. E., Eskelson, C., Sampliner, R. E., & Hartman, B. H. (1986). Identification of alcohol abuse and alcoholism with biological parameters. *Alcoholism: Clinical and Experimental Research, 10*(4), 364–385.

Whipple, S. C., Parker, E. S., & Noble, E. P. (1988). An atypical neurocognitive profile in alcoholic fathers and their sons. *Journal of Studies on Alcohol, 49*(3), 240–244.

Wilkinson, D., & Carlen, P. (1980). Relationship of neuropsychological test performance to brain morphology in amnesic and non-amnesic chronic alcoholics. *Acta Psychiatrica Scandinavica, 62*, 89–102.

Wilson, A., Onstad, G., & Williams, R. (1969). Serum immunoglobulin concentrations in patients with alcoholic liver disease. *Gastroenterology, 57*(1).

Wood, D., Wender, P., & Reimherr, F. (1983). The prevalence of attention deficit disorders, residual type, or minimal brain dysfunction, in a population of male alcoholic patients. *American Journal of Psychiatry, 140,* 95–98.

Zuckerman, M. (1984). Sensation seeking: A comparative approach to a human trait. *Behavior and Brain Sciences, 7,* 413–471.

4

Behavior Genetic Models of Alcohol Abuse

DAVID C. ROWE

To understand the etiology of behavior, we must learn about the relative importance of nature (heredity) versus nurture (environmental) influences. In twentieth century behavioral science, the nature/nurture conflict has flared on many occasions. In his historical review of the child development field, "Your Ancients Revisited," Robert Sears (1975) compared the nature/nurture issue to an earthquake fault producing tremors that shift whole areas of research in new directions. After a period of relative neglect of genetic factors following World War II, there has been a growing interest in the possibility of genetic influence on behavior. Although the first adoptive study of alcohol abuse was undertaken in the 1940s (Roe, 1945), most behavioral genetic research on alcohol has occurred in recent times. Moreover, the antagonism and rancor surrounding the implications of genetic studies has abated. This is primarily due to the recognition by behavioral geneticists that environmental factors must be allowed for in the estimation of hereditary ones. Environmentalists, too, recognize that the traditional family study method inherently confounds heredity and environment (Wachs, 1983). Hence, a need exists for research methods that can scrutinize and separate both kinds of influence. In this chapter, I advocate that alcohol researchers learn about behavioral genetic methods, so that the quality of research on both heredity and environment can be improved.

This chapter aims to educate researchers who work in the field of alcohol abuse about behavioral genetic methods. It will focus on "model fitting" approaches that allow for a separation of genetic and environmental influences; but several subsidiary issues will be addressed. The chapter is intended to inform alcohol researchers about behavioral genetic methods; to guide them to books and articles from which more may be learned; and to entice them to apply these new and powerful methods in their own studies. It is divided into four major sections: in the first, basic behavioral genetic concepts are reviewed, in the second, model fitting procedures are explained and applied to continuous traits; in the third, model fitting is applied to noncontinuous traits; and in the fourth section, the issues of sibling effects and decomposing a correlation are considered. The chapter, however, is not intended as a review of the genetics of alcohol (see Searles, Chapter 1, this volume), and it avoids drawing any conclusion about the heritability of alcohol use and abuse.

BEHAVIORAL GENETIC CONCEPTS

History

In the early 1900s, evolutionary theory was already in existence; and the familial transmission of morphological traits and behavioral traits was recognized. Francis Galton, in the mid-1800s, had already proposed that genetic influence on human behavioral traits could be probed with the twin and adoption study methods (Fancher, 1985). His first adoption study was an attempt to establish the inheritance of intellectual eminence; he compared the adopted offspring of Roman Catholic clergy with the biological relatives of famous Englishmen. As only the latter were themselves eminent, Galton drew the inference that social advantage alone could not produce intellectual eminence. His study, however, was too cursory to provide strong evidence for the genetic inheritance of eminence.

On the other hand, despite these early starts, controversy existed between scientists in the Galtonian tradition, who were concerned with continuous variation, and the newly discovered Mendelian transmission of traits. Mendelian traits were discrete and categorical; and the theory of their variation proposed that the units of inheritance—genes—could vary, but did not blend. Galton, however, wanted to understand the genetics of continuous traits. He invented the correlation coefficient statistic, later perfected by his student, Karl Pearson, to describe familial resemblances. The relationship of continuous variation to categorical Mendelian traits, however, was unclear, and provoked vigorous debate among scholars taking the correlational approach to inheritance (the "biometricians") and those taking the categorical, Mendelian approach. Some scientists, such as Davenport, working at the Cold Spring Harbor Biological Laboratory, sought evidence of Mendelian transmission of a host of human traits: but many behavioral traits cannot be forced into a categorical mold.

R. A. Fisher, holder of the chair formerly occupied by Galton and Pearson at the University of London, and Sewall Wright, developed the "new synthesis" of modern genetics. Their theories provided a unified model of evolutionary change and also reconciled Mendelian and biometrical genetics. Mendelian genetics dealt with genetic variation at a particular locus (position) on human chromosomes. In the simplest genetic system, with a single gene inherited from the father and one from the mother, a maximum of three observable (phenotypic) traits can exist produced by the gene combinations AA, Aa, and aa. If genetic dominance were operating only two traits would be observable because both AA and Aa would appear identical. Yet, Mendelian inheritance could be reconciled with continuous traits if one allowed that genes varying at many loci each contributed slightly to the trait, so that the trait was the summative effect of these many weak and separable gene actions. Indeed, with just four genes, each with an equal frequency of .5 (i.e., half the genes are "A," half "a"), the distribution of a trait already becomes bell-shaped in appearance (see Figure 4.1).

The biometrical geneticists derived mathematically *expected* correlations and variances for such polygenic ("poly" meaning "many" genes) traits. Sewall Wright (1934) invented the method of path analysis—to which most forms of modern linear analysis are heirs—which greatly simplified the derivation of such mathematical expectations. The usual assumptions for these calculations were "random mating," many genes of small individual effects, and equal gene frequencies. The random mating assumption meant an absence of correlation across spouses. This system of mating maximally recombines genes each generation—for example, a tall individual might marry someone who is short and the recombination of their genes will produce a wide range of height in their children. Positive *assortative* mating (i.e., spouse correlation) means that children would resemble their parents

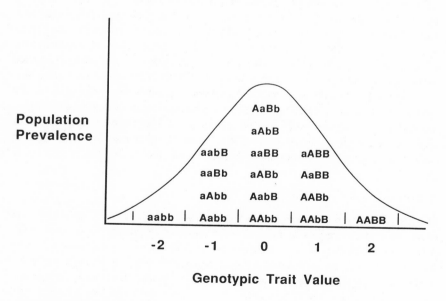

FIGURE 4.1. Population prevalence of genetically determined trait by genotypic trait values (capital letters = .5; lower case letters = −.5).

more so than they would under conditions of "random" mating. For many traits spousal resemblance is greater than that of randomly paired individuals (Buss, 1985). Such correlations, if they are small, have only trivial effects on familial resemblances, often, they can be neglected. Behavioral genetic models, too, can include terms to represent nonrandom mating explicitly (Carey, 1986b). The equal gene frequency assumption was made for convenience of mathematical derivations. When many genes are acting, departures from it are also of small consequence. In a recent issue of the *American Journal of Human Genetics,* Cloninger, Rao, Reich, and Morton (1983) energetically defended path analysis against Karlin, Cameron, and Chakraborty's (1983) criticisms. These articles may be read for a more sophisticated treatment of assumptions in genetic modeling. In sum, just as Mendelian genetics yielded predictions about the proportions of cases in different categories, biometrical genetic theory yielded predictions about familial correlations for continuous traits.

Although theoretical understanding of heredity was achieved early in this century, the physical nature of heredity was not well understood until Watson and Crick published their seminal paper revealing the structure of DNA in 1953. Since the discovery of DNA's structure, breathtaking progress has occurred in the field of molecular genetics. Among these dramatic advances are: breaking the genetic code; gene sequencing; using bacteria as factories to make the products of any gene; and discovering new genetic markers (genes or genetic sequences of known chromosomal location). These advances are still continuing, with a program now initiated to map the human genome with equally spaced "genetic markers" and to sequence the genome (i.e., find the sequence of the millions of combinations of chemical bases in DNA that carry the genetic information). Of these advances, the discovery of multiple genetic markers has the greatest implications for alcohol researchers. These markers permit the localization of the genes involved in Mendelian traits (e.g., Huntington's disease); eventually, they may permit discovery of the genes contributing to polygenic traits. This last enterprise, however, still lies between science and science fiction, and it is too early to anticipate whether it will fail or succeed.

Components of Variations

As discussed earlier, in contrast to other theories in psychology, behavioral genetics rests on a *deductive* theory: population genetics. Given the scientific laws of genetic mechanisms, certain consequences must follow for the trait correlations in biological and nonbiological relatives. Behavioral geneticists attempt to apportion the observed variation in a trait, or the observed correlation among traits, to "latent" components of variation; namely, to "causes" that can be inferred from their effects, but which cannot be themselves measured directly. However, the use of such indirect inferences is not new in science. The planet Neptune was predicted by its gravitational effects on known planets; similarly, different latent components may be discovered by their effects on trait correlations, variances, and other statistics, in research designs of a quasi-experimental nature, such as the comparison of monozygotic (MZ; one egg) twins and dizygotic (DZ; two eggs) twins; or adoptive and nonadoptive siblings. This section defines theoretical (in the sense of mathematically specified) components of variation that constitute parameters in behavioral genetic models. Later, methods of estimating these components will be discussed in the context of research on alcohol use and abuse.

Components of Variation:
Shared and Nonshared Heredity

Genes that vary among individuals are one source of trait variation; genes that are the same for all individuals cannot contribute to trait *variability*, although they may influence species-typical traits (e.g., all people have two rather than four legs). To discover the effects of this genetic variation on behavioral traits, one estimates *heritability*. It is important to emphasize that the concept of heritability applies only to trait variation. Inarguably, both genes and environment—ideally, a beneficent one—are required for physical growth and psychological development. To separate genetic from environmental influences, we must ask a somewhat different question: that is, what contributes more to *differences* among people, differences in environmental exposures, or differences in genetic inheritance. Clearly, given this question, some traits may be more genetically influenced than others. For example, the degree a person speaks in a Bostonian accent will depend on her linguistic environment, with relatively little genetic contribution. On the other hand, variation in physical height depends more on genetic inheritance (e.g., parental height) than on variation in American diets or on variation in other environments. In this example, the latter trait is much more "heritable" (i.e., genetically influenced) than the former.

Technically, heritability can be defined as the ratio of genetic variation to phenotypic (i.e., trait) variation: V_g / V_p. For physical traits, heritabilities exceed .80; for intellectual traits, they range from .40 to .70; and for personality traits, they range from .30 to .50 (Loehlin, Willerman, & Horn, 1988). The estimation of heritability is not without its detractors, who point out, rightly, that this statistic will vary among populations and is subject to the vagaries of sampling error as are all statistics. Such criticisms, however, will apply with equal forcefulness to *any* structural equation model of environmental effects: so that to reject the estimation of one type of influence, heredity, is implicitly to reject estimation of the other, environment. We do not believe scientists want to "throw the baby out with the bath water."

Heredity contributes both to differences among families (the average heredity in a particular family) as well as to differences within families (except for MZ twins, no two people are exactly alike genetically). Hence, some genetic influence is *nonshared*—contributing to differences among family members—whereas other heredity is *shared*—contributing to alikenesses among siblings and other biological relatives. In most discussion of genetic inheritance, however, the concern is with the *total* shared and nonshared effects of heredity on individual differences—namely, with heritability.

Components of Variation: Shared and Nonshared Environment

Environmental differences among families are a possible source of behavioral variation. For example, families differ in social class, structure (single versus two-parent), religion, and on a number of dimensions of parental behavior. Barnes (1984) reported that maternal drinking and low parental nurturance/support were associated with higher levels of alcohol use among children. In behavioral genetic models, such factors can play the role of *shared* environments because they operate to make family members alike in some trait. In the mathematics of behavioral genetics, the shared environmental component always has the ideal role of making family members alike, but different from members of other families. Although no real environmental factor is so pure in its influence, our strategy is to estimate how much trait variation owes to this particular kind of influence—which itself may be a composite of a number of actual environmental treatments.

Other environmental influences operate on each individual uniquely; they are termed *nonshared* environmental influences. Because measurement error is also a unique and idiosyncratic factor, true nonshared influences should be distinguished from mere measurement error—this can be done using information on trait reliability. Categories of nonshared influence include family structure (e.g., birth order); perinatal trauma; the differential treatment of siblings; peer groups; and other extrafamilial factors.

Other Components of Variation

Although heredity, shared family environment, and nonshared environment constitute the main components of the typical behavioral genetic analysis, other apportionments of environmental variation are possible. Sibling mutual imitation may produce trait variation (Carey, 1986a). Sibling effects have some surprising consequences—for example, they will lead to higher trait means for siblings than for single born children.

Effects of heredity can be separated as well. The genetic variation may contain components due to "additive" heredity; due to "dominance"; and due to other "nonadditive" sources (i.e., genetic epistasis). For example, additive variation produces parent–child resemblance; dominance variation does not (e.g., the blue-eyed child of brown-eyed parents). As a heritability coefficient calculated from the twin study method contains both components of genetic variation, it is referred to as a "broad-sense" heritability. Heritability coefficients obtained from designs that exclude MZ twins are typically "narrow-sense" in that they estimate additive-gene effects alone. Sibling effects and the finer levels of genetic analysis are usually not pursued, but there can be occasions when such discriminations are important.

Basic Behavioral Genetic Research Methods

The problem for a behavioral genetic study is to estimate the various contributions of heredity, shared environment, and nonshared environment to trait variation. Once trait variation has been attributed to these theoretical components, a further goal of analysis may be to identify the particular environmental factors involved or the particular genetic factors involved. No responsible person would claim, therefore, that a behavioral genetic study in itself solves the problem of providing a worthy theory of the mechanism of behavioral maintenance and change. Nevertheless, the screening of these theoretical components sets broad limits on the search for these mechanisms. For instance, if *shared* environment contributes little to trait variation, many family environmental factors are thereby eliminated as plausible theoretical explanations. If such factors are important, however, we can focus investigation on the family environment.

Most studies involve some kind of quasi-experimental design, in which family groups differing in the degree of genetic or environmental relatedness are compared. The traditional study usually made use of just one or two kinships. The *family* study method involves comparing the resemblance of biologically related family members. This method unavoidably confounds hereditary and environmental influences. Nevertheless, unless a trait shows some degree of familial transmission, hardly any reason exists for pursuing further behavioral genetic analysis. Hence, parent–child and sibling correlations are important starting points in any study concerned with genetic or environmental "inheritance."

The family study method can be misinterpreted by scholars lacking an informed understanding of genetic principles. It is often noted that, even when traits run in families, affected children will appear in some families in which neither the mother nor the father is affected. Such results are sometimes misinterpreted as evidence *against* a genetic etiology. To the contrary, whenever a trait is polygenic, new cases often will appear when neither parent is affected, just as a very bright child may be born to parents of average IQ.

Another source of misunderstanding concerns the use of the raw or unsquared correlation coefficient as an indicator of "variance explained" rather than the more commonly used squared correlation value. This procedure is correct because we seek to explain the variation of manifest variables in terms of variation in latent, unobserved variables (e.g., shared environment, heredity). Ozer (1985) discussed the mathematical basis for this result, which is identical to the reasons that an unsquared reliability coefficient is interpreted as "reliable" variance explained.

The *twin* study method uses the comparison of identical and fraternal twins. Because MZ twins share twice the genetic similarity of dizygotic DZ twins (100% versus 50%, for genes that vary), they should be more alike for genetically influenced traits than the latter. This comparison rests on the so-called "equal environments" assumption that MZ twins experienced (trait-relevant) environments no more similar than DZ twins experienced. This assumption, like others detailed earlier (e.g., approximately random mating), is necessary for a particular behavioral genetic analysis. Assumptions are the price paid for pursuing a scientific theory; they are unavoidable. Recognizing their importance, scientists have developed methods to evaluate such assumptions as "equal environments," absence of gene × environment interaction, and absence of nonadditivity (Eaves, Last, Young, & Martin, 1978; Plomin, DeFries, and Loehlin, 1977; Scarr & Carter-Saltzman, 1979). For many traits, the twin method's "equal environments" assumption appears reasonable. Whether this sanguine conclusion will extend to socially malleable behaviors such as alcohol use and abuse, however, requires further empirical verification.

The *adoption* study method involves comparisons of the adoptive family, the relinquished children, and the biological parents. As data for the latter are often difficult to obtain, an alternative has been to compare matched groups of adoptive and nonadoptive families. Because, except by coincidence, persons in adoptive families lack any genetic resemblance, the adoptive family method can be used to estimate *shared* environmental influences directly.

MODEL FITTING APPROACHES: CONTINUOUS VARIATION

We can recognize, however, that data from different behavioral genetic designs can be combined into a single analysis so long as the expectations for correlations and other statistics are written in terms of a common set of estimable parameters (e.g., variances, path coefficients). Such methods utilize fully the existing data on a trait and, simultaneously, test various assumptions underlying the model proposed. They are efficient and powerful, assuming the original data are of high quality. Model fitting is done by writing an overdetermined structural equation model (SEM) for kinship correlations or other familial statistics.

An SEM expresses the observed relationships among variables in terms of unobserved, but presumably causal, variables. For example, "heredity" is unobserved because the particular genes producing effects on behavior are unknown. Similarly, family environments may differ in many ways even when no measurements are taken. Path coefficients are numbers relating these unobserved variables to the measured ones. Roughly, they indicate the extent of influence the unobserved variable has on the measured trait. Most structural equation models are "overdetermined" because there are fewer estimated parameters, such as path coefficients, than observed statistics. Overdetermined models are to be preferred because they permit goodness-of-fit tests, that is, the value of the statistics predicted by the model can be compared with the values actually obtained. A nonsignificant statistical test—usually a chi square test—indicates a lack of departure of predicted and observed statistics. In this chapter, the terms "path analytic model" and "structural equation model" are used interchangeably. This follows common practice in the behavioral genetic literature; however, it should be noted that in many fields, the term "path analytic" applies to models containing *only* measured variables—the term "structural equation" model being reserved for models with both measured and "unobserved" variables.

Like ice creams, behavioral genetic models come in a bewildering number of flavors. For the novice, such variety may seem unapproachable; for the expert, it can create the "approach–approach" conflict of trying to choose among attractive alternatives. Although a large number of modeling techniques have been proposed and used, three approaches are in common use: pedigree analysis, "biometrical" models, and path analytic models.

Pedigree analysis is the most complex of the model fitting approaches (Elston, 1981; Morton & MacLearn, 1974). In contrast to path analytic and biometrical models, the pedigree analysis method has the statistical power to distinguish between polygenic influences and major gene influences. Because most pedigree models, however, are designed to analyze parents and their children, they are not ideal for separating family-environmental transmission of a trait from polygenic transmission. Nevertheless, some pedigree models offer parameters to represent the family environments shared by siblings. In pedigree analysis, the data are the scores of each person in the pedigree; these pedigrees may differ from one another in structure (e.g., one family with three children and no grandparents; another with two children and grandparents included). Mathematical equations can be written to represent the expectation for relatives' scores within each pedigree in terms of parameters such as major gene effects, polygenic heritability (h^2), and nonshared environmental effects. The parameters are then estimatable using a maximum likelihood method that calculates values that best fit the observations of each pedigree.

The English school of *"biometrical models"* provides a method of estimating shared environment (c^2), heritability (h^2), and nonshared environment (e^2) (Mather & Jinks, 1971). The data fit by this method can come from a variety of different kinships, such as adoptive families and nonadoptive families; or MZ and DZ twins. Each kinship provides two statistics for fitting—mean squares between and within families. These mean squares are found by conducting a one-way ANOVA on kinship data. For example, if twins are used, the independent variable is families, with levels equal to the number of twin pairs. The fitted statistics are the ANOVA mean squares between pairs and the ANOVA mean squares within pairs. For instance, if MZ twins are used, the MSW represents variation in twin difference scores; hence, its *expectation* can include measurement error and nonshared environmental influence, which operates to make twins unlike, but not heredity, because MZ twins have the same hereditary "score," which is canceled out when twin A's trait score is subtracted from twin B's. Estimation procedures include maximum likelihood methods, such as in the widely used program LISREL (Joreskog & Sorbom, 1983), and weighted least squares methods. Fulker (1981) provides a lucid introduction to biometrical models.

Path analytic approaches constitute a third method of model fitting (Cloninger, Rice, & Reich, 1979; Jencks et al., 1972; Rao, Morton, & Yee, 1974). In contrast to the biometrical modeling approach, the path analytic approach uses as the "raw" data kinship correlations or covariances (e.g., a parent–child correlation), rather than ANOVA mean squares.[1] Like biometrical models, path models can be fit to many different kinships simultaneously. The expectations of the correlations can be obtained from path analytic diagrams. Behavioral geneticists, however, differ in the particular assumptions that are incorporated into their path diagrams. Cloninger et al. (1979) allow family-environment influence to transmit directly from the parental generation to later generations; whereas Jencks et al. (1972) specify that family-environment effects transmit from parental phenotypes to children's environments; and Rao et al. (1974) permit both types of transmission. Loehlin (1978) compared different path analytic models and concluded that, where these models gave different results, it was because of the different assumptions made, rather than because of different estimation procedures or other details. Models from several research groups yielded similar results when assortative mating was assumed to be "phenotypic"— that is, people with similar traits select one another during courtship—and when "equal environments" was assumed for twins and siblings. Behavior is not so well understood to decide unambiguously among alternative models, and the ideal approach is to test several models; and always to be explicit about model assumptions.

An Example of Path Analytic Model Fitting

Data from a study of Finnish twins are used to illustrate the path analytic approach to model fitting. Kaprio, Koskenvuo, and Langinvainio (1984)

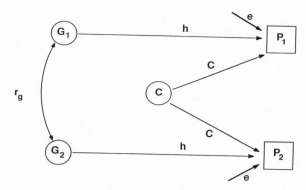

FIGURE 4.2. Path model for twin correlations.

reported data for small samples of MZ twins and DZ twins; their data set combined an adoption design (MZ and DZ twins raised apart) with the traditional twin method (MZ and DZ twins reared together). The twins answered a mailed questionnaire on which they indicated the amount and frequency of beer, wine, and spirits consumed per month, which was scored as grams of alcohol per month. The reared-apart twins had been separated before age 11 years, with little contact after separation; the reared-together twins had been raised in the same family, but now, as adults, were living apart. Because of small sample sizes, it is unwise to draw conclusions about the etiology of alcohol use and abuse, although results here can be used to stimulate the formation of hypotheses.

Figure 4.2 provides a path analytic diagram for twin correlations determined by three latent parameters: shared family environment (C); heredity (G); and nonshared environment plus any measurement error (E). These latent influences determine the observed phenotypes (P) of each twin through the path coefficients c, h, and e, respectively. P_1 is the phenotype (alcohol use) of one twin; P_2 is the phenotype of the other twin. Regardless of rearing conditions, twins' genotypes must correlate +.5 for DZ twins and 1.0 for identical twins. For twins raised apart, however, the shared environmental path, c, equals zero.

Using Wright's rules (Loehlin, 1987), the path diagram can be read to yield the expected values of the twin correlations in terms of path coefficients. Path diagrams consists of "exogenous" variables, without defined causes, and "endogenous" variables, completely explained by the exogenous variables and their own residuals. Only variables of the former type can be connected by double-headed, correlational arrows. The exogenous variables "causally" determine the endogenous ones through single headed arrows. To read such a diagram, one traces all the paths connecting two variables, summing each unique tracing. This path tracing follows Wright's rules:

(a) no loops—each variable enters into a path tracing only once;
(b) no going forward then backward;
(c) a maximum of one curved arrow per path (a rule that cannot be violated in Figure 4.2, but can be in more complex diagrams).

Loehlin (1987) gave an elementary introduction to path analytic methods and provided practice problems, for those who wish to try their hand at deriving path model expectations. Using these rules, the expectations for the four groups in Kaprio et al.'s study are easily found:

(1) MZ twins raised apart: $r = h^2$
(2) MZ twins raised together: $r = h^2 + c^2$
(3) DZ twins raised apart: $r = .5h^2$
(4) DZ twins raised together: $r = .5h^2 + c^2$

Lastly, the remaining variation that represents nonshared environment and measurement error can be estimated:

(5) $e^2 = 1 - (c^2 + h^2)$

Although Wright's rules can be used to derive expectations for this model, and for other models like it, it should be cautioned that in some situations, these rules fail to give proper expectations. The most common of these is the case where *assortative* mating is present. Assortative mating can impose a correlation on endogenous variables that violates the ordinary path reading rules. In this situation, the correct path expectations can be derived using matrix algebra method, however (Carey, 1986b).

Estimation

Estimation was done using the method of Rao et al. (1974). Correlations were first z-transformed. The z-transformed correlations follow an approximately normal distribution. Using statistical theory, Rao and his colleagues derived the likelihood function for independent, normally distributed variables—namely, for the independent correlations from different kinships. This likelihood was equivalent to the chi square function shown below:

$$\chi^2 = \Sigma (z_i - \mathbf{z}_i)^2 / s_i^2$$

where z_i is the z-transformed correlation coefficient for the ith kinship group; $\mathbf{z}_i$ is the z-transformed, expected correlation for the ith kinship group, calculated from the equations given earlier; and s^2 is the variance of the z_i coefficients (i.e., $1/(N_i - 3/2)$, where N_i is the number of twin pairs). The summation is over the number of kinships ($k = 4$ kinships). This formula is similar to a "least squares" estimation, because the numerator is simply the squared deviation of the observed z coefficient from the one predicted. Each squared difference, however, is weighted by $1/s_i^2$, so that a relatively large kinship (hence, a smaller variance) contributes *more* to the chi square. In our example, this formula indicates that the outcome of model fitting will be determined more by twins reared together than reared apart.

An iterative search computer program was used to fit this path model. It started with trial values of the parameters and adjusted them until the value of the chi square was minimized (Loehlin, 1987, p. 229). Parameter values yielding this minimum chi square also constitute maximum likelihood estimates of their population values.

Table 4.1 presents the path analytic results from fitting Kaprio et al.'s twin data set. Three models were compared: Model I, including both the hereditary (h) and shared-environment (c) parameters; Model II, including just the hereditary parameter; and Model III, including just the environmental parameter. The number of degrees of freedom for the chi square test was the number of correlations (4) minus the number of parameters.

First, consider the results for males. The model fitting procedure strongly rejected the purely genetic model ($\chi^2 = 16.7$, df = 3, $p < .01$). The reason for this failure was clearly evident in the predicted correlations: this model estimated a correlation for MZ twins raised apart of .712, which was greater than the one obtained (.045). A purely environmental model

TABLE 4.1. Path Analytic Model Fits to Alcohol Consumption Correlations

Group	r	No. pairs	Predicted Correlations, χ		
			Model I	Model II	Model III
			Males		
MZA	.045	13	.351	.712	0
MZT	.851	23	.795	.712	.659
DZA	.121	33	.175	.356	0
DZT	.550	60	.620	.356	.659
χ^2			2.6	16.7	6.6
			Females		
MZA	.055	16	.502	.682	0
MZT	.912	24	.794	.682	.553
DZA	.108	55	.251	.341	0
DZT	.315	71	.543	.341	.553
χ^2			15.0	23.3	25.7

Model I: $h_m = .592$, $c_m = .667$; $h_f = .709$, $c_f = .54$.
Model II: $h_m = .884$; $h_f = .826$.
Model III: $c_m = .812$; $c_f = .744$.

(Model III) fit more satisfactorily: ($\chi^2 = 6.6$, df $= 3$, $p > .05$). Yet, Model I, combining both parameters, provided an even better fit than the environmental one. Models I and III can be compared by subtracting their chi square values (e.g., χ^2 Model III $- \chi^2$ Model I $= 4.0$) and degrees of freedom (e.g., $3 - 2 = 1$ df) and then by evaluating the statistical significance of this chi square. If it is significant, then the addition of a parameter, h, has improved the model's fit statistically. As $\chi^2 = 4$ was significant ($p < .05$), Model I, combining hereditary and environmental parameters, was superior to Model III, consisting of only the shared-environment parameter. Inspecting the predicted correlations from Model I shows that, except for the MZA group, the obtained and estimated values are close. The MZA discrepancy (.045 vs. .351), however, occurs where the sample size is small (N pairs $= 13$), creating the conditions for sampling variation in the value of the correlation coefficient. To complete the apportionment of variation, nonshared environmental influences, including measurement error, can be estimated from these results. As the total variation is 100%, the nonshared component can be obtained by subtraction: ($100 - c^2 - h^2 = 21\%$).

In contrast to the males, no model was able to provide a statistically adequate result for females' alcohol consumption pattern. Because the models were rejected, we do not have a theoretical explanation for females' alcohol consumption. Moreover, the problem could lie either in the design and execution of Kaprio's study or in the assumptions of our model. Design problems can include subject attrition, nonnormality in the alcohol consumption variable for females, or sampling variation that produces a Type II statistical error. This behavioral genetic model assumes approximate normality to the observations; where observations are nonnormal, often they can be mathematically transformed to yield a distribution closer to the normal. However, Kaprio's article lacks information on the distribution of alcohol consumption scores. Another alternative is that our genetic–environment theory of females' alcohol consumption is wrong. If so, a different model may be proposed to account for the females' data, such as one postulating an environmental effect unique to MZ twins that produces behavioral resemblance in MZ twins raised together exceeding that of the other kinships.

The features of genetic modeling for testing specific hypotheses with respect to the etiology of alcohol use and abuse have been reviewed above. The model builder must first write a path diagram that is consistent internally, that obeys the scientific laws of heredity, and that contains theoretically interesting parameters, such as the shared-environment parameter (c). Second, the model builder must have a method of estimation that extracts from a data set these parameter estimates. Finally, she needs a statistical "goodness-of-fit" test to decide whether the predicted statistics lie reasonably close to the obtained ones. For males, the genetic heritability of alcohol consumption was estimated at $h^2 = 35\%$ and its environmental "heritability" at $c^2 = 44\%$. Although the latter result may seem natural to many scientists, it is quite rare to discover family-environment effects in behavioral genetic studies (Rowe, 1987). These results encourage us to investigate family influences on alcohol consumption, although, as we shall see later, the environmental familial resemblance may be due to sibling mutual interaction, rather than to parental treatments or modeling.

MODEL FITTING: DISCONTINUOUS VARIATION

In the previous section, we apportioned a continuous trait to different sources of variation. The methods just outlined apply to the many continuous variables used in alcohol research, such as alcohol consumption per month. Such variables, however, tend to represent mainly the normal range of drinking behavior. Serious alcohol abuse, and clinically diagnosable alcoholism, are relatively rare conditions. For this reason, in clinical studies it becomes inefficient to take random samples. Instead, one typically identifies individuals who display a condition, called the *probands,* and then one locates their immediate relatives. The risk to relatives is calculated as the concordance coefficient. If 100 alcoholic men were sampled, and 25 of their brothers were alcoholic, the pairwise concordance coefficient would be .25 (25 / 100). In studies where a proband may be potentially sampled twice—for example, his name might appear in two sets of hospital records—concordance is computed using the *proband* method, but its interpretation is still as the risk to relatives.[2]

This section presents a discussion of methods of placing data collected using the proband study method into the standard behavioral genetic framework of "multifactorial threshold (MFT)" models (Falconer, 1965; Reich, Cloninger, & Guze, 1975). The advantage of MFT models is that they can be used to attribute categorial trait variation to different determinants, such as genetic inheritance and family environment. These methods also avoid many of the pitfalls of interpreting concordance risks.

The main problem of concordance risks is that they are not measures of statistical association. Thus, the concordance risk fails to indicate how *strongly* family members resemble one another for a particular trait. For example, consider the case in which MZ twins have a concordance risk of 30%. At first glance, this concordance appears to represent a strong association. However, the strength of relationship will depend on the prevalence of the disorder in the general population; if it is rare, then identical twins will resemble one another. On the other hand, suppose the concordance risk referred to is a common behavior problem, such as bed-wetting in male children, with a hypothetical prevalence near 30% among boys. In this latter example, the *correlation* of male twins would be near zero!

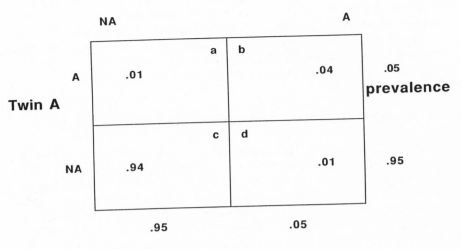

FIGURE 4.3. Association for concordance risk.

The correct interpretation of a concordance coefficient is indicated by Figure 4.3. In the figure, NA and A symbolize "not affected" and "affected" twins, respectively. The illustration shows the four kinds of twin pairs that may exist in the population: (1) both twins affected (cell b); (2) twin A affected but not twin B (cell a); (3) twin B affected but not twin A (cell d); and (4) both twins unaffected (cell c). This, therefore, shows the strength of association between finding the disorder in one twin and finding it in the other. A proband study, however, just samples cases where one twin is already affected; and where the co-twin may or may not have been affected.

The concordance coefficient, then, is the probability that the co-twin is affected, *given* an affected proband (i.e., $P(A_c/A_p)$). By Bayes' theorem, the probability that both a proband and co-twin are affected is:

$$(6) \quad P(A_c \cap A_p) = P(A_p) \ [P(A_c/A_p)]$$

where $P(A_p)$ is just the prevalence of the disorder in the population. Using this information, one can complete Figure 4.3 to translate a concordance into all the data needed to compute a measure of association. For example, in Figure 4.3, the concordance was assumed to be .80, and the population prevalence of the disorder was assumed to be .05 (i.e., 5%). Hence, the proportion of twin pairs in which both proband and co-twin were affected was .04 (.05 × .8). From these values, the remaining cells of the 2 × 2 illustration can be filled from the marginals (which must sum to 1.0, or

100%). In the figure, a strong twin association existed for the hypothetical disorder. Using the phi statistic—the correlation coefficient of categorical variables—the correlation was $\phi = .79$.

The assumptions of the MFT model, however, make the tetrachoric correlation, not ϕ, the appropriate measure of association as the underlying variables are continuous. The MFT model requires the assumption that the actual environmental and genetic determinants of a manifest behavior possess a normal distribution, which is referred to as a *liability*. The liability concept is consistent with polygenic theory, in that many genes with small effects probably influence most traits. The presence or absence of a disorder, however, is clearly a categorical variable. To connect this (unobserved) liability with the overt categories, a concept of a threshold is used. Individuals who have liabilities exceeding the threshold will display the trait. Thus, the population prevalence is the tail of the normal curve that exceeds the threshold value, as shown by Figure 4.4 *center*. A second normal curve can be used to represent the risk to the relatives of probands, where *concordance* risk is the area under the normal curve exceeding the threshold (see Figure 4.4 *right*). The *tetrachoric* correlation, computed from these normal curves, represents the correlation of relatives' liabilities. The tetrachoric correlation can be estimated from a data set using maximum likelihood methods; or, conveniently, it can be read off Gottesman and Carey's (1983, p. 39) Figure 1 to about 6% accuracy. The tetrachoric correlation (Figure 4.3) equals .99, considerably greater than its ϕ coefficient, which made no assumption about the existence of a liability.

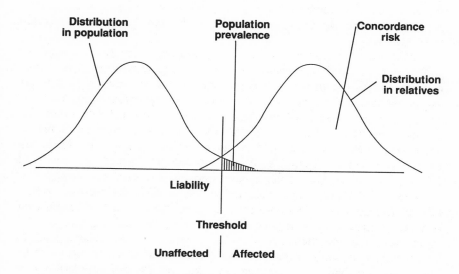

FIGURE 4.4. Multifactorial threshold model of a categorical trait.

TABLE 4.2. Twin Tetrachoric Correlation for Alcoholism[a]

| | | | Tetrachoric r's | | |
Group	No. pairs	Concordance	1%	5%	10%
MZ Twins	271	26.3	.70	.54	.39
DZ Twins	444	11.9	.48	.24	.06
		h^2	44%	40%	66%
		c^2	22%	14%	−27%

[a]*Source*. U.S. Veterans Twin Study (Hrubec & Omenn, 1981).

Tetrachoric correlations can serve to correct several misinterpretations of concordance data. Concordances, unfortunately, are sometimes viewed as though they were a measure of association; but the conclusion that a twin group with a greater concordance will show more "association," i.e., behavioral resemblance, may be wrong. For example, Kaprio et al. (1984) reported probandwise concordance (PbC) risks for heavy drinking in male MZ twins raised apart (PbC = 81.8) and in female MZ twins raised apart (PbC = 73.7). Heavy drinking was defined as drinking (on at least one occasion in the past month) 5 bottles of beer, a bottle of wine, or half a bottle of hard liquor. Heavy drinking was more common in men than women, with a prevalence of about 5% in women and about 30% in men. Despite the greater male than female concordance risks, the MZA's tetrachoric correlations were nearly *equal* in both sexes ($r > .95$, N(pairs) ≤ 25). In general, when population prevalences differ across groups, concordance risks are probably useless for group comparisons because different concordance risks may have similar liability correlations.

Tetrachoric correlations can be used to provide estimates of heritability and common family-environment effects using equations that express liability correlations in terms of behavioral genetic parameters. It is important to recognize, however, that this model fitting method provides estimates of genetic and environmental influence on the liability rather than on the overt trait. Table 4.2, for example, provides an estimate of the tetrachoric correlations for alcoholism under various assumptions about population prevalence. Falconer's (1960) estimate of heritability was used: $h^2 = 2(r_{MZ} - r_{DZ})$. Shared family environment was estimated as $r_{MZ} - h^2$. As shown, for population prevalences of 1% to 10%, the estimate of heritability increased, from 44% to 66%, whereas the estimate of shared environment decreased and finally, unrealistically, became negative ($-.27$). Note that even with these relatively *low* estimates of concordance risk, the heritability of alcoholism can be substantial, on the order of half of all liability variation. Note, too, that the more realistic 1%–5% population prevalence figures for alcoholism suggest a relatively small effect of family environment, especially in comparison to genetic transmission. Similarly,

Gottesman and Carey (1983) analyzed twin concordances from Kaij's (1960) Swedish study in terms of tetrachoric correlations; they found that heritabilities increased, and *shared* environmental effects decreased, when a progressively more severe criterion was applied to the diagnosis of alcoholism. Their article also gives further enlightenment on the problems of interpreting concordance risks.

Estimation

General methods of estimating behavioral genetic parameters from categorical data have been developed. Rao and his colleagues developed an estimation method based on maximum likelihood theory (Rao, Morton, Gottesman, & Lew, 1981). Rao's log-likelihood function is based on maximizing the likelihood of the obtained sample concordance risks in the various kinships. These sample concordances, in turn, are expressible as functions of the tetrachoric correlation coefficients, which, in their turn, are expressible as functions of behavior genetic parameters, such as h^2 (i.e., heritability). Their maximum likelihood estimation procedure provides a likelihood ratio goodness-of-fit test.

DeFries and Fulker (1985) developed an estimation method using ordinary least squares multiple regression:

$$(7) \quad C = B_1 P + B_2 r + A$$

where C is the co-twin's predicted score, P is the proband's score, r is the coefficient of (genetic) relationship ($r = 1$ for MZ twins; .5 for DZ twins or siblings), and A is the regression constant. The regression weight, B_1, measures twin similarity, independent of zygosity; B_2 provides a test of genetic etiology similar to that of differential twin concordances. DeFries and Fulker discussed the use of these regression coefficients to estimate heritability, and also provided an extended regression model that estimates both shared environmental influences and heritability. Their approach also permits one to decide whether probands constitute an extreme group, drawn from a normally distributed risk liability, or a group qualitatively different from the general population. Alcohol researchers lacking a background in maximum likelihood estimation procedures may find the approach of De Fries and Fulker (1985) to be especially helpful.

Considering the lessons of this section as a whole, alcohol researchers would be well-advised to calculate the tetrachoric correlation equivalents of concordance risks. To accomplish this goal, it would be desirable to have accurate information on the true population prevalences of different forms of alcohol abuse; to use uniform diagnostic criteria across different studies so that data from various kinships can be justifiably combined; and to employ a method of modeling that provides estimates of and significance tests for important parameters.

RECENT ADVANCES

Advances in behavior genetic modeling permit the exploration of sibling effects and components of correlation (or covariance). In this section, these new developments will be briefly introduced.

Sibling Mutual Imitation Effects

Alcohol usage increases markedly during early adolescence. In American culture, the context for early drinking is usually the peer group. Peers are seen as major influences on the development of drinking habits (Kandel, 1980). Family studies of alcohol use and abuse, however, tend to overlook the family member who is most similar to one's peer: a sibling. Although parental use of alcohol may provide a model that promotes (or deters) usage by children, siblings can serve the same modeling function and also influence one another in other ways.

The behavioral genetic contribution to understanding sibling influence is to provide quantitative models of the effects that sibling mutual imitation, or contrast, may have on the development of a behavioral trait. Just as with the models presented earlier, consequences of sibling effects have been derived for variances and correlations in different kinships (Carey, 1986a; Eaves, 1976).

These derivations show that, under proper assumptions, sibling effects can have a pronounced impact, detectable as changes in variances and correlations. "Mutual imitation" refers to a situation in which sibling A's behavior directly influences sibling B's; then the siblings switch roles, and B's behavior rebounds back to influence A. In the case of *imitation*, where there is a positive effect of one sibling on the other, sibling correlations will increase over time as the process continues. However, as the sibling mutual influence parameter, symbolized as a, takes a value < 1, sibling mutual imitation effects die out over time and reach a limiting value. In his model, Carey assumed some initial sibling resemblance due to heredity. According to Carey's model, sibling mutual imitation had several effects: (1) to increase the sibling correlation, (2) to increase the sibling correlation more in large families with interacting sets of siblings than in small families, and (3) to increase trait variance in families of two or more children in comparison to families with just single-born children. Similarly, mutual imitation can increase trait means. Applied to alcohol use, mutual imitation may lead to single-born children having a lower prevalence of alcohol use than children with siblings. Such a prediction may seem counterintuitive, but it follows from the mathematics of Carey's model.

Another sibling effects model was applied to Kaprio's et. al.'s twin correlations for alcohol consumption, presented earlier. Eaves' (1976) model, as shown in Figure 4.5, takes a relatively simple path analytic form because it

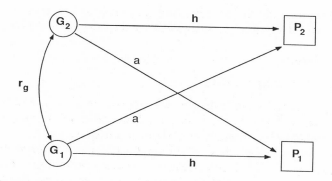

FIGURE 4.5. Path model of joint hereditary and sibling influences.

contains the fiction that one siblings' genotype (G) can directly influence the others phenotype (P) through the path coefficient *a*. By this stratagem, his path model is *recursive*, meaning that all causality flows in one direction; in contrast, Carey's models were nonrecursive (i.e., bidirectional causal flow). From Figure 4.5, the expected twin correlation can be derived:

$$(8) \quad r_{\text{twin}} = r_g h^2 + 2ah + r_g a^2$$

where *a* is the sibling influence path coefficient, *h* is the genetic path coefficient, and r_g is the coefficient of genetic relationship ($r_g = 1.0$ for MZ twins; .50 for DZ twins). In the case of twins reared apart, terms involving sibling mutual influence, naturally, would disappear from this equation.

Using Rao et al.'s (1974) methods described previously, these theoretical expectations were fitted to the alcohol correlations from Kaprio et al.'s (1984) study of MZ and DZ twins raised apart and MZ and DZ twins raised together. For females, the parameter estimates reached unreasonable values ($h = -.051$; $a = 1.0$). For males, however, the model produced reasonable parameter estimates ($h = .19$; $a = .73$), with an excellent overall fit ($x^2 = .36$, df = 2, $p > .9$). Because this model was not nested within the heredity–shared environment model, its chi square (.36) cannot be compared statistically with the one from the latter model (2.6). Nevertheless, its quality of fit was clearly superior.

These results illustrate an important point: in structural equation modeling, a closely fitting model fails to eliminate other models. To decide between adequate models, we need additional information beyond mere statistical criteria. Research designs can be developed to explore whether siblings close in age and twins strongly influence one another's alcohol consumption; or whether the environmental effects are truly something shared in general by siblings, such as social class or parental models of alcohol use.

Components of Correlation

Previously, we have described behavioral genetic methods, in which a single trait score was available for each person. Most studies of alcohol, however, are multivariate. They produce correlations among variables of different explanatory status. For example, Cloninger (1987) theorized that alcoholics differ from others in their combination of three continuously distributed personality traits: harm avoidance, reward dependence, and novelty seeking. Physiological markers, such as brain evoked potentials, have been employed in studies of alcoholism. Another set of measures may be indexes of environmental treatments, measured for each individual in a study. Such multiple measurements can be analyzed using multivariate behavioral genetic methods.

To explore etiology, the *correlation* of personality traits or neurophysiological traits can be apportioned to genetic, nonshared-environment, and shared-environment components. The path diagram of Figure 4.6 demonstrates how the correlation of trait 1 and 2 can be apportioned to latent components.

$$(9) \quad r_{12} = h_1 h_2 r_g + c_1 c_2 r_{se} + e_1 e_2 r_{nse}$$

where r_g is the genetic correlation of the traits genotypes ($0 < r_g < 1$), r_{se} is the correlation of shared environments, and r_{nse} is the correlation of nonshared environments, which affect each individual uniquely. The path coefficients are h, c, and e, respectively.

The genetic correlation, r_g, is the degree to which some loci are involved in the determination of both traits. For instance, height and weight are correlated through common genetic effects on body size, even though some genes may influence weight (or height) alone. Influence can also flow through correlated, shared environments. For example, exposure to lead (SE_1) may correlate with brain evoked responses (trait 1); and it may correlate with exposure to high rates of drinking (SE_2), affecting trait 2, alcohol use. Hence, a "social class" process could induce correlations environmentally through the environments that siblings may share.

Finally, environmental effects unique to each individual can induce correlations within individuals. This last pathway may be best understood by considering a hypothetical situation in which the sibling correlations for trait 1 and trait 2 were zero. Despite a lack of family resemblance, a trait may still correlate within individuals. For example, the twin correlation for handedness is very low; yet, handedness certainly would correlate with

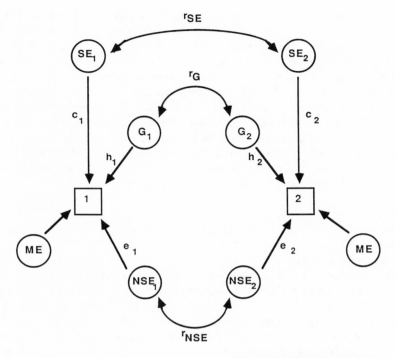

SE = shared environment
NSE = nonshared environment
G = genotype
ME = measurement error

FIGURE 4.6. Path model of correlation between two traits.

preference for right- or left-handed scissors. In the alcohol area, perinatal insults might influence susceptibility to alcohol by inducing brain damage; yet, because perinatal events occur relatively randomly across families, they would show low sibling correlations. Hence, they would produce within-person correlations through the nonshared-environment pathway. In sum, the aim of a behavior genetic analysis of *correlation* is to partition the total correlation within person to those theoretical influences on traits with which we were already familiar.

Estimation

Details of the estimation of path coefficients and correlations in multivariate designs are beyond the scope of this chapter. Two different approaches have been developed that use the computer program LISREL to measure these parameters and their standard errors (Boomsma & Molenaar, 1986; Ho, Baker, & Decker, 1988). These approaches rely on recasting the behavioral genetic models into LISREL matrices. The products of these matrices then will reproduce the correct mathematical expectations for correlations (or covariances). Even without a background in behavioral genetics, researchers familiar with LISREL modeling can readily cast the path analytic models into a LISREL framework. Baker (1986) developed a method of path analysis for tetrachoric correlations among several variables. Hence, her method is useful for noncontinuous data. The main advantage of all these multivariate approaches is that they may restrict the number of competing explanation for obtained results—one can see the whole picture, and not ignore the inevitable dependencies among variables.

CONCLUSIONS

The modeling approach offers an advantage over other methods of conceptualizing etiology in that it forces the researcher to derive the *consequences* of a theory. Research on behavioral development, however, often seems trapped at the level of our everyday psychology; models are stated in verbal form, and their implications are not well understood. For example, the idea that social class differences among families may influence personality development is an old one. The model builder, however, takes this theory and derives from it certain consequences—for instance, that siblings, who share family experiences, should be more alike than nonsiblings. And secondly, she attempts to remove hereditary confounds, which may inadvertently create the appearance of *environmental* social class effects. The great benefit of such modeling attempts is that they are like a corrective lens that can change the theoretical preconceptions leading to erroneous impressions of causality; in this respect, the absence of shared-environment effects on many personality traits—leading to the conclusion that familial resemblances are due solely to shared heredity (see Rowe, 1987)—is really one of the unassimilated discoveries of modern behavioral genetics.

For the alcohol researcher, we have reviewed the main elements of behavioral genetic methods. All the methods provide a partitioning of etiological effects to shared-environment, nonshared-environment, and hereditary determinants. Further apportionment to single gene effects, components of genetic variation, and sibling effects is possible. Both the modeling of continuous and categorical traits share the same basic features: collecting data on different kinships, expressing correlations (or other statistics) in terms of the model; and using a method of estimating model parameters and testing goodness-of-fit. Modeling is not a panacea nor a substitute for good theory; but the interplay between theory, on the one hand, and testing the fit of the theory against data, on the other, will eventually lead to a more complete understanding of human behavior. Alcohol researchers and behavioral geneticists, whenever feasible, should cooperate in the search for etiological processes—a joint venture worth toasting.

NOTES

1. A natural relationship exists between path analytic and "biometrical" model expectations. Using a path diagram, the expectation for the total variance of a phenotype and the correlation of phenotypes can be derived. The expectation for within-pair variation can be obtained by subtracting the expectation for the correlation from the total variance of the phenotype. The expectation for the correlation is set equal to $\sigma_b{}^2$, the between pair variance; and the expectation for the within pair variance is set equal to $\sigma_w{}^2$, the within pair variance. Expectations for mean squares in various kinships can be derived by expressing the mean squares in terms of these two variances, for example:

$$\text{Mean Square Between} = 2\sigma_b^2 + \sigma_w^2$$

$$\text{Mean Square Within} = \sigma_w^2$$

2. In the probandwise method, the concordance is given by the formula: $PC = 2c / [2c + (2 - a)d]$, where PC is probandwise concordance, c is the number of concordant pairs, d is the number of discordant pairs, and a is the probability that both members of a pair were independently ascertained as probands. The probandwise concordance is greater than the pairwise value and provides the correct conditional probability of finding an affected relative, given an affected proband.

REFERENCES

Baker, L. A. (1986). Estimating genetic correlations among discontinuous phenotypes: An analysis of criminal convictions and psychiatric-hospital diagnoses in Danish adoptees. *Behavior Genetics, 16,* 127–142.

Barnes, G. M. (1984). Adolescent alcohol abuse and other problem behaviors: Their relationships and common parental influences. *Journal of Youth and Adolescence, 13,* 329–348.

Boomsma, D. I., & Molenaar, P. C. M. (1986). Using LISREL to analyze genetic and environmental covariance structure. *Behavior Genetics, 16,* 237–250.

Buss, D. M. (1985). Human mate selection. *American Scientist, 73,* 47–51.

Carey, G. (1986a). Sibling imitation and contrast effects. *Behavior Genetics, 16,* 319–341.

Carey, G. (1986b). A general multivariate approach to linear modeling in human genetics. *American Journal of Human Genetics, 39,* 775–786.

Cloninger, C. R. (1987). Neurogenetic adaptive mechanisms in alcoholism. *Science*, 236, 410–416.

Cloninger, C. R., Rao, D. C., Reich, T., & Morton, N. E. (1983). A defense of path analysis in genetic epidemiology. *American Journal of Human Genetics, 35,* 733–756.

Cloninger, C. R., Rice, J., & Reich, T. (1979). Multifactorial inheritance with cultural transmission and assortative mating. II. A general model of combined polygenic and cultural inheritance. *American Journal of Human Genetics, 31,* 176–198.

DeFries, J. C., & Fulker, D. W., (1985). Multiple regression analysis of twin data. *Behavior Genetics, 15,* 467–473.

Eaves, L. J., Last, K. A., Young, P. A., & Martin, N. G. (1978). Model fitting approach to the analysis of human behavior. *Heredity, 41,* 249–320.

Eaves. L. (1976). A model for sibling effects in man. *Heredity, 36,* 205–214.

Elston, R. C. (1981). Segregation analysis. In H. Harris & K. Hirschhorn (Eds.), *Advances in human genetics.* Vol. 11 (pp. 63–120). New York: Plenum.

Falconer, D. S. (1960). *Introduction to quantitative genetics.* New York: Ronald Press.

Falconer, D. S. (1965). The inheritance of liability to certain diseases. *Annals of Human Genetics, 29,* 51–76.

Fancher, R. E. (1985). *The intelligence men: Makers of the IQ controversy.* New York & London: W. W. Norton.

Fulker, D. W. (1981). The genetic and environmental architecture of psychoticism, extraversion, and neuroticism. In H. J. Eysenck (Ed.), *A model for personality* (pp. 88–122). New York: Springer Verlag.

Gottesman, I. I., & Carey, G. (1983). Extracting meaning and direction from twin data. *Psychiatric Developments, 1,* 35–50.

Ho, H., Baker, L. A., & Decker, S. N. (1988). Covariation between intelligence and speed of cognitive processing: Genetic and environmental influences. *Behavior Genetics, 18,* 247–261.

Hrubec, Z., & Omenn, G. S. (1981). Evidence of genetic predisposition to alcoholic cirrhosis and psychosis. *Alcoholism: Clinical and Experimental Research, 5,* 207–215.

Joreskog, K. G., & Sorbom, D. (1983) LISREL V and LISREL VI: Analysis of Linear structural relationships by maximum likelihood and least squares methods. Uppsala: University of Uppsala.

Jencks, C., Smith, M., Acland, H., Bane, M. J., Cohen, D., Gintis, H., Heyns, B., & Michelson, S. (1972). *Inequality: A reassessment of the effect of family and schooling in America.* New York: Basic Books.

Kandel, D. B. (1980). Drug and drinking behavior among youth. *Annual Review of Sociology, 6,* 235–285.

Kaprio, J., Koskenvuo, H. & Langinvainio, H. (1984). Finnish twins reared apart. IV: Smoking and drinking habits. A preliminary analysis of the effect of heredity and environment. *Acta Geneticae Medicae et Gemellologia, 33,* 425–433.

Kaij, K. (1960). *Alcoholism in twins.* Stockholm: Almqvist & Wiksell.

Karlin, S., Cameron, E. C., & Chakraborty, R. (1983). Path analysis in genetic epidemiology: A critique. *American Journal of Human Genetics, 35,* 695–732.

Loehlin, J. C. (1978). Heredity-environment analysis of Jenck's IQ correlations. *Behavior Genetics, 8,* 415–436.

Loehlin, J. C. (1987). *Latent variable models: An introduction to factor, path, and structural analysis.* Hillsdale, NJ: Erlbaum.

Loehlin, J. C., Willerman, L., & Horn, J. M. (1988). Human behavior genetics. *Annual Review of Psychology, 39,* 101–133.

Mather, K., & Jinks, L. J. (1971). *Biometrical genetics: The study of continuous variation.* Chapman & Hall: London.

Morton, N. E., & MacLean, C. J. (1974). Analysis of family resemblance. III. Complex segregation analysis of quantitative traits. *American Journal of Human Genetics, 26,* 489–503.

Ozer, D. J. (1985). Correlation and the coefficient of determination. *Psychological Bulletin, 97,* 307–315.

Plomin, R., DeFries, J. C., & Loehlin, J. C. (1977). Genotype-environment interaction and correlation in the analysis of human behavior. *Psychological Bulletin, 84,* 309–322.

Rao, D. C., Morton, N. E., Gottesman, I. I., & Lew, R. (1981). Path analysis of qualitative data on pairs of relatives: Application to schizophrenia. *Human Heredity, 31,* 325–333.

Rao, D. C., Morton, N. E., & Yee, S. (1974). Analysis of family resemblance. II. A linear model for familial correlation. *American Journal of Human Genetics, 26,* 331–359.

Reich, T., Cloninger, C. R., & Guze, S. B. (1975). The multifactorial model of disease transmission: I. Description of the model and its use in psychiatry. *British Journal of Psychiatry, 127,* 1–10.

Roe, A. (1945). The adult adjustment of children of alcoholic parents raised in foster homes. *Quarterly Journal of Studies in Alcohol, 5,* 378–393.

Rowe, D. C. (1987). Resolving the person-situation debate: Invitation to an interdisciplinary dialogue. *American Psychologist, 42,* 218–237.

Sears. R. R. (1975). Your ancients revisited: A history of child development. In E. M. Hetherington (Ed.), *Review of child development research* (Vol. 5). Chicago: University of Chicago Press.

Scarr, S., & Carter-Saltzman, L. (1979). Twin method: Defense of a critical assumption. *Behavior Genetics, 9,* 527–542.

Wachs, T. D. (1983). The use and abuse of environment in behavior-genetic research. *Child Development, 54,* 396–407.

Watson, J. D., & Crick, F. H. C. (1953). Molecular structure of nucleic acids: A structure for deoxyribose nucleic acid. *Nature, 171,* 737–738.

Wright, S. (1934). The method of path coefficients. *Annals of Mathematical Statistics, 5,* 161–215.

PART II

FAMILY PROCESSES

5

Impact of the Family on Adolescent Drinking Patterns

GRACE M. BARNES

The family, as the basic social unit of society, can be expected to exert powerful influences on the development of social behaviors such as adolescent drinking. A child's first exposure to and experiences with alcohol are likely to be in the context of the family. It is commonly known that alcohol problems run in families, that is, alcoholic parents are much more likely than those without alcohol problems to have children who develop alcoholism (e.g., Cotton, 1979). Some explanations for this phenomenon involve genetic theories of the development of alcoholism (e.g., Goodwin, 1984; Schuckit, 1987). However, biological vulnerability for alcoholism at best explains a portion of the variance in some severe types of alcoholism, especially among sons of male alcoholics. Biological vulnerability does not explain adolescents' decisions to begin using alcohol or the variations in adolescent drinking patterns, from abstention to moderate use to problem drinking. Thus, even with a family history of alcoholism, the process of becoming an alcoholic has been characterized by Zucker and Gomberg (1986) as occurring in a social world and being influenced by a biopsychosocial process. Furthermore, biological vulnerability to alcoholism does not offer adequate explanations for the strong correlations between alcohol abuse, illicit drug use, and other problem behaviors in both male and female adolescents. On the other hand, there is strong theoretical and empirical evidence showing the importance of parent–child relationships and socialization in the family on the development of a wide range of adolescent behaviors, including alcohol abuse, illicit drug abuse, and delinquency. Even given genetic predispositions to the development of some types of alcoholism, most young people, nevertheless, grow up in families where alcohol is more or less available, where family members hold certain attitudes and expectations about alcohol, and where adults serve as role models for various types of drinking behaviors. In addition to the direct

137

learning of alcohol-related behaviors in the family, parents are powerful agents of socialization more generally conceived. Thus, parenting behaviors, particularly support (nurturance) and control (discipline), can be expected to exert important influences on the development of adolescent behaviors including drinking behaviors.

THEORETICAL BASIS

This chapter will provide a broad conceptual framework for examining the empirical findings relating family factors to the development of adolescent drinking. Figure 5.1 is a model for organizing the vast amount of descriptive and theoretical research that examines both the influences on the family as well as the family's impact on adolescent drinking behavior. This model has been influenced by early theoretical formulations of Parsons (1955a,b) in which the American family was viewed in the context of per-

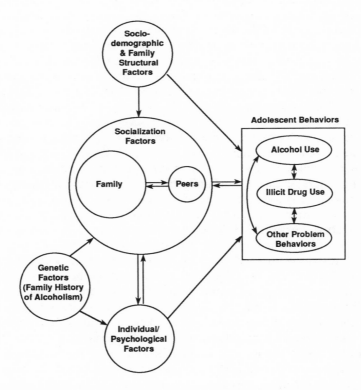

FIGURE 5.1. Model of the development of adolescent drinking behaviors.

sonality and social structure. According to Parsons, socialization of children is a basic and irreducible function of the family. This function of the family is on behalf of personality, since, according to Parsons, the human personality is not "born" but must be "made" through the socialization process within the family. This process of socialization is the internalization of the cultural system so that the child can learn to carry out the roles required of him/her in an achievement-oriented society. Family socialization is of critical importance in this theoretical scheme because it is the consensual basis for maintaining social order—or, relating this concept to our present concern with adolescent drinking behavior, socialization within the family is of critical importance to the development of nonproblem behavior, including nonproblem drinking.

In the model presented in Figure 5.1, family socialization is seen as the link between individual factors (psychological and biological) and the larger culture (including sociodemographic and structural factors). In this model, the young person learns social behaviors, including drinking behaviors, during the socialization process by ongoing interactions with significant others—parents, older siblings, and peers who play an increasingly important role during adolescence. However, parent–child relationships are seen as particularly potent and primary, occurring early in development. Furthermore, parent–child interactions may serve as a basis for the adolescents' choice of friendships with peers. In their extensive review of the parent–child interaction literature, Maccoby and Martin (1983) note that the parent–child bond is unique among human relationships. The tie is enduring throughout the child's development; and even during the child's adulthood, the tie is seldom severed completely as, for example, divorce may sever a marriage bond. Maccoby and Martin (1983) further note that the parent–child bond is unique in its initial asymmetry with the inherent differential power and competence between parents and children. While there are undoubtedly bidirectional effects, whereby adolescents' behaviors affect parental behaviors (which will be discussed later), nonetheless, most of the existing theory and empirical research supports a "social mold" perspective with parents exerting powerful influences on the development of their children (Peterson & Rollins, 1987).

In addition to the general theory described above, the model in Figure 5.1 draws upon previous theoretical work specifically related to the development of adolescent drinking; but the current model focuses much more on the centrality of the family and the socialization process as a nexus for other social, psychological, and biological influences which may contribute to adolescent drinking behavior.

Jessor and Jessor (1977) and Jessor (1987) explain the development of adolescent problem drinking within an overall problem behavior theoretical framework. Problem behavior theory aids in the specification and explanation of alcohol abuse, illicit drug abuse, and other problem behaviors as interrelated phenomena. The theory says that drinking behavior is learned behavior and as such it is shaped by the norms and expectations of the larger culture and by particular experiences a young person has in the context of everyday life (Jessor, 1987). The primary focus of problem-behavior theory is on three systems of psychosocial influence: the personality system, the perceived environment system, and the behavior system. Explanatory variables reflect either "instigations" to problem behavior or "controls" against it, together constituting a "proneness" or "risk" for problem behaviors. Proneness in the personality system includes lower value on academic achievement, higher value on independence, greater tolerance of deviance, and lesser religiosity. Proneness in the perceived environment system includes lower compatibility between parent and friends' expectations, greater influences from friends than parents, greater friends' approval for problem behavior, and greater friends' models for problem behavior. Proneness in the behavior system includes greater involvement in other problem behaviors, such as delinquency, illicit drug use, and less attendance at church. The structure of problem-behavior theory takes into account demographic and social structure variables and aspects of parental and peer socialization as antecedent variables related to the three systems of personality, environment, and behavior.

The theoretical perspective modeled in Figure 5.1 is also consistent with the developmental framework of Zucker (1976, 1979) which links four classes of influences to the development of drinking behavior in adolescence and early adulthood. The first of these classes of influences are sociocultural and community influences, including, for example, socioeconomic status of the family, ethnicity, and drinking specific factors such as availability of alcohol. Primary and secondary group influences, that is, parental and peer interactions, are presented in Zucker's model as two additional classes of influence. Intraindividual influences are Zucker's fourth class of influences on the development of drinking behaviors with this group, including such factors as temperament, genetic influences, and attitudes and beliefs about alcohol.

The model proposed in Figure 5.1 for the development of adolescent drinking behaviors incorporates many of the components of the theoretical perspectives described above. However, for the present purpose of discussing family influences on adolescent drinking, the model shows the socialization process, particularly within the family, as being a central focus for the development of drinking behaviors, other substance use, and other problem behaviors. Furthermore, the model shows the socialization process as being the focal point for the integration of other important influences on drinking. For example, the individual's genetic and psychological characteristics are acted upon and shaped in the process of interaction within the family. Thus, in this model, individual factors that may be related to adolescent behaviors will be moderated or enhanced in the interaction process within the family. Similarly, sociodemographic factors may show relationships to alcohol use and other adolescent behaviors, but these structural variables are given meaning in the family interaction process. Thus, sex roles and age-specific behaviors, for example, are developed in the socialization process within the family and also, during adolescence, within the peer group.

PATTERNS OF ADOLESCENT ALCOHOL USE AND ABUSE—RELATIONSHIPS TO OTHER PROBLEM BEHAVIORS

Much of the research designed to determine family and other antecedents of adolescent drinking has begun with a description of the prevalence and correlates of drinking patterns and alcohol-related problems in youth. Studies using large representative samples of secondary school students, carried out over more than two decades, have consistently shown that the majority of young people drink at least occasionally and a significant minority of young people drink heavily and experience various alcohol-related problems (e.g., Barnes & Welte, 1986b; Blane & Hewitt, 1977; Rachal et al., 1975, 1980). While most adolescent drinking is not legally sanctioned and alcohol abuse among teenagers is recognized as a serious social problem, nonetheless, the extent of adolescent drinking is not surprising given that the majority of adults also drink alcoholic beverages and a significant number drink heavily (Hilton, 1988). Within a social learning perspective, teenagers are being socialized by their parents and other models into adult behaviors, including drinking behaviors. Thus, the drinking patterns of adolescents can be expected to reflect the drinking patterns of adults in the same sociocultural context. Table 5.1 is an empirical example of this notion.

Data on drinking patterns of adults in New York State and secondary school students in New York State are presented here from two independent, large representative samples. In the adult study, adults were selected for analysis if they had 12- to 17-year-old children in their households. These are then adults who would likely be similar to the parents of the secondary school students in the second sample. Despite the age differences in the samples, the methodological differences in drinking questions, and modes of administration of the survey instruments (interview vs. questionnaire), the findings for drinking are remarkably similar in the two samples: 71% of the secondary school students in New York State are drinkers and 78% of the adults are drinkers. Of the students 13% are characterized as heavier drinkers and 11% of the adults with 12- to 17-year-old children are so classified. (Heavier drinking is defined as consuming an average of over two drinks per day.) The rates of heavier drinking for both groups of males are also very similar—18% for adult males and 17% for adolescent males. This similarity in patterns between independent samples

TABLE 5.1. Comparison of Drinking Patterns of Adults in NYS Who Have Adolescents in Their Households with Drinking Patterns of NYS Secondary School Students

Drinking levels	Drinking of NYS adults who have 12- to 17-year-old children in their households (1986) (N = 1,120)			Drinking among NYS 7th–12th grade students (1983) (N = 27,335)		
	Males	Females	Totals	Males	Females	Totals
Abstainer	17%	26%	22%	26%	32%	29%
Light-moderate drinker (no more than 2 drinks/day)	65%	69%	67%	57%	59%	58%
Heavier drinker (over 2 drinks/day)	18%	6%	11%	17%	10%	13%
Totals	100%	101%[a]	100%	100%	101%[a]	100%

[a]Rounding error.

of young people and adults living in the same geographic area has been shown previously in other samples, along with similarities between adolescents and parents in reports of availability of alcohol in the home and reasons for drinking (Barnes, 1981). The direct relationships between adolescents' and their own parents' behaviors will be examined below in more detail. These overall patterns of drinking, however, do support the notion that drinking among adolescents is learned social behavior which is to a great extent a model of the drinking of adults in the society.

Furthermore, early learning with regard to alcohol use may have long-term effects on an individual's drinking behaviors. Using data from a 1978 household sample of employed adults in metropolitan Detroit, Parker and Harford (1987) found that adult children with heavy-drinking parents had a higher percentage of dependent problem drinking than those without heavy-drinking parents. (The dependent problem drinking scale included withdrawal symptoms, loss of control, and behavior symptomatic of episodes of intoxication.) Also, adult children with low status occupations were found to have a higher percentage of dependent problem drinking than those with high status occupation. While the study design did not allow the investigators to disentangle genetic processes from social processes, nonetheless, the findings indicate that having heavy-drinking parents and a low status occupation seem to put sons and daughters at elevated risk for alcohol-related problems.

The long-term consequences of early alcohol experiences were also evidenced in a representative sample of over 6,000 adults in New York State (Barnes & Welte, 1988). In this study, age of first drink and age of first becoming drunk on alcohol were both good predictors of current drinking, regardless of the adult's current age. Thus, for every age cohort, including older adults who were decades removed from their first drinking experiences, the finding was consistent—the earlier individuals reported beginning to drink alcohol, the more likely they were to be current heavier drinkers.

In terms of adolescent outcome behaviors noted in Figure 5.1, the model also shows that alcohol use is related to both illicit drug use and other problem behaviors. This has been a consistent finding in numerous empirical studies (e.g., Barnes, 1984; Barnes & Welte, 1986a; Donovan & Jessor, 1985; Jessor & Jessor, 1977). More specifically, adolescents who are heavier drinkers are more likely than other young people to be frequent marijuana users. Similarly, the more often adolescents use marijuana and other illicit substances, the more likely they are to be heavier drinkers (Frank et al., 1985). These substance abuse behaviors are also strongly linked to various delinquent activities, school problems, and other interpersonal conflict. Jessor and associates have described alcohol abuse, illicit drug abuse, and delinquency as a system of interrelated behaviors constituting a problem behavior syndrome (Donovan & Jessor, 1985; Jessor, 1987; Jessor & Jessor, 1977). Furthermore, this syndrome of behaviors may have common antecedents in the family, such as inadequate socialization within the family (Barnes, 1977; Barnes, 1984; Barnes, Farrell, & Cairns, 1986; Kandel, 1983).

FAMILY SOCIODEMOGRAPHIC FACTORS AS INFLUENCES ON ADOLESCENT DRINKING

It is well beyond of the scope of this work to review the vast number of sociodemographic factors which have been related to variations in drinking behaviors. Age, sex, race, ethnicity, religion, and socioeconomic status, for example, have all been linked to drinking in adults (e.g., Barnes & Welte, 1988) and in adolescents (e.g., Barnes & Welte, 1986b; Welte & Barnes, 1987). While these factors may be directly related to the development of adolescent drinking behaviors, it is also very likely that these same variables affect the ongoing socialization process within the family which in turn has a significant impact on adolescent drinking (Figure 5.1). For example, it has been shown that black and Hispanic youth have lower rates of drinking than white adolescents, but minority youth experience more alcohol-related problems per ounce of alcohol consumed than their white counterparts (Welte & Barnes, 1987). Explanations for these variations may lie within the family structure or the family socialization process whereby cultural values and expectations are transformed into roles and behaviors; but there are virtually no empirical studies that focus on minority family factors as they affect developing adolescent drinking.

As another example, Jessor and Jessor (1977) independently assessed mothers' ideology in terms of religiosity, tolerance of deviance, and traditional beliefs, providing a linkage between sociocultural factors and socialization influences. They clearly found that the more religious, conventional, and traditional the mother, the lower the incidence of adolescent problem behaviors, including problem drinking and illicit drug use. Thus, in considering family influences on the development of adolescent drinking, it is important to take into account critical sociocultural characteristics of the family as well.

FAMILY STRUCTURAL FACTORS RELATED TO ADOLESCENT DRINKING

One-Parent Versus Two-Parent Families

The relationships between marital disruption and alcohol abuse in adults have been demonstrated (e.g., McCrady, 1982); however, few studies have examined the interaction of parental marital status and parental drinking patterns on adolescent drinking behaviors. Burnside, Baer, McLaughlin, and Pokorny (1986) examined this issue in a large sample of secondary school students. Their findings indicate that adolescents in single and step-parent families reported more alcohol use than adolescents from intact families when considering both frequency and quantity of alcohol use. In addition, parents in nonintact families were reported to have higher levels of alcohol use than other parents. Adolescent alcohol use was significantly correlated with parental alcohol use. After adjusting adolescent alcohol use for parental alcohol use as a covariate, the finding of greater alcohol use by adolescents in non-intact families remained.

Barnes and Windle (1987), in a study of high school students, also reported a tendency for adolescents living with both natural parents to have fewer alcohol-related problems when compared to those adolescents living with either a single parent or a parent and a stepparent. The findings were even stronger for illicit drug use among adolescents. Selnow (1987) examined substance usage for youngsters in single-parent and two-parent families considering as well the influences of parent–child relationships. The parental relations index was comprised of the respondents' general outlook toward relationships with parents (e.g., how well you get along with mother and father) and perceptions of intimacy with custodial parent(s) (e.g., how often you talk to them about really good or bad news). In two separate studies of large samples of school children, similar findings were evident. There was greater substance use among young people living in single-parent households. Respondents who reported better relationships with parents had significantly less substance use. However, the parental relationships variable had a stronger relationship to substance use than did single- versus two-parent household. A conclusion to be drawn from this work is that improved parental relationships may go a long way to offsetting the disadvantages of living in a single-parent home.

Family Size, Sibling Spacing, and Birth Order

Family structural characteristics may affect adolescent outcomes directly or through the influence they exert on parent–child relationships in the socialization process. Three components of family structure have been repeatedly addressed in the socialization literature—family size (or sibling number), sibling spacing (or child density), and birth order. Generalizations derived from the theoretical and empirical literature (e.g., Peterson & Rollins, 1987) can be posed for each of these components. Regarding family size, as the sibling number increases, the family becomes more complex in terms of role relationships and may experience increasing levels of frustration. Thus, as sibling numbers increase, parents may exert more coercive control attempts and less supportive behaviors toward the child, resulting in more adolescent problem behaviors. A commonly held assumption in this same literature is that wider spacing of children is most effective for parental socialization attempts. More specifically, as average spacing between children increases, it is expected that parents are able to relax their discipline and exhibit higher levels of supportive behaviors, again resulting in more positive adolescent outcomes. The third generalization regarding family structure deals with birth order. A number of investigators have found that first-borns, compared to later-borns, receive more parental nurturance, overall attention, and achievement pressure (e.g., review of Peterson & Rollins, 1987).

Family structural variables also have been related to the development of drinking behaviors, especially the development of alcoholism in adult males. In general, these factors have not been systematically examined in the development of adolescent drinking behaviors, simultaneously taking into account family interaction factors. Zucker (1976) reviewed social structural characteristics of families as they related to drinking behaviors. Overall there was evidence of a preponderance of larger families in the backgrounds of alcoholics. Zucker noted that plausible explanations for this finding involved the family-interaction network, such that larger families are more likely to show diluted socialization effects, more authoritarian discipline, looser parental controls, and greater sibling rivalry. Blane and Barry (1973), in their early review of birth order and alcoholism, concluded that in families with two or more children, there were consistently more last-born men than first-born men who became alcoholic. Family size interacts with birth order in that the overrepresentation of last-borns was more pronounced with large family size. In a later study these investigators found that among later-born, male alcoholics having at least two older siblings, the second older sibling was more often a sister than a brother (Blane & Barry, 1975). This led to the conclusion that alcoholism in men may represent sex-role conflict, especially in the expression of dependency needs. Thus, sibling sex is another family structural factor to be taken into consideration in family research on the development of alcohol abuse.

The findings between birth order and alcohol abuse are more equivocal in studies of young nonalcoholic or female samples (e.g., Blane & Barry, 1975; Zucker & Van Horn, 1972). Considering the methodological problems of unrepresentative samples, uncontrolled variables, and lack of control groups, other reviewers have concluded that there is very little solid evidence pointing to the relationship between birth order and alcoholism (Steinglass & Robertson, 1983) or the relationship between birth order and other substance abuse (Stagner, 1986). Nonetheless, birth order is still considered in clinical work and research on the development of alcoholism. For example, Wegscheider (1981) has characterized birth order positions in the children of alcoholics (i.e., first-born as Hero, second-born as Scapegoat, etc.) suggesting that each birth position carries a particular risk for psychosocial development. Another recent empirical example was an examination of birth order effects in intact families with three children of second-generation alcoholics (Keltner, McIntyre, & Gee, 1986). This study showed a consistent pattern of first-borns having significantly less exaggerated psychopathology (as measured by MMPI scores) than both groups of later-borns. One explanation for this was that later-born children of alcoholic parents experience increasingly disrupted home life with parental socialization skills progressively deteriorating over the years. What is becoming clear is that family research dealing with birth order as a structural factor affecting adolescent outcomes must also statistically control for the effects of sibling size, spacing, and sex of siblings (Kidwell, 1981).

PARENTAL SOCIALIZATION FACTORS

Parents as Models for Developing Adolescent Drinking Behavior

A child's first experiences with alcohol are likely to be within the context of the family where parents serve as role models for how to drink, for what occasions drinking is appropriate, and for what reasons alcohol is consumed. Kandel (1983) describes two processes related to the influence of significant others on adolescents' drinking and other substance use, both of which are consistent with the social learning perspective (e.g., Bandura, 1977; Maccoby & Martin, 1983). The first process is imitation, in which young people model their own behaviors after those of significant others.

Thus, adolescents are more likely to drink when their parents drink. The second process Kandel (1983) describes is social reinforcement whereby adolescents internalize definitions and exhibit behaviors and values approved by significant others. Kandel, Kessler, and Margulies' (1978) data support the modeling theory in that mothers' and fathers' use of hard liquor was found to be a moderately good predictor of initiation into hard liquor usage by their adolescents. Kandel et al. (1978) further showed that the drug behaviors of parents (and peers) were consistently more important than their drug-related beliefs and values as predictors of transitions in adolescent drug use. This suggests that adolescent socialization may take place more through a modeling effect than through social reinforcement, although values and prescriptions do play some role.

In a 1978 national study of adolescent drinking behaviors, Rachal et al. (1980) asked adolescents for their perceptions of their parents' drinking behavior. Parents' drinking and teenagers' drinking were found to be generally similar, with abstaining adolescents more likely than drinking adolescents to come from homes where parents were also abstainers. Similarly, heavier-drinking adolescents were likely to have parents who drank regularly. Adolescents' perceptions of their parents' approval or disapproval of teenage drinking were also related to their own drinking behavior, with adolescents whose parents disapproved of their drinking being less likely to drink; and adolescents whose parents were perceived as generally approving of alcohol use more likely than other young people to be heavier drinkers.

Harburg, Davis, and Caplan (1982) also found that offspring tend to imitate their perception of their parents' drinking, particularly that of the same-sex parent. However, when parental drinking behavior was perceived as extreme, either abstaining or heavy, the imitation dropped off. These authors found as did Barnes, Farrell, and Cairns (1986) that while abstaining parents had a high proportion of abstaining children, they also had relatively high proportions of heavy-drinking children. This may be related to earlier findings by Globetti (e.g., 1972) of drinking by teenagers in abstinence communities. In these southern U.S. communities, most of the adolescents abstained from alcohol in conformance to the norms of parents, church, and community. However, when young people did drink, they were at a high risk for a variety of alcohol-related problems and related deviant behaviors. This may be due to rebellion of children from strict parental control and conflict with the peer group and community norms which tolerate drinking. Some social learning proponents might say that these young people with abstaining parents have not been taught to drink moderately when they do drink. However, the reason this subgroup begins to drink, when other children of abstaining parents abstain, is not clear.

Parental modeling of alcohol use is an important factor in adolescents learning to drink, but it does not provide a complete explanation for adolescent drinking behavior (Barnes, Farrell & Cairns, 1986). Both parental and adolescent drinking behaviors may be a function of a number of other family factors including quality of family relationships and critical family life events as well as other agents of socialization, including older siblings and the adolescent's peer group.

Parental Support and Control Attempts

There is a sizable body of theoretical and empirical research that shows the importance of specific aspects of parental socialization, particularly support and control, for the development of a wide variety of childhood behaviors including cognitive development, achievement, aggression, and social competence (e.g., Rollins & Thomas, 1979). The *support construct* has been defined by Rollins and Thomas (1979) as parental behaviors toward the child, such as praising, encouraging, and giving physical affection, which indicate to the child that she or he is accepted, approved of, and loved. The *control construct* has been defined as parental behaviors toward the child which are intended to direct the child's behavior in a manner acceptable to the parent. Control attempts can range from coercive parental actions such as hitting, threatening, and yelling to inductive control attempts, such as parents explaining why the adolescent should not have done something and how they expect the child to behave in the future. Control attempts may also consist of explicit parental rules for adolescent behavior, including curfews, rules about homework, dating, dress, and so forth.

The overall theory of parental support and control attempts (e.g., Rollins & Thomas, 1979) would indicate that high levels of parental support and moderate levels of overall parental control are associated with nonproblem behaviors. Most studies of adolescent drinking have not systematically measured these constructs, nor have they examined the joint effects of parental support and control attempts. Nonetheless, isolated findings from many studies note significant relationships between aspects of parental socialization factors and adolescent drinking behaviors. Related to the support construct, the profiles of excessive adolescent alcohol users indicate that they are more likely to feel alienation from than closeness to their families (Wechsler & Thum, 1973); and to feel rejection in the relationship with both their mothers and fathers (Prendergast & Schaefer, 1974). Similarly, Zucker and Barron (1973) found mothers of problem-drinking sons to exhibit more expressive rejection in their relationships with their adolescents. Potvin and Lee (1980) found that parental support influenced conformity-commitment in adolescents, which in turn had an inverse effect on drinking and illicit drug use. (Potvin and Lee's support scale was similar to the construct described above and included physical signs of affection, listening, and other descriptions of the parent as emotionally expressive and loving. Conformity-commitment was determined based on the importance of family, church, and school in life influences over peer influences.)

Kandel et al. (1978) found that closeness to parents shielded adolescents from initiation into hard drug use. In fact, parental influences, especially the quality of adolescent–parent relationships, explained the largest amount of variance in the most severe stage of illicit substance use. Later work by Kandel and Andrews (1987) also confirmed that the quality of the parent–child bond makes an important contribution to restraining adolescents from using drugs. Closeness between parents and child had a significant effect in determining frequency of alcohol use, frequency of marijuana use, and initiation into marijuana use.

Related to the control construct described above, singular findings from a number of types of studies have documented inadequacies in parental control among problem drinkers and alcoholics. Prendergast and Schaefer (1974) found that excessive drinking among high school students was strongly correlated with lax parental controls. Dishion and Loeber (1985), in a study of 7th and 10th grade boys and their families, measured parent monitoring (e.g., knowledge of the child's whereabouts, time spent with parents, and who the child goes to with problems) as well as inept parent discipline (not following up on commands and inconsistency in disciplining). The finding indicated that less parental monitoring and less parental discipline were related to increased adolescent alcohol consumption among the boys in the study. Holmes and Robins (1987) in a case-control study from the general population found childhood disciplinary experiences to be a significant factor in the development of alcoholism and depression. Unfair, inconsistent, and harsh discipline by parents predicted both alcohol and depressive disorders independently of the influences of parental psychiatric history, the respondent's sex, and childhood behavior problems. Having been frequently punched or hit with a belt, stick, or similar object differentiated both depressives and alcoholics from controls. High proportions of parents of depressives and alcoholics were reported to usually use harsh physical punishment to discipline their children, exceeding greatly the rates of controls. Other aspects of punishment differentiating alcoholics from controls were inconsistent punishment, that is, parents threatened to punish but did not carry out their threats, and parental punishment in front of other people. Holmes and Robins (1987) note that many of the parental practices that were perceived as unfair and cruel by their offspring appeared to have had long-term adverse effects.

Brook, Whiteman, and Gordon (1983) found that family factors, particularly parental alcohol and illicit drug use and parental warmth and aspects of parental control, were related to stages of adolescent drug use, that is, from no use, to use of legal substances, to use of marijuana, and use of other illicit drugs. Furthermore, inadequate family relations were associated with higher stages of drug use even after controlling for demographic factors, personality factors, and peer relations. More specifically, inadequate family socialization was related to stages of alcohol and illicit drug use regardless of the existence of a non-drug-prone personality or the influence of a conventional peer group. Thus, this work supports the contention that adolescent socialization experiences within the family are predisposing factors for substance abuse.

Williams and Klerman (1984), in a review of family background characteristics of female alcoholics, noted a greater likelihood among female alcoholics as compared with other women to have grown up in unstable family environments, with greater disruption in terms of separation and divorce, economic distress, and parental abuse or neglect. Socialization experiences of alcoholic women were poor, with erratic and lax discipline, a lack of affection from parents, and limited responsiveness to the child's needs, which is consistent with earlier case reports concerning the socialization experiences of children of alcoholics (Burk, 1972; Hecht, 1973). Furthermore, Williams and Klerman note that it appears likely that the description of female alcoholics' experiences in their families of origin are recreated in their own families of procreation, and that the cycle of family disruption and alcoholism is often continued into the next generation.

Barnes, Farrell, and Cairns (1986) examined the interaction of both support and control and found evidence for high parental support and moderate parental control as determinants of nonproblem drinking in a general population sample of adolescents. However, it was clear in their work that the most important parental factor of the two is parental support, which consistently shows a strong positive relationship to nonproblem adolescent behaviors (Barnes, 1984; Barnes, Farrell, & Windle, 1987). In findings from a high school sample, Barnes and Windle (1987) reported that parental control, as measured by the number of parental rules for adolescent behaviors, showed a negative linear relationship to adolescent alcohol abuse and related problem behaviors; that is, the more specific rules parents had for adolescent behavior (as described above), the lower the reported number of adolescent alcohol problems, incidents of illicit drug use, and deviant acts. Thus, this measure of control was not curvilinear in its relationship to adolescent outcome, as was the more general control dimension (Barnes, Farrell & Cairns, 1986; Rollins & Thomas, 1979). It may be that having clear, up-front rules or expectations for adolescent behavior is conceptually different from after-the-fact parental punishment attempts. Much more systematic work is required regarding control aspects of parental socialization and their relationship to adolescent outcomes.

Peer Socialization Factors

The peer group is another important agent of socialization during the period of adolescence and it can be expected that peer influences interact with family influences in their relationships to the development of adolescent drinking and related behaviors. Where parent–child interaction is problematic, adolescents are likely to withdraw from the family and rely more heavily on the influence of peer subcultures. Empirical data has shown that adolescents who value peer opinions, as opposed to those of their parents, for important life decisions and values are at a high risk for alcohol abuse, illicit drug use, and other problem behaviors (Barnes & Windle, 1987). Furthermore, Barnes, Farrell, and Windle (1987) used structural equations to model the interrelationships among parental socialization factors, parent/peer orientation, and problem behaviors among adolescents. Their data fit a model showing that parental support was inversely related to problem behaviors by a direct effect, as well as by an indirect effect via its influence on peer versus parent orientation.

Similarly, Kandel and Andrews (1987) found that parental variables, such as parental closeness, discourage drug use both directly and through their impact on peer-related variables, especially the choice of non-drug-using friends. Peers contribute significantly to adolescent socialization and drug use by enhancing or vitiating the parental effects (Kandel, 1980). Adolescents with close relationships with parents are less likely to associate with deviant peers. Thus, parents influence the kinds of friendships developed by their children and these friendships become important as far as subsequent drug use or nonuse is concerned (Kandel & Andrews, 1987).

Other investigators have likewise found relationships between parental and peer socialization factors as they relate to adolescent problem behaviors. Brook, Whiteman, and Gordon (1983) found that poor socialization experiences, particularly a lack of maternal positive reinforcement, when accompanied by friends' drug use, resulted in high levels of drug use among adolescents. Dishion and Loeber (1985) also found that parental monitoring has an indirect effect on adolescent substance use by increasing the likelihood that the youngster spends time with deviant peers, which led the authors to conclude that adolescent delinquency and drug use are outcomes of disrupted family processes and exposure to deviant peers.

Sibling Influences in the Development of Adolescent Drinking

One of the most neglected areas of research regarding family influences on the development of adolescent drinking is the relationship of siblings, particularly older siblings, in the initiation and continuation of substance use among adolescents. In fact, siblings may constitute a potentially powerful combination of peer and family socialization agent. In a sample of young adult men in the United States, Clayton and Lacy (1982) found a significant positive relationship between perceived siblings' drug use and respondents' own use and intentions to use. The investigators concluded that siblings may constitute a special category of peer influence in terms of social learning or modeling of substance use behaviors and in terms of drug availability. Brook, Whiteman, Gordon, and Brenden (1983) examined older brother's influence on younger sibling's drug use in a sample of 9th and 10th grade students. Having an older brother who used marijuana had a significant effect on the adolescent's substance use, even after peer influence was controlled. In one study where independent information was obtained from both adolescents and their older siblings (Needle et al., 1986), it was found that adolescent's frequency of drug use was predicted by older sibling and peer substance use, each being significant after controlling for the other. Furthermore, older siblings, like peers, were frequently found to be sources of drugs and companions in the use of substances with their younger siblings. Thus, in addition to examining the relative effects of parents and peers on developing adolescent alcohol use and abuse, more research is needed regarding siblings as peer/family agents of socialization into substance use.

FAMILY SYSTEM IN THE DEVELOPMENT OF ADOLESCENT DRINKING

While much of the literature dealing with family influences on adolescent behaviors is focused on the parent–child dyad, the family system is recognizably complex and other family interactions may influence parental socialization and, thereby, influence adolescent outcomes. Barber has recently shown, using structural equation analysis, that the quality of marital relations has a direct effect on adolescent self-esteem as well as an indirect effect via parental support (Barber, 1987). Thus, it is expected that higher marital quality would result in more positive parenting and in more positive adolescent outcomes.

There is a lack of empirical research relating family systems theory to adolescent alcohol misuse (Mayer, 1986), although family systems concepts as related to the families of adult alcoholics have been developed in the literature (e.g., see reviews by Jacob, 1987; Steinglass & Robertson, 1983) and can be extended to the development of adolescent drinking. From a family systems perspective, the drinking behavior of an adolescent may be symptomatic of other family problems, including problematic styles of interacting and communicating. Most family systems theorists agree that important variables are cohesion, adaptability (flexibility), and communication clarity (e.g., Walsh, 1982). *Cohesion*, which ranges from overinvolvement or enmeshment to disengagement, is defined as the emotional bonding that family members have toward one another. *Flexibility* refers to the ability of the family to alter roles and rituals in response to situational stress or developmental changes (Olson et al., 1983). *Communication clarity* refers to the degree to which the members make use of ambiguous or "paradoxical" communication (Broderick & Pulliam-Krager, 1979). Problems in these family process dimensions can result in a variety of counternormative coalitions between family members. Minuchin (1974) describes the development of coalitions; for example, where husband–wife conflict may result in one parent (often the mother) forming a coalition with the child against the father. In another instance, owing to marital conflict, a child can be the target of what Vogel and Bell (1960) have called "scapegoating." In this latter example, the mother and father form a coalition focusing criticism on the child as a source of family problems and thereby diverting attention from their own marital difficulties.

The combined effect of these family systems variables and parental socialization factors have not been systematically studied as they relate to the development of adolescent drinking behaviors. However, it is likely that parental socialization, i.e., support and control dimensions, may be a function of overall family cohesion, adaptability, and communication, and that both family systems variables and socialization variables would have a combined effect on adolescent substance abuse behaviors. Furthermore, the "pile up" of family life events (e.g., marital conflict, divorce, death, financial problems) also has been linked to drinking (Linsky, Straus, & Colby, 1985; Moos & Moos, 1984). Families who have problematic functioning along the dimensions of cohesion and adaptability are likely to abuse alcohol as a means of coping with critical family events and consequently, these parents are likely to provide inadequate socialization (support and control) for developing children.

There is some empirical support for these hypothesized relationships as related to adolescent drinking. Gantman (1978) compared the family interaction patterns among families with normal, emotionally disturbed, and drug-abusing adolescents. The normal families displayed clearer communication, more cooperation, more decision-making, greater sensitivity among members, and less scapegoating. Many of these family systems variables have been explored in families with an alcoholic parent. Filstead, McElfresh, and Anderson (1981) measured aspects of family environment, including cohesion, expressiveness, and conflict. A comparison between alcoholic and "normal" families (each having a child aged 9 or older) revealed significant differences between the groups. Alcoholic families perceived their family environments to be less cohesive and less expressive, with more conflict as compared to "normal" families. West and Prinz (1987), in a review of the literature on relationships between parental alcoholism and childhood psychopathology, conclude that parental alcoholism is associated with a heightened incidence of child symptoms of psychopathology, including substance abuse and delinquency. However, major methodological problems exist and it is difficult to infer causal pathways. It seems plausible that the presence of an alcoholic parent severely disrupts family interaction, which in turn causes child psychopathology; but which critical aspects of disrupted family functioning still have to be isolated. According to the authors, increased marital discord could be the influential factor, but other possibilities include disrupted family routine, inadequate parental guidance and nurturance, and modeling of maladaptive coping styles.

The disruption of family rituals is one interesting aspect of family functioning which has been well documented (Wolin & Bennett, 1984) and related to the development of alcohol problems in children of alcoholics. Wolin, Bennett, Noonan, and Teitelbaum (1980) have shown that when one or both parents in a family are alcoholics, their children are more likely to become alcoholics if family rituals—the dinner time, evenings, holidays, weekends, vacations, and visitors—are disrupted during the period of heaviest parental drinking. They describe the family ritual as "a symbolic form of communication which, owing to the satisfaction that family members experience through its repetition, is acted out in a systematic fashion over time. Through their special meaning and their repetitive nature, rituals contribute significantly to the establishment and preservation of a family's collective sense of itself. Rituals stabilize family life by clarifying expected roles, delineating boundaries within and without the family, and defining rules so that all members know that 'this is the way our family is' " (p. 201).

FUTURE RESEARCH DIRECTIONS

Integration of Multiple Theoretical Approaches

In terms of conceptualization and explanation of developing adolescent drinking, there needs to be more integration of family theory into empirical research efforts. Multiple theoretical perspectives are called for, drawing upon, for example, social learning theory (Abrams & Niaura, 1987; Bandura, 1977), family interaction and socialization theoretical perspectives (Maccoby & Martin, 1983; Peterson & Rollins, 1987; Sadava, 1987), and family systems theory (Walsh, 1982). Individual factors and family sociocultural factors interact, finding a focus within the context of the family interaction/socialization process. This multivariate process results in a significant impact upon developing adolescent drinking patterns. Theoretical and empirical research models must be designed to take into account the combined effects of multiple factors which influence adolescent drinking.

General Population Samples of Adolescents and Their Families

Much of our understanding of the patterns of adolescent drinking comes from school samples. While these studies have been of tremendous benefit in defining and describing the problem of adolescent alcohol abuse, they generally contain sparse information on parent–child interactions and other family factors. Furthermore, most school samples do not include independent assessments from parents as well as from adolescents. Another significant proportion of the literature on alcohol problems in youth comes from small samples of "deviant" youth in select institutional settings. This can be important work for defining relationships for further study, but it is also important to determine what types of families are effective in socializing children for non-problem-behavior patterns.

Another large body of literature that includes family factors comes from retrospective studies of adult alcoholics which show that chronic inebriates' family socialization experiences were significantly deficient, contributing to poor social adjustment in adolescence and adulthood (Park, 1962; Pittman & Gordon, 1958). While retrospective studies of alcoholics have added to the literature on alcohol and the family, inherent in their design are the problems of reconstructing the past, that is, loss of memory by the alcoholics, difficulties in separating antecedent factors from the effects of the disease, and second-hand information on parental behaviors. The problem with case reports is that there are often not adequate control groups and it is uncertain whether the observed relationships are unique to alcoholics. Thus, there is a need for more prospective studies using representative general population samples of adolescents and their family members to assess family influences on the full range of adolescent drinking (and nondrinking) behaviors.

Furthermore, it is important for studies to include sufficient numbers of respondents in theoretically important population subgroups. For example, there is a serious lack of data on the relationships between family structural factors, parental socialization factors, and adolescent drinking in comparative studies of white, black, and other minority adolescents. Most observations about adolescent drug use have been based on white samples (Brunswick, Merzel, & Messeri, 1985), yet it is known that drinking patterns are different among white and minority adolescents (e.g. Barnes & Welte, 1986b; Welte & Barnes, 1987). Similarly, numerous studies have examined the development of alcoholism in males, drawing heavily upon the father's history of alcoholism. On the other hand, childhood socialization research has focused primarily on mothers' influences on children, often ignoring fathers' roles in this process. There needs to be a more balanced examination of mothers' and fathers' influences on both sons and daughters.

Parallel Studies of General Population Families and Alcoholic Families

While systematic studies of the development of adolescent drinking in representative samples of families are vitally important, there is a critical need for rigorous parallel studies among children of alcoholic parents. Standardized measures assessing socialization experiences, family structure, and family systems properties are important to undertake in alcoholic families since these family properties may serve to prevent or encourage the transmission of alcoholism in children with a family history of alcoholism.

Along with these parallel studies within alcohol-problem families and non-alcoholic-problem families, multiple measurement approaches should be used. For example, in addition to survey methodologies, it is important to directly study parent–child interactions whether in the home or laboratory settings.

Longitudinal Designs

Most of the work dealing with family factors in adolescent drinking behavior has been carried out at a single point in time. Longitudinal approaches are critically important in attempting to understand the time sequence of "causal links" in the development of adolescent behaviors. In terms of socialization practices and adolescent drinking behaviors, the primary direction of causation is assumed to be from parents to children. However, it has become increasingly recognized that the parent–child system may be bidirectional in terms of influence processes (Belsky, Hertzog, & Rovine, 1986). Thus, while there is strong evidence that parental factors are critical in the development of adolescent behaviors, it must also be taken into account that some children may initiate problem behaviors which lead to negative parental socialization practices and negative family environments. Only through longitudinal designs can we begin to untangle these cause and effect relationships. This applies to the area of peer influences on adolescent drinking as well. It appears that peer influences affect drinking after many family influences have had an impact on adolescent behavior; however, in longitudinal designs, tests can be made of whether or not negative peer influences occurred first and produced deterioration in family relations. Adolescent alcohol abuse and related problem behaviors will undoubtedly have additional deteriorating effects on existing family relationships and these changes can be assessed most accurately through study at multiple points of time.

REFERENCES

Abrams, D. B., & Niaura, R. S. (1987). Social learning theory. In H. T. Blane & K. E. Leonard (Eds.), *Psychological theories of drinking and alcoholism* (pp. 131–178). New York: Guilford.

Bandura, A. (1977). *Social learning theory.* Englewood Cliffs, NJ: Prentice-Hall.

Barber, B. K. (1987). Marital quality, parental behaviors, and adolescent self-esteem. *Family Perspective, 21,* 301–319.

Barnes, G. M. (1977). The development of adolescent drinking behavior: An evaluative review of the impact of the socialization process within the family. *Adolescence, 12,* 571–591.

Barnes, G. M. (1981). Drinking among adolescents: A subcultural phenomenon or a model of adult behaviors. *Adolescence, 16*(61), 211–229.

Barnes, G. M. (1984). Adolescent alcohol abuse and other problem behaviors: Their relationships and common parental influences. *Journal of Youth and Adolescence, 13,* 329–348.

Barnes, G. M., Farrell, M. P., & Cairns, A. L. (1986). Parental socialization factors and adolescent drinking behaviors. *Journal of Marriage and the Family, 48,* 27–36.

Barnes, G. M., Farrell, M. P., & Windle, M. (1987). Parent–adolescent interactions in the development of alcohol abuse and other deviant behaviors. *Family Perspective, 21,* 321–335.

Barnes, G. M., & Welte, J. W. (1986a). Adolescent alcohol abuse: Subgroup differences and relationships with other problem behaviors. *Journal of Adolescent Research, 1,* 79–94.

Barnes, G. M., & Welte, J. W. (1986b). Patterns and predictors of alcohol use among 7–12th grade students in New York State. *Journal of Studies on Alcohol, 47,* 53–62.

Barnes, G. M., & Welte, J. W. (1988). *Alcohol use and abuse among adults in New York State.* Buffalo, NY: Research Institute on Alcoholism.

Barnes, G. M., & Windle, M. (1987). Family factors in adolescent alcohol and drug abuse. *Pediatrician—International Journal of Child and Adolescent Health, 14,* 13–18.

Belsky, J., Hertzog, C., & Rovine, M. (1986). Causal analysis of multiple determinants of parenting: Empirical and methodological advances. In M. Lamb, A. Brown, & B. Rugoff (Eds.), *Advances in developmental psychology,* Vol. 4 (pp. 153–202). Hillsdale, NJ: Erlbaum.

Blane, H. T., & Barry, H., III (1973). Birth order and alcoholism: A review. *Quarterly Journal of Studies on Alcohol, 34,* 837–852.

Blane, H. T., & Barry, H., III (1975). Sex of siblings of male alcoholics. *Archives of General Psychiatry, 32,* 1403–1405.

Blane, H. R., & Hewitt, L. E. (1977). *Alcohol and youth—An analysis of the literature 1960–1975.* Rockville, MD: National Institute on Alcohol Abuse and Alcoholism.

Broderick, C. B., & Pulliam-Krager, H. (1979). Family process and child outcomes. In W. R. Burr, R. Hill, F. I. Nye & I. Reiss (Eds.), *Contemporary theories about the family,* Vol. 1. New York: The Free Press.

Brook, J. S., Whiteman, M., & Gordon, A. (1983). Stages of drug use in adolescence: Personality, peer, and family correlates. *Developmental Psychology, 19,* 269–277.

Brook, J. S., Whiteman, M., Gordon, A. S., & Brenden, C. (1983). Older brother's influence on younger sibling's drug use. *The Journal of Psychology, 114,* 83–90.

Brunswick, A. F., Merzel, C. R., & Messeri, P. A. (1985). Drug use initiation among urban black youth: A seven-year follow-up of developmental and secular influences. *Youth & Society, 17,* 189–216.

Burk, E. D. (1972). Some contemporary issues in child development and the children of alcoholic parents. In F. A. Seixas, G. S. Omenn, E. D. Burk, & S. Eggleston (Eds.), *Nature and nurture in alcoholism.* Annals of the New York Academy of Sciences.

Burnside, M. A., Baer, P. E., McLaughlin, R. J., & Pokorny, A. D. (1986). Alcohol use by adolescents in disrupted families. *Alcoholism: Clinical and Experimental Research, 10,* 274–278.

Clayton, R. R., & Lacy, W. B. (1982). Interpersonal influences on male drug use and drug use intentions. *The International Journal of the Addictions, 17,* 655–666.

Cotton, N. S. (1979). The familial incidence of alcoholism. *Journal of Studies on Alcohol, 40*(1), 89–116.

Dishion, T. J., & Loeber, R. (1985). Adolescent marijuana and alcohol use: The role of parents and peers revisited. *American Journal of Drug and Alcohol Abuse, 11,* 11–25.

Donovan, J. E., & Jessor, R. (1985). Structure of problem behavior in adolescence and young adulthood. *Journal of Consulting and Clinical Psychology, 53,* 890–904.

Filstead, W. J., McElfresh, O., & Anderson, C. (1981). Comparing the family environments of alcoholic and 'normal' families. *Journal of Alcohol and Drug Education, 26,* 24–31.

Frank, B., Lipton, D., Marel, R., Schmeidler, J., Barnes, G., & Welte, J. (1985). *A double danger: Relationships between alcohol use and substance use among secondary school students in New York State.* Buffalo, NY: Research Institute on Alcoholism.

Gantman, C. (1978). Family interaction patterns among families with normal, disturbed, and drug-abusing adolescents. *Journal of Youth and Adolescence, 7,* 429–440.

Globetti, G. (1972). Problem and non-problem drinking among high school students in abstinence communities. *The International Journal of the Addictions, 7,* 511–523.

Goodwin, D. W. (1984). Studies of familial alcoholism: A growth industry. In D. W. Goodwin, K. T. Van Dusen, & S. A. Mednick (Eds.), *Longitudinal research in alcoholism.* Boston: Kluwer-Nijhoff.

Harburg, E., Davis, D. R., & Caplan, R. (1982). Parent and offspring alcohol use—Imitative and aversive transmission. *Journal of Studies on Alcohol, 43,* 497–516.

Hecht, M. (1973). Children of alcoholics are children at risk. *American Journal of Nursing, 73*(10), 1764–1767.

Hilton, M. E. (1988). Trends in U.S. drinking patterns: Further evidence from the past 20 years. *British Journal of Addiction, 83,* 269–278.

Holmes, S. J., & Robins, L. N. (1987). The influence of childhood disciplinary experience on the development of alcoholism and depression. *Journal of Child Psychology and Psychiatry, 28,* 399–415.

Jacob. T. (1987). Alcoholism: A family interaction perspective. In C. P. Rivers (Ed.), *Alcohol and addictive behavior—Nebraska Symposium on Motivation,* Vol. 34 (pp. 159–206). Lincoln, NE: University of Nebraska Press.

Jessor, R. (1987). Problem-behavior theory, psychosocial development, and adolescent problem drinking. *British Journal of Addiction, 82,* 331–342.

Jessor, R., & Jessor, S. L. (1977). *Problem behavior and psychosocial development—A longitudinal study of youth.* New York: Academic Press.

Kandel, D. B. (1980). Drug and drinking behavior among youth. *Annual Review of Sociology, 6,* 235–285.

Kandel, D. B. (1983). Socialization and adolescent drinking. In O. Jeanneret (Ed.), *Alcohol and youth, child health and development,* Vol. 2 (pp. 66–75). Basel: S. Karger.

Kandel, D. B., & Andrews, K. (1987). Processes of adolescent socialization by parents and peers. *The International Journal of the Addictions, 22,* 319–342.

Kandel, D. B., Kessler, R. C., & Margulies, R. Z. (1978). Antecedents of adolescent initiation into stages of drug use: A developmental analysis. In D. B. Kandel (Ed.), *Longitudinal research on drug use* (pp. 73–99). Washington, DC: Hemisphere.

Keltner, N. L., McIntyre, C. W., & Gee, R. (1986). Birth order effects in second-generation alcoholics. *Journal of Studies on Alcohol, 47,* 495–497.

Kidwell, J. S. (1981). Number of siblings, sibling spacing, sex, and birth order: Their effects on perceived parent-adolescent relationships. *Journal of Marriage and the Family, 43,* 315–332.

Linsky, A. S., Straus, M. A., & Colby, J. P., Jr. (1985). Stressful events, stressful conditions and alcohol problems in the United States: A partial test of Bale's Theory. *Journal of Studies on Alcohol, 46*(1), 72–80.

Maccoby, E. E., & Martin, J. A. (1983). Socialization in the context of the family: Parent-child interaction. In E. M. Hetherington (Ed.), *Handbook of child psychology, Volume IV, Socialization, personality, and social development* (pp. 1–101). New York: Wiley.

Mayer, J. E. (1986). Adolescent alcohol misuse: A family systems perspective. In C. M. Felsted (Ed.), *Youth and alcohol abuse: Readings and resources* (pp. 52–62). Phoenix, AZ: Oryx.

McCrady, B. S. (1982). Marital dysfunction: Alcoholism and marriage. In E. M. Pattison & E. Kaufman (Eds.), *Encyclopedic handbook of alcoholism* (pp. 673–695). New York: Gardner.

Minuchin, S. (1974). *Families and family therapy.* Cambridge, MA: Harvard University Press.

Moos, R. H., & Moos, B. S. (1984). The process of recovery from alcoholism: III. Comparing functioning in families of alcoholics and matched control families. *Journal of Studies on Alcohol, 45*(2), 111–118.

Needle, R., McCubbin, H., Wilson, M., Reineck, R., Lazar, A., & Mederer, H. (1986). Interpersonal influences in adolescent drug use—The role of older siblings, parents, and peers. *The International Journal of the Addictions, 21,* 739–766.

Olson, D. H., McCubbin, H. I., Barnes, H., Larsen, A. S., Muxen, M. J., & Wilson, M. A. (1983). *Families, what makes them work?* Beverly Hills, CA: Sage.

Park, P. (1962). Problem in drinking and role deviation: A study in incipient alcoholism. In D. J. Pittman & C. R. Snyder (Eds.), *Society, culture and drinking patterns.* New York: Wiley.

Parker, D. A., & Harford, T. C. (1987). Alcohol-related problems of children of heavy-drinking parents. *Journal of Studies on Alcohol, 48,* 265–268.

Parsons, T. (1955a). The American family: Its relations to personality and to the social structure. In T. Parsons & R. F. Bales, *Family, socialization and interaction process* (pp. 3–33). New York: The Free Press.

Parsons, T. (1955b). Family structure and the socialization of the child. In T. Parsons & R. F. Bales, *Family, socialization and interaction process* (pp. 35–131). New York: The Free Press.

Peterson, G. W., & Rollins, B. C. (1987). Parent-child socialization. In M. B. Sussman and S. K. Steinmetz (Eds.), *Handbook of marriage and the family* (pp. 471–507). New York: Plenum.

Pittman, D. J., & Gordon, C. W. (1958). *Revolving door—A study of the chronic police case inebriate*. Glencoe, IL: The Free Press.

Potvin, R. H., & Lee, C. F. (1980). Multistage path models of adolescent alcohol and drug use. *Journal of Studies on Alcohol, 41*, 531–542.

Prendergast, T. J., Jr., & Schaefer, E. S. (1974). Correlates of drinking and drunkenness among high-school students. *Quarterly Journal of Studies on Alcohol, 35*, 232–242.

Rachal, J. V., Guess, L. L., Hubbard, R. L., Maisto, S. A., Cavanaugh, E. R., Waddell, R., & Benrud, C. H. (1980). *Adolescent drinking behavior: The 1974 and 1978 national sample studies*. Research Triangle Park, NC: Research Triangle Institute.

Rachal, J. V., Williams, J. R., Brehm, M. L., Cavanaugh, B., Moore, R. P., & Eckerman, W. C. (1975). *A national study of adolescent drinking behavior, attitudes and correlates*. Springfield, VA: National Technical Information Service.

Rollins, B. C., & Thomas, D. L. (1979). Parental support, power, and control techniques in the socialization of children. In W. R. Burr, R. Hill, F. I. Nye, & I. L. Reiss (Eds.), *Contemporary theories about the family*, Vol. 1 (pp. 317–364). New York: The Free Press.

Sadava, S. W. (1987). Interactional theory. In H. T. Blane & K. E. Leonard (Eds.), *Psychological theories of drinking and alcoholism* (pp. 90–130). New York: Guilford.

Schuckit, M. A. (1987). Biological vulnerability to alcoholism. *Journal of Consulting and Clinical Psychology, 55*, 301–309.

Selnow, G. A. (1987). Parent–child relationships and single and two parent families: Implications for substance usage. *Journal of Drug Education, 17*, 315–326.

Stagner, B. H. (1986). The viability of birth order studies in substance abuse research. *The International Journal of the Addictions, 21*, 377–384.

Steinglass, P., & Robertson, A. (1983). The alcoholic family. In B. Kissin & H. Begleiter (Eds.), *The pathogenesis of alcoholism—Psychosocial factors* (pp. 243–307). New York: Plenum.

Vogel, E. F., & Bell, N. W. (1960). The emotionally disturbed child as a family scapegoat. In N. W. Bell & E. F. Vogel (Eds.), *A modern introduction to the family*. New York: Free Press.

Walsh, F. (1982). *Normal family processes*. New York: Guilford.

Wechsler, H., & Thum, D. (1973). Teenage drinking, drug use and social correlates. *Quarterly Journal of Studies on Alcohol, 34*, 1220–1227.

Wegscheider, S. (1981). *Another chance: Hope and health for the alcoholic family*. Palo Alto, CA: Science and Behavior Books.

Welte, J. W., & Barnes, G. M. (1987). Alcohol use among adolescent minority groups. *Journal of Studies on Alcohol, 48*, 329–336.

West, M. O., & Prinz, R. J. (1987). Parental alcoholism and childhood psychopathology. *Psychological Bulletin, 102,* 204–218.

Williams, C. N., & Klerman, L. V. (1984). Female alcohol abuse: Its effects on the family. In S. C. Wilsnack & L. J. Beckman (Eds.), *Alcohol problems in women: antecedents, consequences, and intervention* (pp. 280–318). New York: Guilford.

Wolin, S. J., & Bennett, L. A. (1984). Family rituals. *Family Process, 23,* 401–420.

Wolin, S. J., Bennett, L. A., Noonan, D. L., & Teitelbaum, M. A. (1980). Disrupted family rituals—A factor in the intergenerational transmission of alcoholism. *Journal of Studies on Alcohol, 41,* 199–214.

Zucker, R. (1976). Parental influences on the drinking patterns of their children. In M. Greenblatt & M. A. Schuckit (Eds.), *Alcoholism problems in women and children* (pp. 211–238). New York: Grune & Stratton.

Zucker, R. (1979). Developmental aspects of drinking through the young adult years. In H. Blume and M. Chafetz (Eds.), *Youth, alcohol & social policy* (pp. 91–146). New York: Plenum.

Zucker, R., & Barron, F. H. (1973). Parental behaviors associated with problem drinking and antisocial behavior among adolescent males. In M. Chafetz (Ed.), *Proceedings of the first annual alcoholism conference of the National Institute on Alcohol Abuse and Alcoholism, Research on alcoholism: clinical problems and special populations.* Rockville, MD: NIAAA.

Zucker, R. A., & Gomberg, E. S. (1986). Etiology of alcoholism reconsidered— The case for a biopsychosocial process. *American Psychologist, 41,* 783–793.

Zucker, R., & Van Horn, H. (1972). Sibling social structure and oral behavior; Drinking and smoking in adolescence. *Quarterly Journal of Studies on Alcohol, 33,* 193–197.

6

When Children Change: Research Perspectives on Children of Alcoholics

JEANNETTE L. JOHNSON* and JON E. ROLF

INTRODUCTION

At the present time, school-age and adult children of alcoholics receive much attention from the scientific research community. One body of research studies the transmission of alcoholism in the offspring of alcoholics (Cloninger, Reich, & Wetzel, 1979; NIAAA, 1985). Another emphasizes the search for psychobiological markers of vulnerability (Begleiter & Porjesz, 1988), and a third examines psychosocial characteristics of children of alcoholics (Russell, Henderson, & Blume, 1985). Each of these three approaches hypothesizes that individual differences between children of alcoholics and children of nonalcoholics influence later maladaptive behaviors, such as academic, career, or relationship failures. Data from each approach increasingly find support for the belief that children of alcoholics are at risk for a variety of problems that may include behavioral, psychological, cognitive, or neuropsychological deficits. Other chapters in this volume summarize genetic and psychobiological research on children of alcoholics. In this chapter, we address the body of research emphasizing psychosocial variables.

Not surprisingly, the emerging findings of psychosocial studies of children of alcoholics have yet to present a consistent picture of collective risk and individual vulnerabilities. Thus, a unified concept of psychosocial

*Dr. Johnson is the Project Director for the Panel on High Risk Youth with the Committee on Child Development Research and Public Policy. Her opinions reflect her own views which are not necessarily those of the Committee or the National Research Council or the National Academy of Sciences.

maladaptation for children of alcoholics has not yet emerged. To be fair, part of this lack of clarification about psychosocial maladaptation in children of alcoholics is due to the many ways children can develop and change across time and circumstances. In infants, the change and developmental progression of psychosocial skills may be apparent from day to day. In children, other changes in these same areas may be visible from month to month; and later still, many changes continue to occur throughout adulthood.

The developmental process confounds most simple explanations of why some behaviors of children of alcoholics are either different from or identical to the behaviors of children of nonalcoholics. For the researcher and the clinician, recognizing the dynamic process of development creates special problems, such as understanding the stability and instability of salient behavior traits across time or the continuity and discontinuity of developmental changes. Intraindividual variations in quantitative (e.g., hormonal fluctuations of puberty) and qualitative (e.g., increases in cognitive capacity) developmental changes also complicate explanations of psychosocial maladaptation in children of alcoholics.

To clarify psychosocial maladaptation in children of alcoholics, we must first understand them in the context of normal development. Therefore, we begin with a selective overview of the research on children of alcoholics and with a discussion of a developmental theory of change and its application to children of alcoholics. In a third section we illustrate our attempts to incorporate developmental principles in research on children of alcoholics by outlining a comprehensive approach to psychosocial assessment. We conclude the chapter by discussing some implications of developmental models to future research with children of alcoholics.

Selective Review of the Literature

Early reviews of the research on children of alcoholics revealed that many of the early studies were of two types: either clinical observations or research that used a variety of samples and methods to examine a large range of dependent variables (Chafetz, Blane, & Hill, 1971; El-Guebalay & Offord, 1977; Jacob, Favorini, Meisal, & Anderson, 1978; Wilson & Orford, 1978; Warner & Rosett, 1975; Watters & Theimer, 1978). Owing to the diversity and increasing complexity of contemporary research on children of alcoholics, current literature reviews typically classify the research into four groups of studies: heritability, the fetal alcohol syndrome, alcoholic families, and high risk research (Adler & Raphael, 1983; Corder, McRee, & Rohrer, 1984; Russell, Henderson, & Blume, 1985; Sher, 1987). After briefly discussing the first three, we turn most of our attention to the fourth group, high risk research, with an emphasis on psychosocial studies.

Heritability

The pathway by which the genetic diathesis is expressed is currently a subject of great interest (Begleiter, 1988). Many studies of related individuals (e.g., families, twins, or adopted out siblings) support a genetic theory of alcoholism transmission (Amark, 1951; Cotton, 1979; Kaij, 1960; Schuckit, Goodwin, & Winokur, 1972). In particular, the greater influence of the biologic versus the adoptive family in the development of alcoholism has fostered the idea of genetic transmission (Goodwin, 1976). In one representative study, male adoptees with alcoholic biologic fathers were four times as likely to become alcoholic than those without, although relationships with alcohol misuse in the adoptive parents were not observed (Cadoret, Cain, & Grove, 1980). Goodwin (1985) reports that the prevalence of alcoholism among both male (25%) and female (5 to 10%) relatives of alcoholics exceeds the estimated population prevalence for alcoholics, which are 3% to 5% for men and 0.1% to 1% for women.

Fetal Alcohol Syndrome

The second group of studies consists of those investigating the teratogenic effects of maternal alcohol use. These studies report strong relationships between in utero alcohol exposure and later childhood problems such as minor physical anomalies, hyperactivity, mental retardation, and EEG anomalies (Abel, 1980, 1981, 1982; Jones & Smith, 1973; Ulleland, 1972). The critical observation in these early studies was the identification of the fetal alcohol syndrome (FAS). Jones and Smith (1973) first described the FAS as a cluster of four characteristics occurring in the offspring of mothers who drank excessively during pregnancy: central nervous system dysfunction, abnormal facial features, behavioral deficits, and growth deficiency. Since that time, research has confirmed Jones and Smith's observations and elaborately described the adverse effects of maternal alcohol abuse on the fetus.

Alcoholic Families

A third group of studies highlights different aspects of the alcoholic family environment and family interaction (Steinglass, Bennett, Wolin, & Reiss, 1987). Family studies view children from a family illness perspective with regard to the dynamics of the illness and its effects on family functioning. Family studies involve two separate areas of research (Bennett & Wolin, 1986; Johnson & Bennett, 1989): the impact of alcoholism upon the families generally and the impact of alcoholism on the adult children of alcoholics specifically. These studies typically conclude that the transmission of alcoholism is complex and involves multiple genetic, psychological, sociological, and cultural interactions (see Bennett & Wolin, Chapter 7, this volume).

High Risk Research

Concepts of risk originate from the epidemiological emphasis on patterns of disease occurrence (Lilienfield & Lilienfield, 1980). Individuals are at risk for disease, disability, or disorder and a child is considered at high risk if there is a greater likelihood that he or she will develop a disorder compared to a randomly selected child from the same community. Studies of children at risk examine precursors to behavioral outcomes, attributes of vulnerable and stress-resistant individuals, and the interactions that predict successful and unsuccessful adaptation (Masten & Garmezy, 1987). Children at risk for behavior disorders, for example, are those with (NIMH, 1978): (1) deviant parents, especially those parents with psychotic and criminal histories; (2) chronic aggressive behavior disorders; (3) very severe social, cultural, economic, and nutritional deprivations; and (4) physical, temperamental, or intellectual handicaps. The diversity of risk factor research has also shown that children are at risk for cognitive and behavioral problems if they are living in poverty (Furstenberg, Brooks-Gunn, & Morgan, 1987), experiencing multiple stressors (Rutter, 1981), or born to adolescent mothers (Brooks-Gunn & Furstenberg, 1986). The studies of Norman Garmezy and his students and colleagues exemplify the application of the high risk paradigm to children at risk for schizophrenia (Garmezy, 1974a,b; Watt, Anthony, Wynne, & Rolf, 1984).

Risk and Protective Factors

In any individual, the presence of risk or protective factors increases or decreases, respectively, the expression of the disorder; thus, they are statistically associated with higher or lower rates of the disorder. Risk factors are those environmental or genetic agents that have demonstrated or presumed potency to increase the expression of risk in the individual. Sources of risk factors range from the presence of certain biological or psychological features in the family background (such as alcoholism or schizophrenia) to characteristics of the physical environment (such as malnutrition). Thus, they increase the likelihood of future maladaptation. An environmental risk factor, for example, could be the continuous, close contact with an abusive parent; consequently, the child has an increased probability of exposure to deviant thinking and behavior, marital conflicts, and abusive communications. Developmental lags (failure to acquire normal developmental milestones within the normal age range) or dysfunctional social behavior (failing to interact successfully with peers) are the possible expressions of the risk factor.

Conversely, protective factors increase the likelihood for future positive adaptation, especially when stressful life events challenge the individual. Kandel and Mednick (1988), for example, have shown that IQ may be a potential protective factor for individuals who are at risk for antisocial behavior. For the child of an alcoholic, a possible protective factor could be a positive nonalcoholic role model actively involved in the child's life.

Potential Psychosocial Risk Factors in Children of Alcoholics

In addition to the powerful influence of biology, psychosocial risk factors may also increase the likelihood of alcoholism or maladaptive behavior in children of alcoholics. These children are vulnerable because of their exposure to their psychopathological or alcoholic parental models. Increased exposure to such environmental factors produces an increased risk for developing a variety of psychosocial and psychopathological disorders (see review by West and Prinz, 1987). We discuss three potential psychosocial risk factors below: cognition, personality, and adaptation.

Cognition. Many researchers consider deficits in cognitive processes to be potential risk factors for psychosocial maladaptation or alcoholism. It is a logical choice for intensive study because cognitive processes are fundamental to human adaptation at all stages of development; they can be uniformly measured across developmental stages, and they may show sufficient continuity to be measurable as predictive traits. Extensive research has documented cognitive deficits in detoxified chronic alcoholics; there is some recovery of functioning after varying periods of abstinence from alcohol, but deficits continue to persist in some individuals (Cermak & Ryback, 1976; Parsons, 1983; Parsons & Farr, 1981; Ryan & Butters, 1983; Yohman, Parsons, & Leber, 1985). Although cognitive deficits could be the long-term, long-lasting effects of alcohol abuse, this line of research suggests that impaired cognitive capacities may exist in high risk individuals before the actual onset of alcohol abuse.

To date, research provides suggestive, but inconclusive, evidence that cognitive deficits exist in children of alcoholics (see review by West & Prinz, 1987). Some studies of academic performance report lowered functioning in children of alcoholics (Hughes, 1977; Knop, Teasdale, Schulsinger, & Goodwin, 1985). Others (Rimmer, 1982), however, find no statistically significant differences between children of alcoholic, nonalcoholic, or depressed parents.

Studies of intellectual functioning, separate from academic performance, are also inconsistent. Descriptions of significantly lowered levels of intellectual functioning in children of alcoholics confirm hypotheses about cognitive deficits in children of alcoholics (Aronsen, Kyllerman, Sabel, Sandin, & Olegard, 1985; Bennett, Wolin, & Reiss, 1988; Ervin, Little, Streissguth, & Beck, 1984; Gabrielli & Mednick, 1983; Steinhausen, Gobel, & Nestler, 1984). Tarter, Jacob, and Bremer (1989) recently suggested that an anterior cerebral dysfunction was responsible for the observed cognitive deficits in children of alcoholics. Other data dispute these conclusions (Herjanic, Herjanic, Wetzel, & Tomelleri, 1978; Johnson & Rolf, 1988; Kern et al., 1981; Tarter, Hegedus, Goldstein, Shelly, & Alterman, 1984). One study examined academic ability, intellectual functioning, and perceptions of cognitive competence in homogeneous samples of children of recovering alcoholics (Johnson & Rolf, 1988). They did not find statistically significant group differences on cognitive performance tasks (IQ and academic achievement). However, there were significant differences in the measures requiring mothers and children to rate their perceptions of cognitive abilities. Compared to nonalcoholic families, children of alcoholics and their mothers underestimated their cognitive abilities. The authors suggested that negative perceptions of cognitive competence may affect motivation, self-esteem, and academic performance.

Taken together, studies of cognitive functioning in children of alcoholics have not identified any one cognitive pattern that distinguishes children of alcoholics from children of nonalcoholics. The evidence, however, is provocative. Werner's (1986) research shows that cognitive deficits may not characterize children of alcoholics as a whole. In a subsample of her longitudinal study of Hawaiian children, she compared children of alcoholics with problems (e.g., repeated or serious delinquencies or mental health problems requiring treatment) to children of alcoholics without problems. She showed that children of alcoholics with problems scored lower on verbal and quantitative cognitive measures. She suggests that only a subgroup of children of alcoholics are at risk for cognitive deficits. In this light, the question can be asked, Why are some children of alcoholics protected from cognitive deficits and some not?

Personality. Current arguments endorse the notion that in order for alcoholism or psychosocial maladaptation to develop in children of alcoholics, a combination of certain personality traits must be present. Tarter (1988) argues that certain types of personality and heritable behavioral dispositions, such as temperament, may predispose children of alcoholics toward alcoholism. He suggests that antisocial and neurotic personality characteristics interact with temperamental variables (e.g., activity level, emotionality, and sociability) to reduce or increase the expression of vulnerability toward substance abuse in children of alcoholics. Cloninger, Sigvardsson, and Bohman (1988) extend this argument to suggest that susceptibility to alcoholism may be governed by neurobiological mechanisms interacting with childhood personality. They reported that high novelty-seeking and low harm-avoidance childhood characteristics are strongly related to adult alcohol abuse.

Gender-related personality issues are also studied to identify potential risk factors. In a survey of 860 undergraduates, Berkowitz and Perkins (1988) found gender-related personality differences in children of alcoholics that were distinct from children of nonalcoholics. Reports of self-depreciation (defined as depression and low self-esteem) were more frequent in female children of alcoholics than in female children of nonalcoholics. Male children of alcoholics rated themselves as more directive (seeking of leadership positions), independent, and reliant on others than did the male children of nonalcoholics. However, males and females in both groups responded similarly on measures of impulsiveness, lack of tension, other-directedness, directiveness, the need for social support, and sociability.

General Studies of Adaptation. Many studies, best described as generalized studies of adaptation, examine behaviors such as adjustment, affect, self-esteem, and interpersonal awareness. Jacob and Leonard (1986) suggest that, overall, children of alcoholics are not as impaired on these measures as the clinical literature suggests. For example, Kammeier (1971) reported that, other than school absenteeism, adolescents from alcoholic families were similar to adolescents from nonalcoholic families. Callen and Jackson (1986) also reported that, with the exception of personal satisfaction, adolescent children of active alcoholics were similar to adolescent children of recovered alcoholics. Adolescent children of active alcoholics reported that they were not as happy with their lives as those adolescents living with recovering parents.

Other studies examine depression, self-concept, and response to stress. Clair and Genest (1987) reported that college-age children of alcoholics perceived the problems they faced as beyond their control. Compared to children of nonalcoholics, they also used more emotion-focused than problem-focused coping strategies; they were also more prone to depression. Moderator variables (e.g., level of familial dysfunction or social support) contributed to the individual's level of present functioning. It is noteworthy, however, that most of the children of alcoholics in this study were performing at normal, or even above normal, levels of functioning. Similarly, Rolf, Johnson, Israel, Baldwin, and Chandra (1988) and Roosa, Sandler, Beals, and Short (1988) report that school-age children of alcoholics show more depressive affect than normal controls.

Earls, Reich, Jung, and Cloninger (1988) recently reported on the frequency of psychopathology in children of alcoholics. Results from extensive structured interviews with 75 children aged 6 through 17 showed that children of alcoholics were diagnosed more frequently with a behavioral disorder, an attention deficit disorder with hyperactivity, an oppositional disorder, or a conduct disorder. An earlier study (Haberman, 1966) corroborates this by showing that children of alcoholics present more frequently with behavioral problems similar to those included among the constellation of behaviors associated with these psychiatric disorders.

Bennett, et al. (1988) provide convincing data showing that children from intact alcoholic families function less successfully on aggregate measures of emotional and behavioral functioning. They compared a homogeneous sample of 64 children of alcoholics to 80 children of nonalcoholics on an extensive psychosocial battery which included measures of self-concept, behavior problems, and psychiatric symptomatology. Children of alcoholics scored significantly lower on 6 of the 13 measures of behavioral and emotional functioning.

Summary

The most compelling data from the psychosocial literature suggest that children of alcoholics *might* have more problems than children of nonalcoholics. To date, research has not unraveled the intricacies of these problems or the nature of their impact. The inconsistencies among reports of psychosocial maladaptation in children of alcoholics have fostered a closer examination of the research techniques used to gather the data. Much of this research has been criticized for being methodologically weak (Earls et al., 1988; El-Guebaly & Offord, 1977, 1979; Johnson, in press; Sher, 1987). These weaknesses impair our ability (1) to distinguish true psychosocial risk factors from transient psychosocial risk factors and (2) to determine which maladaptive behaviors specifically distinguish children of alcoholics from children of nonalcoholics. Specificity, in this case, refers to the ability of the data to distinguish between potential subgroups of children of alcoholics (e.g., children of alcoholics with problems vs. children of alcoholics without problems) or to differentiate children of alcoholics from other children who have undergone crises unrelated to alcoholism, especially children from other dysfunctional families (e.g., divorce) or children with other problems (e.g., chronic illness). The following section argues that it is not only poor methodology which prevents us from answering specific research questions about children of alcoholics, but that the normal developmental changes inherent in childhood complicate our research questions, designs, and interpretations.

CONCEPTS OF DEVELOPMENTAL CHANGE

Normative Change

Whether they grow up in alcoholic or nonalcoholic homes, children face the challenge of each developmental stage with whatever resources they inherit, the ones provided by their environment, and the ones they intentionally or unintentionally develop themselves. Maturational and environmental interactions influence developmental changes in every domain, whether learning the social customs of the culture, advancing through puberty, or finishing homework. Rates of change in one developmental domain are not always consistent with rates of change in other developmental domains, so that in some children, for example, biological development may be more advanced than social development.

Developmental research describes behavioral changes that occur with increases in chronological age (Spiker, 1966). Developmental consequences are conceived in terms of the way such changes fit into an overall developmental sequence. Change and progression through the developmental sequence are viewed as both a dynamic quantitative and qualitative process. When change is quantitative, it is additive; as children grow, they think, feel, and learn more. When change is qualitative, it is unique; as children grow, they think, feel, and learn differently. Movement through the developmental sequence is often described as the progression from one stage of development to the next. Stage theory has been used to describe psychosexual, moral, affective, and emotional development. Progression through each stage is generally viewed as movement from less mature to more mature functioning. Cognitive developmental changes, for example, have been elaborately described by Piaget (1963) as a series of stages that are hierarchical and invariant in their order.

What is the process by which children change? There are many theories and descriptions of developmental sequences, but fewer theories about how these changes come about. While some questions about Piaget's stage theory remain unresolved (Sigel, Brodzinsky, & Golinkoff, 1981), his constructivist theory of equilibrium addressing the process of change enjoys wide acceptance (Neimark, 1985). Equilibration accounts for the changing and transformational character of how children and adults come to know the world in which they live. Coming to know the world and acting on this knowledge is an important component of Piaget's (1970, 1971) genetic epistemological model which views development as the gradual transformation and interplay of biological and logical structures. Self-monitored adaptation to events, people, and objects in the environment facilitates equilibrium, or a balance, between oneself and the environment.

Equilibration through self-regulated interaction is accomplished through two processes, assimilation and accommodation. Assimilation and accommodation occur automatically and often without the conscious awareness of the individual, enabling the child to incorporate new sensory and motoric experiences to already present cognitive structures.

Novel experiences are changed, or assimilated, to facilitate their incorporation into already present cognitive structures. In the process of assimilating new experiences, however, existing cognitive structures must adjust. This is done through the second adaptive function, accommodation.

Through these biologically determined processes, development occurs through constantly changing structures which absorb (assimilate) novel experiences. Thus, development is seen as a self-generated or self-constructed cycle in which actions and thoughts feed back upon their initial cognitive organization; this feedback changes those original structures that originally set the entire process into action.

During normal developmental changes, physical appearances transform, cognitive abilities alter quantitatively and qualitatively, and biological and psychological functioning undergo rapid and sometimes dramatic fluctuations. Even for children of nonalcoholics, one particularly vulnerable time of developmental fluctuation is adolescence. Characterized by unique biological and psychosocial integrations and newly acquired cognitive developmental capacities (i.e., formal operational thinking), adolescence becomes a particularly stressful stage of the life cycle (Lerner & Foch, 1987; Hamburg, 1974).

As a result of new cognitive developmental skills, coupled with an increase in personal independence, adolescence is a developmental transition period when most youths begin to experiment with many varieties of behavior (including those involving drugs and sex). Adolescence, therefore, becomes a time of increased risks for significant emotional problems (e.g., episodes of serious anxiety or depression) and health impairing behaviors (eating disorders, substance abuse, and withdrawal from supportive relationships). In children of alcoholics, adolescent experimentation may also interact with family history as they strive to adapt to normal developmental challenges.

Developmental Models for Studying Children of Alcoholics

To better understand the interplay between adaptive and maladaptive processes across the life span in children at risk, an integrative perspective combining biological, psychobiological, and psychosocial paradigms from developmental and clinical theories is necessary (Rolf & Read, 1984). Combining both perspectives has been done with children at risk for schizophrenia through the theoretical model of developmental psychopathology. This model can also be applied to children at risk for alcoholism.

Developmental psychopathology synthesizes the paradigms from both normal developmental psychology and psychopathology in order to study the continuities and discontinuities of behaviors over time. Developmental psychologists typically select for study persons undergoing normative developmental transitions which challenge their adaptive capacities. On the other hand, clinical research uses high risk paradigms to maximize confidence in assuming initial risk status and for observing variation in developmental adaptation. Together, the two approaches overlap when high risk subjects are studied during developmental transitions and, especially, when nonnormative stressful life events (such as physical abuse or long-term parental absence) coincide with the normative transition.

Developmental psychopathology shifts the focus from describing what psychopathology is to how it emerges and transforms over time (Cowan, 1988). In research with children of alcoholics, we can also shift our focus from describing what alcoholism or psychosocial maladaptation is to how it emerges and transforms over time. Shifting the focus will enable us to understand the self-generated transformations that risk factors must undergo in order to maintain equilibrium in the developing child. Prospectively studying pubertal youths at high risk for alcoholism who live in families experiencing parental divorce would be of this type.

The inconsistent picture of psychosocial maladaptation in children of alcoholics could simply be the incomplete tracking of the transformation of one risk factor with another or the interplay between risk and protection. Thus, identifying etiological pathways toward alcoholism or the stability of psychosocial maladaptation may not occur through the understanding of between-group differences, but through understanding the fluctuating developmental trajectories of intraindividual differences. When cognitive differences are observed in children of alcoholics, do we label it as a deficit or merely a developmental delay? It could be a deficit in a between-group research design, or a delay in a within-group research design.

Answering this question relies on our understanding of the developmental trajectories of specific risk factors in children of alcoholics. Psychosocial maladaptation could: (1) start in childhood and continue through to adulthood (early maladaptation will predict later maladaptation); (2) not be present in childhood, but start in adolescence and continue through adulthood (certain experiences occurring in critical periods will predict later maladaptation); (3) bypass childhood and adolescence altogether and start in adulthood (early adaptation will not predict later maladaptation); or, (4) start in childhood, disappear during adolescence, and reappear once again in adulthood (certain experiences occurring in critical periods will predict later maladaptation). Each developmental trajectory involves continuing adaptation to developmental challenges, but if the developmental challenge overstresses the organism at a particularly vulnerable period, psychological resources break down causing other structures to change in order to maintain equilibrium, thus causing a developmental delay or a permanent deficit.

Developmental theories view maladaptation as a consequence of the failure to cope with developmental challenges. There are many challenges in a child's life: first entry to school, new siblings, parental alcoholism. Individuals who have not reached the appropriate developmental level are more likely to exhibit maladaptation at early stages of social challenge (Phillips, 1966). Such may be the case with adolescent children of alcoholics when normal adolescent experimentation challenges psychosocial processes. Normal adolescent experimentation may significantly alter the timing and experience of normative life choice points in children who are also at biological risk.

Most adolescents experience depression, anxiety, or social alienation. Normally adaptive children cope with the stresses of adolescent transitions and begin to express age-related behavior tendencies. Many of them will show transient behavior disorders, yet very few will become alcoholic, engage in seriously delinquent activities, or perform so poorly in school that they are considered academically deficit. How is it that some children of alcoholics can engage in normative experimentation while others go beyond the normative range?

We can better understand psychosocial maladaptation if we study the behavior as it changes. Either we study individual children as they change (i.e., longitudinally), those children who are already in a transitional phase (i.e., puberty), or use age as a significant dependent variable for interpreting our results. In any case, a comprehensive view of the individual child is necessary. Since adaptation involves complex processes resulting from the interplay of personal and environmental factors, prospective research requires that some of the risk and protective variables be both initially identifiable and subsequently observable over time. From the literature, we have some clues about what to include in our multivariate assessment.

ASSESSING PSYCHOSOCIAL CHANGE

Understanding the nature of the changes which contribute to psychosocial maladaptation in children of alcoholics requires the adoption of research techniques that reveal the details of the interchanges occurring across time. Because traditional techniques have not solved the problems of understanding continuity, we present below a practical application of developmental theory to the assessment of psychosocial changes in children of alcoholics. These measures provide sufficient information to show how changes occur and how they preserve or modify existing structures. We use information from a project completed at the intramural program of the National Institute on Alcohol Abuse and Alcoholism (Protocol 83-AA-204, Principal Investigator, Jeannette Johnson) designed to characterize the behavioral and developmental patterns of the children of alcoholics with the use of multivariate measures of developmentally relevant risk and protective factors. We discuss below the two components we believe most practical for understanding psychosocial changes in children of alcoholics—parent and child assessments—but we first begin by acknowledging the pivotal role that interpersonal interaction plays in assessing children.

Interpersonal Interaction

Testing children of alcoholics can be stressful for both subject and experimenter alike. It is heartbreaking to read answers to sensitive and personal questions when they have been written by a sad and lonely 12-year-old. It is trying and tiring to keep a hyperactive child on task when assessing intelligence; it requires unflagging persistence. How do the experimenter's feelings affect the scoring and interpretation of qualitative data when they have had a positive or negative experience with the target child?

Another interpersonal challenge is the ability or inability of the experimenter to elicit a positive motivational response from the child. In children, motivational patterns influence the establishment, maintenance, and attainment of achievement goals (Dweck, 1986). The relationship between the experimenter and the subject critically influences the type and quality of the data obtained, especially during a lengthy research session requiring answers to sensitive questions or frustrating problem-solving tasks. The child's confidence in the experimenter is all too often dependent upon who examines the child and the manner in which the questions are asked.

The research setting itself can be a stressful developmental challenge to some young children. For an uncooperative adolescent, it may be an opportunity for social disengagement. In a good testing session, our goal is a measure of the child's response to the task at hand, not his or her response to the situation or the skill of the experimenter.

Assessment of Parents

Reasons for Participation. Why do parents allow their children to participate in research? Parental approval for their child's participation in research provides a glimpse at potential sample biases. For both normal control and alcoholic parents, parents allow their children to participate for a variety of reasons. Some parents: (1) are concerned about their children's behavior and desire feedback from the research psychological assessment; (2) are concerned about their parenting styles and want information about parenting techniques; (3) need the reimbursement; or (4) have free time on their hands. We must acknowledge the possible effects that parental participation has on the type of sample we select.

Changing Patterns of Parental Alcoholism

Assessment of children of alcoholics typically begins with the determination of parental alcohol abuse. Even though the most commonly studied alcoholic family is the intact, paternal alcoholic household, there are multiple combinations of adult alcoholic relationships resulting from divorce, stepparenting, cohabitation, and single parenting. Parents manifest not only different combinations of and types of alcoholism, but combinations that change over time.

Throughout the child's lifetime, the changing pattern of parental alcoholism affects childhood experiences. Table 6.1 is a partial list of potential variables related to parental drinking which may influence the outcome of the offspring. Multiple marriages, changeable cohabitation arrangements, and sporadic periods of single parenting occur in a single child's lifetime. Sometimes the changing partners are alcoholic, sometimes not.

Moreover, alcoholism may co-occur with other drug dependencies at different times during adulthood. As the popularity of abusable substances changes over time, abuse or dependence will not be limited to one class but will involve several different classes of substances. Polysubstance abusers constitute the major proportion of patients at chemical dependency treatment centers (Meller, Keafer, & Widmer, 1986). Substance abuse coupled with alcoholism complicates future etiological studies of children at risk for alcoholism. What types of childhood environmental experiences accompany parental dual dependency? Some evidence about the effects of dual dependency shows that alcoholic opiate addicts report more disruptive

TABLE 6.1. Types of Variables Related to Parental Drinking Which May Influence Child Outcome

Cultural

    Legal drinking age
    Acceptance of child drinking in the community
    Ethnicity

Family

    Degree of marital conflict
    Ability of other family members to provide substitute parenting
      for the child
    Degree to which the family is organized around the drinking
    Presence of violence in the home
    Acceptance of child drinking within the home

Parent

    Type and severity of alcoholism
    Gender of the alcoholic parent
    The number of years parent was an alcoholic
    Recent treatment history
    Extent of psychopathology or criminality

Child

    Child's relationship with the nonalcoholic parent
    Child's age at onset of parent's drinking
    Gender
    Child's constitutional factors
    Perception of growing up in an alcoholic home
    Presence of exposure to prenatal maternal drinking

childhood events than nonalcoholic addicts (Kosten, Rounsaville, & Kleber, 1985), but we still know very little about children of polysubstance abusers (Johnson, 1990).

Type of Alcohol Abuse

Although common sense tells us that different types of alcoholic drinking can differentially affect children's behavior, many studies nevertheless do not differentiate the type or severity of parental alcoholism. From the child's point of view, the type and severity of parental drinking may affect the parent–child interaction in very important ways (Jacob & Leonard, 1986). For example, binge drinkers may differ from daily drinkers in the extent to which they do or do not satisfy the caretaking needs of their child, in the administration of positive or negative affective reinforcement, and in the level of disruption in the family.

It is possible that severity or type also influences the nonalcoholic's well-being (e.g., the mother), thereby influencing her parenting as well. Research on the relationship between parenting practices and social competency in children shows that hostile, inconsistent parenting predicts the development of socially incompetent (aggressive) behavior in children (Baldwin, 1955; Eron, 1982; George & Main, 1979). On the other hand, warm, responsive parenting is related to socially competent behavior in children (Baumrind, 1967; Bryant & Crockenberg, 1980). Certain parenting styles, such as how much time the mother spends monitoring her young adolescent's behavior, are also associated with conduct disorder in childhood (Patterson & Stouthamer-Loeber, 1984). Parenting is not a singular activity; it is also embedded in the context of the mother–father relationship. How well this relationship works will also affect parenting styles.

The type of parental alcoholism also influences the type of environmental experiences available to the child. Type 1 alcoholics (minimal criminality associated with isolated or mild problems with alcohol) provide different home environments compared to the home environments provided by Type 2 alcoholics (severe criminality associated with recurrent, moderate, or severe problems with alcohol) (Cloninger, Sigvardsson, & Bohman, 1981). At the very least, the alcoholic parent may invite different types of adult friends into the home, depending upon the type of parental alcoholism. The patterns of Type 1 and Type 2 alcoholic drinking can contribute to variations in parental absence (e.g., treatment or imprisonment), the possibility of adult antisocial behavior role models in the home, and differences in parent–child interactions.

Assessment of Children

Psychosocial maladaptation is a complicated, multifactorial problem that is best assessed with several replicable and quantifiable procedures. Because complex behavior is multiply determined, multivariate assessment may increase predictive power and our understanding of potentially understudied risk factors. Recognizing that this approach also provokes methodological and statistical problems (e.g., too many measures capitalize on chance) the perfect balance is between enough measures and too few.

Measures of psychosocial maladaptation in children of alcoholics should be relevant to outcome behavior in order to provide data on the roles that developmental processes and maturational changes have on the emergence of psychosocial maladaptation. Achenback and McConaughy (1987) recommend the following psychometric principles to aid in measurement decisions: (1) employ standardized procedures; (2) use multiple, aggregate items to sample each aspect of functioning; (3) use normative reference groups for individual comparisons with age appropriate levels; and (4) use psychometrically sound assessment procedures which are reliable and valid. We provide below examples of psychosocial assessment which incorporate these recommendations.

Informant Reports

Ideally, objectively measured behavior in one situation should correlate with objectively measured behavior in another. Thus, finding that children of alcoholics are impulsive on a given laboratory experiment may highlight our understanding of their performance at home or in the classroom. However, Mischel (1968) argues that single observations of behavior, whether in the laboratory or elsewhere, may be so situationally unique as to be incapable of establishing reliable generalizations that hold during even the most minor situational variations. To resolve this, it is necessary to collect measures of childhood behavior from different sources of information.

Separate sources of information on children include peer ratings, parental reports (both mother and father), teacher reports, self-reports, clinical observations, and experimenter performance evaluations (e.g., laboratory testing). It is likely that some differences in children's behavior may depend on who fills out the report, and some differences may not. Disagreements between mother's and father's reports of their child's behavior, for example, provide important clinical information about both the child and the parent. Reports about children's behavior may vary because the child may vary his or her behavior toward different individuals. On the other hand, reports may vary because different individuals may elicit the problem behavior themselves or, alternatively, have a lower tolerance for it.

Example of parental reports which satisfy most of the psychometric principles recommended by Achenback and McConaughy (1987) are provided in Table 6.2. The Child Behavior Checklist (CBCL; Achenbach & Edelbrock, 1983) is a checklist comprised of 113 behavior problems and 20 competence items designed to be reported by parents of children aged 4 to

TABLE 6.2. Parental Reports of Behavior

Domain	Measure
Behavioral	Child Behavior Checklist
	Connor's Parent Questionnaire
Birth history	Garmezy Developmental Questionnaire
Stress	Life Events Questionnaire

16. The items on the CBCL have been factor analyzed separately by sex for the age strata corresponding to preschool, grade school, and high school and have been normed according to clinic and nonclinic samples. The CBCL's factoring according to sex and age provides primary and secondary factor T-scores which are interpreted according to their percentile deviation from the reference groups. The Parent Questionnaire (PQ; Goyette, Connors, & Ulrich, 1978) is a 93-item checklist of symptoms often related to childhood behavior disorders. Parents rate their child's symptoms on a 4-point scale with the lowest score referring to "not at all" and the highest score referring to "very much." The Life Events Questionnaire is a questionnaire designed to measure the parent's perception of stress in his child's life (Garmezy, 1981). Finally, the Garmezy Developmental Questionnaire is an interview which asks about the parent's retrospective assessment of his child's attainment of developmental milestones (e.g., walking, talking, etc.) (Garmezy, 1981).

Together these assessments provide a comprehensive report of childhood behaviors. The CBCL measures the empirically derived syndromes which are listed in Table 6.3. In addition, the Parent's Questionnaire measures conduct disorder, anxiety, impulsive-hyperactive, learning problems, psychosomatic symptoms, perfectionism, antisocial behavior, and muscular tension. The PQ is highly correlated with several of the CBCL behavioral syndromes. The advantage of the PQ is that it takes less time to complete than the CBCL. The qualitative responses derived from the Garmezy Developmental Questionnaire provide data on the attainment of developmental milestones which can then be compared to previously published behavioral norms.

Behavioral Assessment

How do you operationally define a source of risk for a child given the possibility of multiple risks which may interact at any point in time with the child's genetic and environmental constitution? Risk and protective factors can be separated into two primary domains: individual and contextual. Within the individual domain are two clusters: psychological (personality, cognitive, affective, social), and biological (health, maturation, physiological, and sensory motor). Within the contextual domain are separate levels of variables for the macroenvironment, peers, school, and home.

Included in this list of risk factors are the endless possibilities for interaction. Any single factor can be considered a risk or protective factor, depending upon its interaction with other factors. For example, in the social domain, social skills that are usually considered risk factors are those that render the child unpleasant, difficult, or aggressive. Social skills that are usually considered protective factors are those that lead the child to be friendly, well liked, and socially adept. Precocious puberty is an example of a biological risk factor that would place a friendly, mature looking, yet socially inexperienced, adolescent with an older peer group and expose the child to experiences beyond the appropriate developmental period. Con-

TABLE 6.3. Behavioral Syndromes of the Child Behavior Checklist[a]

Group	Internalizing syndromes	Mixed syndromes	Externalizing syndromes
Boys aged 4–5	Social Withdrawal Depressed Immature Somatic Complaints	Sex Problems	Delinquent Aggressive Schizoid
Boys aged 6–11	Schizoid or Anxious Depressed Uncommunicative Obsessive-Compulsive Somatic Complaints	Social Withdrawal	Delinquent Aggressive Hyperactive
Boys aged 12–16	Somatic Complaints Schizoid Uncommunicative Immature Obsessive-Compulsive	Hostile Withdrawal	Hyperactive Aggressive Delinquent
Girls aged 4–5	Somatic Complaints Depressed Schizoid or Anxious Social Withdrawal	Obese	Hyperactive Sex problems Aggressive
Girls aged 6–11	Depressed Social Withdrawal Somatic Complaints Schizoid-Obsessive		Cruel Aggressive Delinquent Sex problems Hyperactive
Girls aged 12–16	Anxious-Obsessive Somatic Complaints Schizoid Depressed Withdrawal	Immature Hyperactive	Cruel Aggressive Delinquent

[a]From Achenbach and Edelbrock (1983), page 16. © 1983 T. M. Achenbach. Reproduced by permission.

versely, a timely staging of puberty with psychosocial skill attainment could be considered more protective since the child would be gradually learning appropriate social behaviors at the appropriate developmental level.

Choosing developmentally relevant assessments which are appropriate for these measurement domains is challenging. First, lengthy test batteries require more time to administer to younger children than to older children. To keep their attention and motivation, many breaks are needed. The experimenter's facility with young children is a mandatory requirement for efficacious, productive research sessions. Secondly, many measures of behavioral processes in childhood are just now establishing norms. This is due, in part, to the recent advances in understanding behavioral development in different behavioral domains over the course of a child's lifetime. Third, children of differing ages and sex exhibit different types of behaviors for the same behavioral label. Achenbach and Edelbrock's (1983) detailed analysis of aggression in boys between the ages of 6 and 18 shows that similarities in aggressive behavior for all boys include: argues, is cruel to others, demands attention, disobeys at home, exhibits jealousy, fights, attacks people, screams, is stubborn, moody, sulks, has a temper, is loud, talks excessively, teases, threatens, and swears. However, aggressive behavior for boys ages 6 to 11 (but not for boys aged 12 to 18) includes: brags, has poor peer relations, lies and cheats, is unliked, shows off, and disobeys at school. Included as aggressive behavior for boys aged 12 to 18 (but not for boys aged 6 to 11) is: feels persecuted, suspicious, impulsive, hyperactive, and nervous.

How do you measure the same behavioral syndrome in children if it takes different forms at different ages? Aggression in 7-year-olds is very different from aggression in 15-year-olds. Separate forms of the same test

TABLE 6.4. Multivariable Assessment of Childhood Global Behaviors

Behavioral domain	Measures
Contextual	
Macroenvironment	Hollingshead 4-Factor Index
School	Wide Range Achievement Test—Revised
Home	Home Environment Interview for Children
Individual	
Cognition	WISC-R or WAIS-R
Affect	Children's Depression Inventory
	How I Feel Questionnaire
Psychiatric symptomatology	Diagnostic Interview for Children
Alcohol and drug history	Modified MAST
Stress	Life Events Questionnaire
Self concept	Youth Self Report
	Perceived Competence Scale for Children

must be designed which reflect age-appropriate questions and age-related changes in behavior. However, if statistical analyses reveal within-group age-related differences, how do you know it is not due to the test form? For this reason, we must have confidence in our tests and measurements and choose reliable and valid assessments of childhood behavior that have established sound psychometric properties.

Some choices for psychosocial assessment are outlined in Table 6.4. The tests identified in Table 6.4 measure those behaviors identified in Table 6.5. Academic ability and intellectual functioning are measured by the Wide Range Achievement Test—Revised (WRAT-R; Jastak & Wilkinson, 1984) and the Wechsler Intelligence Scale for Children—Revised (or the WAIS-R for adolescents above 16 years). Self-concepts and competence are measured by the Perceived Competence Scale for Children (Harter, 1983), a 36-item self-report questionnaire, and the Youth Self Report (Achenbach & Edelbrock, 1987), a self-report filled out by 11- to 18-year-olds designed to assess competence and behavior problems. Clinical functioning is assessed with the Diagnostic Interview for Children and Adolescents (Herjanic & Reich, 1982; Reich, Herjanic, Welner, & Ghandy, 1982), a structured psychiatric interview for children. Affect is measured by the Children's Depression Inventory (CDI; Kovacs, 1983; Kovacs & Beck, 1977) in youths up to 15 years; those aged 16 years and older complete the Beck Depression Inventory (BDI; Beck & Beck, 1972; Beck & Beamesderfer, 1974). Home environment and family functioning can be assessed by

TABLE 6.5. Dependent Variables

Behavioral domain	Factor labels/Dependent variables
Macroenvironment	SES
School	Standard Scores for reading, writing, and arithmetic
Home	Effects of parental drinking on children, parents as role models, negative life events, parental abuse and neglect, sibling relations, positive parent–child relations, coping skills, parent–child conflict, marital conflict
Cognition	Verbal, Performance, Full Scale IQ plus individual subtest scores
Affect	Depression, State/Trait Anxiety
Psychiatric symptomatology	DSM-III-R diagnoses
Alcohol and drug history	Frequency of use/abuse
Self-concept/Competence	Scholastic competence, social acceptance, athletic competence, physical appearance, behavior conduct, and self worth
	Total competence, School competence, Activities
Stress	Positive, Negative, Ambiguous stress

TABLE 6.6. Problem Scales from the Youth Self Report[a]

Group	Internalizing syndromes	Mixed syndromes	Externalizing syndromes
Boys	Depressed Unpopular	Somatic Complaints Self-Destructive/ Identity Problems Thought Disorder	Aggressive Delinquent
Girls	Somatic Complaints Depressed	Unpopular Thought Disorder	Delinquent Aggressive

[a]From Achenbach and Edelbrock (1987), page 19. © 1987 T. M. Achenbach. Reproduced by permission.

the Home Environment Interview for Children (Reich & Earls, 1982). Stress is measured by the Life Events Questionnaire (Garmezy, 1981). Self-concept and competence can be measured by the Perceived Competence Scale for Children (Harter, 1983) and the Youth Self Report (YSR; Achenback & Edelbrock, 1987). Like the CBCL, the YSR is a measure of empirically derived behavior syndromes (Table 6.6).

To illustrate the usefulness of a multivariate psychosocial assessment battery, and how we can incorporate developmental principles in data interpretation, the following section presents examples from research conducted during 1984–1987 by the authors under Protocol 83-AA-204 at the National Institute on Alcohol Abuse and Alcoholism in Bethesda, MD.

Examples of Psychosocial Assessment

An example of multidimensional research embracing a developmental perspective can be found in one of the authors' studies of minor children of alcoholics. The purpose of the study was to assess any problems of adaptation in children at risk for alcoholism while controlling for some of the methodological problems in previous studies. The alcoholic parent probands were carefully chosen to qualify for multiple diagnostic criteria for alcoholism while also avoiding two sampling biases. First, the alcoholic parent must have been in a longstanding recovering status to ensure that our measures of current family functioning and child adjustment would not be masked by an ongoing or recent episode of pathological drinking or detoxification. Second, the biological mothers must also have reported no alcoholic or problem drinking while pregnant with the offspring to be studied to avoid possible teratogenic effects or residuals of subtle cases of the fetal alcohol syndrome. We avoided a third bias in the detection of deficits in the children primarily as a function of socioeconomically impoverished rearing environments by choosing proband and control families who were white and middle class.

Previous reports (Johnson & Rolf, 1988; Rolf et al., 1988) have presented descriptions of the sampling strategy and demographic characteristics and also some of our own findings of the similarities and differences in adaptive functioning between matched offspring groups which contained 50 children of alcoholics and 48 children of nonalcoholics aged 6 to 18 years. There were no significant differences in SES, age, sex, IQ, or substance abuse between the two groups (see Johnson & Rolf, 1988). Both groups of children were from relatively middle class, white suburbs of Washington, D.C.

In brief, our findings presented a pattern of normal intellectual aptitudes and academic achievement, but with significant child and parent underestimates of these cognitive skills for the children of alcoholics (Johnson & Rolk, 1988). Rolf et al. (1988) also reported that both the children of alcoholics and their mothers reported more depressive affect than the children of nonalcoholics.

Data on the subjects were obtained from three sources: (1) an extensive multimethod assessment battery for the child; (2) extensive diagnostic interviews and self-report questionnaires on psychosocial functioning provided by the mother; and (3) rating scales completed by the child's teacher at school. The measures used assessed the domains of adaptive functioning listed in Tables 6.4 and 6.5. In addition, several laboratory assessments of electrophysiologic functioning were also employed. Our purpose in reporting here some preliminary new findings from this study is to discuss how multimethod studies can detect possible developmental patterns of risk for maladaptation which may or may not be predictive of future problems.

Table 6.7 shows how informant reports can provide information on the differences between the two groups. In addition, it also illustrates how the mother's report differs from the child's report of behavior. The relationships between the behavioral syndromes identified by the Youth Self Re-

TABLE 6.7. Relationship between the Youth Self Report and the Child Behavior Checklist for Boys Aged 12–16[a]

	Sons of alcoholics	Sons of nonalcoholics
Aggression	.31	.55[*]
Delinquency	.03	.57[*]
Depression	.19	.98[*]
Internalizing	.28	.29
Externalizing	.31	.55[*]
Somatic	−.11	−.09

[a]Each correlation is the mother's report (CBCL) correlated with her son's report (YSR) for the identified behavioral syndrome.

[*]$p<.05$.

port and Child Behavior Checklist show that sons of nonalcoholics and their mothers agree more frequently with each other than sons of alcoholics and their mothers.

In Table 6.8, we present the correlations between 48 dependent variables and age separately for children of alcoholics and children of nonalcoholics (males and females combined). Overall, correlations with age are frequently inversely related or negligible for children of alcoholics (26 negative correlations) (compared to 13 negative correlations for children of non-alcoholics). Thus, as age increases, many scores decrease for children of alcoholics. Exaggerated differences in correlations with age between children of alcoholics and children of nonalcoholics can be seen in affect (state anxiety, depression (z score)) and self- or parental reports of competence (e.g., social withdrawal).

How does development proceed in children of alcoholics? Do children of alcoholics simply get more depressed, more anxious, or more delinquent as they grow older? These correlations indicate that age plays a significant role in the development of psychosocial maladaptation in children of alcoholics. Obviously, some intervening variables or combinations of variables interact to change the developmental process in children of alcoholics. Conversely, some intervening variables may interact to protect the child of an alcoholic from maladaptive outcome. Until we understand the parameters of this trajectory, we cannot answer a fundamental question: do we see developmental deficits or delays in children of alcoholics?

FUTURE QUESTIONS

The purpose of this chapter has been to provide some comments on the state of the psychosocial research in children of alcoholics and to suggest how impediments to progress in this field might be overcome using models from developmental psychology. Much of the psychosocial research on children of alcoholics has been criticized for methodological weaknesses. Sher (1987) addresses many of these methodological problems in his comprehensive overview of the literature. In this chapter, we argue that these weaknesses are compounded by the lack of attention to developmental processes which occur during normal growth.

In much of the psychosocial research on children of alcoholics normal developmental differences and predicted changes in children's performance are often ignored. Thus, subjects of wide age ranges, both sexes, and differing cognitive developmental stages are combined into a single group. Developmental research shows that children of different ages are qualitatively and quantitatively different; they think and feel and act according to differences in cognitive and affective stages of development.

Developmental research has also shown that early family experience plays a key role in the development of social skills and status among peers in the

TABLE 6.8. Relationships between Age and Dependent Variables

	Children of alcoholics	Children of nonalcoholics
WRAT-SS Reading	−.14	.06
WRAT-SS Spelling	−.24	−.11
WRAT-SS Arithmetic	−.31	.35
Verbal IQ	−.11	−.13
Performance IQ	.00	−.13
Full Scale IQ	−.09	−.15
Anxiety—State	.54	.07
Anxiety—Trait	.24	.22
Locus of Control	−.18	−.27
Youth Self Report:		
Competence—Activities	.06	.10
Competence—Social	.07	.37
Somatic Complaints	.28	.04
Depression	.22	.14
Unpopular	−.17	−.03
Thought Disorder	.15	.13
Aggression	.11	.11
Delinquent	.26	.27
Self Des./ID Problems	−.31	.16
Other Problems	−.05	.07
Internalizing	.13	.06
Externalizing	.13	−.01
Depression (Z score)	.21	.01
Child Behavior Checklist:		
Aggression	−.03	.17
Anxious—Obsessive	−.30	.15
Cruel	.05	.33
Delinquent	.02	.17
Depressed	−.05	.19
Depressed—Withdrawal	−.09	.06
Hostile—Withdrawal	−.07	.06
Hyperactive	.26	.27
Immature	−.30	−.06
Immature—Hyperactive	−.35	−.17
Obsessive—Compulsive	.15	.04
Schizoid	−.05	−.01
Schizoid—Anxious	−.18	.76
Schizoid—Obsessive	−.25	−.89
Sex Problems	−.34	−.91
Social Withdrawal	−.09	.40
Somatic Complaints	.07	.10
Uncommunicative	.17	−.06
Internalizing	.02	.27
Externalizing	.02	.35
Competence—Activities	−.26	.17
Competence—Social	−.35	.15
Competence—School	−.23	.12
Life Events—Positive	.07	.19
Life Events—Negative	−.08	.13
Life Events—Ambiguous	−.07	.17

school (Maccoby & Martin, 1983). The degree to which alcoholism impacts on parent–child relationships and family environment will likely show variable outcomes among individuals. Behavior patterns, social interactions, and relationships first occur within the context of the family. Learning appropriate or inappropriate interaction styles from these initial parent–child interactions can influence behavior in other settings, especially school. Forehand, Long, Brody, and Fauber (1986) report that both academic performance and externalizing problem behaviors in school are related to and predicted by the parent–adolescent relationship, especially conduct disorder scores and grade point average. Hess and Holloway (1984) and MacDonald and Parke (1984) both suggest that school achievement and social functioning are related to the parent–child relationship. Childhood externalizing behaviors are related to problematic home environments more often than internalizing or anxiety difficulties (Emery, 1982).

The implications for psychosocial research on children of alcoholics are twofold. First, we can select a developmental trajectory to study. To understand the interplay between adaptive and maladaptive processes in children of alcoholics across the life span, we can assess these processes: (1) as they occur (longitudinally), (2) in the child who is undergoing transitional periods of development (i.e., adolescence), or (3) with children who are challenged by nonnormative stresses (e.g., parental separation).

Secondly, psychosocial maladaptation and risk for alcoholism in children of alcoholics may be comparatively unique, but until we identify the trajectories of adaptive and maladaptive behavior we will be unable to answer the question of whether we observe a true deficit or a developmental delay. It may be that maladaptation in children of alcoholics is only identified through specific developmental trajectories. Children of alcoholics may evince a psychosocial maladaptive pattern which is only observable across time. As developmental challenges increase or as task demands become more complex, psychosocial maladaptation in certain children may become more pronounced. Similarly, by observing how children of alcoholics make decisions to drink and then engage in substance abusing behavior, we may discover that children of alcoholics do not simply drink more at earlier ages compared to their same-age cohort; but they may drink differently, at different ages, with different results. It is conceivable that at some later date we may define a developmental substance abuse disorder distinct from the substance abuse disorders of adulthood.

One of the most important questions about psychosocial adaptation in children of alcoholics asks how we describe adaptive behavior in these children. Werner (1986) describes resilient children as those who actively solve problems, perceive experiences constructively, gain positive attention, and use faith to maintain meaning in their lives. We can find many examples of resilience in the literature. Huckleberry Finn was the son of an alcoholic.

Even after being locked in a cabin and escaping the drunken beatings of his father, his adventurous spirit was not suppressed. We can find the same resilient spirit in Anne Shirley, an orphaned girl who finally finds a home in Green Gables. "While we are bewitched by Anne's turn of phrase, we are also led to admire her courage. We wonder how she overcame her earlier life of almost constant hardship to develop her resilience and her determination to taste life to its fullest" (Shapiro, 1987, p. xvi).

How can we operationalize "determination" and "spirit" in our research on children of alcoholics? To identify these traits as protective factors is certainly necessary, but not sufficient. To shift our focus, perhaps we can understand the interplay of risk and protective factors by asking three seminal questions: (1) which problems tend to persist during development, and which do not; (2) which early problems or combinations of problems predict later disorders; and (3) which behaviors are normative and age-appropriate and which are not? (Verhulst & Althaus, 1988).

Acknowledgments. The authors thank Victoria Brewington for her helpful comments on the manuscript, Sybil Paige for manuscript preparation, and Dr. David Newlin for his encouragement and support. The data reported in this chapter were collected at the National Institute on Alcohol Abuse and Alcoholism in Bethesda, MD under Protocol 83-AA-204. We thank Dr. Michael Eckardt for his support.

REFERENCES

Abel, E. L. (1980). The fetal alcohol syndrome: Behavioral teratology. *Psychological Bulletin*, 29–50.

Abel, E. L. (1981). Behavioral teratology of alcohol. *Psychological Bulletin, 90*, 564–581.

Abel, E. L. (1982). Consumption of alcohol during pregnancy: A review of effects on growth and development of offspring. *Human Biology, 54*, 421–453.

Achenbach, T. M., & Edelbrock, C. (1983). *Manual for the child behavior checklist.* USA. Queen City Printers, Inc.

Achenbach, T. M., & Edelbrock, C. (1987). *Manual for the youth self-report and profile.* Burlington, VT: University of Vermont Department of Psychiatry.

Achenbach, T. M., & McConaughy, S. H. (1987). *Empirically based assessment of child and adolescent psychopathology: Practical applications.* Newbury Park, CA: Sage Publications.

Adler, R., & Raphael, B. (1983). Children of alcoholics. *Australian and New Zealand Journal of Psychiatry, 17*, 3–8.

Amark, C. (1951). A study in alcoholism: Clinical, social-psychiatric and genetic investigations. *Acta Psychiatrica et Neurologica Scandinavica, Suppl. 70*, 1–283.

Aronson, M., Kyllerman, M., Sable, K. G., Sandin, B., & Olegard, R. (1985). Children of alcoholic mothers: Developmental, perceptual and behavioral characteristics as compared to matched controls, *Acta Paediatrica Scandinavia, 74,* 27–35.

Baldwin, A. L. (1955). *Behavior and development in childhood,* New York: Dreyden.

Baumrind, D. (1967). Child care practices anteceding three patterns of preschool behavior. *Genetic Psychology Monographs, 75,* 43–88.

Beck, A. T., & Beamesderfer, A. (1974). Psychological measurements in psychopharmacology. In P. Pichot (Ed.), *Modern problems in pharmacopsychiatry,* Vol. 7, (pp. 151–169). Paris: Karger.

Beck, A. T., & Beck, R. W. (1972). Screening depressed patients in family practice: a rapid technique. *Postgraduate Medicine, 52,* 81–85.

Begleiter, H. (1988). The genetics of alcoholism: Introduction to the Symposium. *Alcoholism: Clinical and Experimental Research, 12*(4), 457.

Begleiter, H., & Porjesz, B. (1988). Potential biological markers in individuals at high risk for developing alcoholism. *Alcoholism: Clinical and Experimental Research, 12*(4), 488–493.

Bennett, L. A., & Wolin, S. J. (1986). Daughters and sons of alcoholics: Developmental paths in transmission. *Alcoholism: Journal on Alcoholism and Related Addictions, 22*(1), 3–15.

Bennett, L. A., Wolin, S. J., & Reiss, D. (1988). Cognitive, behavioral, and emotional problems among school-age children of alcoholic parents. *American Journal of Psychiatry, 145*(2), 185–190.

Berkowitz, A., & Perkins, H. W. (1988). Personality characteristics of children of alcoholics. *Journal of Consulting and Clinical Psychology, 56*(2), 206–209.

Brooks-Gunn, J. & Furstenberg, F. (1986). The children of adolescent mothers: Physical, academic, and psychological outcomes. *Developmental Review, 6,* 225–251.

Bryant, B. K., & Crockenberg, S. B. (1980). Correlates and dimensions of prosocial behavior: A study of female siblings with their mothers. *Child Development, 51,* 529–544.

Cadoret, R. J., Cain, C. A., & Grove, W. M. (1980). Development of alcoholism in adoptees raised apart from alcoholic biologic relatives. *Archives of General Psychiatry, 37,* 561–563.

Callan, V. J., & Jackson, D. (1986). Children of alcoholic fathers and recovered alcoholic fathers: Personal and family functioning. *Journal of Studies on Alcohol, 47*(2), 180–182.

Cermak, L. S., & Ryback, R. S. (1976). Recovery of verbal short-term memory in alcoholics. *Journal of Studies on Alcohol, 37,* 46–52.

Chafetz, M. E., Blane, H. T., & Hill, M. J. (1971). Children of alcoholics. Observations in a child guidance clinic. *Quarterly Journal of Studies on Alcohol, 32,* 687–698.

Clair, D., & Genest, M. (1987). Variables associated with the adjustment of offspring of alcoholic fathers. *Journal of Studies on Alcohol, 48*(4), 345–355.

Cloninger, C. R., Bohman, M., & Sigvardsson, S. (1981). Inheritance of alcohol abuse: Cross fostering analysis of adopted men. *Archives of General Psychiatry, 38,* 861–868.

Cloninger, C. R., Reich, T., & Wetzel, R. (1979). Alcoholism and affective disorders: Familial associations and genetic models. In D. W. Goodwin & C. K. Erickson (Eds.), *Alcoholism and affective disorders: Clinical, genetic, and biochemical studies* (pp. 57–86). New York: SP Medical & Scientific Books.

Cloninger, C. R., Sigvardsson, S., & Bohman, M. (1988). Childhood personality predicts alcohol abuse in young adults. *Alcoholism: Clinical and Experimental Research, 12*(4), 494–505.

Corder, B. F., McRee, C., & Rohrer, H. (1984). A brief review of literature on daughters of alcoholic fathers. *North Carolina Journal of Mental Health, 10*(20), 37–43.

Cotton, N. S. (1979). The familial incidence of alcoholism: A review. *Journal of Studies on Alcohol, 40,* 89–116.

Cowan, P. (1988). Developmental psychopathology: A nine-cell map of the territory. *New directions for child development, 39,* 5–30.

Dweck, C. S. (1986). Motivational processes affecting learning. *American Psychologist, 41*(10), 1040–1048.

Earls, F., Reich, W., Jung, K., & Cloninger, C. R. (1988). Psychopathology in children of alcoholic and antisocial parents. *Alcoholism: Clinical and Experimental Research, 12*(4), 481–487.

El-Guebalay, N., & Offord, D. R. (1977). The offspring of alcoholics, a critical review. *American Journal of Psychiatry, 134,* 357–365.

El-Guebalay, N., & Offord, D. R. (1979). On being the offspring of an alcoholic; an update. *Alcoholism: Clinical and Experimental Research, 3,* 148–157.

Emery, R. E. (1982). Interparental conflict and the children of discord and divorce. *Psychological Bulletin, 92,* 310–330.

Eron, L. (1982). Parent–child interaction, television violence, and aggression in children. *American Psychologist, 37,* 197–211.

Ervin, C., Little, R., Streissguth, A., & Beck, D. (1984). Alcoholic fathering and its relation to child's intellectual development: A pilot investigation. *Alcoholism: Clinical and Experimental Research, 8,* 362–365.

Forehand, R., Long, N., Brody, G. H., & Fauber, R. (1986). Home predictors of young adolescents' school behavior and academic performance. *Child Development, 57,* 1528–1533.

Furstenberg, F., Brooks-Gunn, J., & Morgan, S. P. (1987). *Adolescent mothers in later life.* Cambridge, UK: Cambridge University Press.

Gabrielli, W., & Mednick, S. (1983). Intellectual performance in children of alcoholics. *Journal of Nervous and Mental Disease, 171,* 444–447.

Gabrielli, W. F., Mednick, S. A. Volavka, J., Pollock, V. E., Schulsinger, F., & Itil, T. M. (1982). Electroencephalograms in children of alcoholic fathers. *Psychophysiology, 19,* 404–407.

Garmezy, N. (1974a). Children at risk: The search for the antecedents of schizophrenia. Part 1. Conceptual models and research methods. *Schizophrenia Bulletin, 1* (Experimental Issue No 8), 14–90.

Garmezy, N. (1974b). Children at risk: The search for the antecedents of schizophrenia: Part 2. Ongoing research programs, issues, and intervention. *Schizophrenia Bulletin, 1* (Experimental Issue No. 9), 105–125.

Garmezy, N. (1981). *Project Competence: Studies of stress resistant children.* University of Minnesota, (N. Garmezy, Principal Investigator; A. Tellegen, V. T. Devine, Co-Investigators), with support from the National Institute of Mental Health and the William T. Grant Foundation.

George, C., & Main, M. (1979). Social interactions of young abused children: Approach, avoidance, and aggression. *Child Development, 50,* 306–318.

Goodwin, D. W. (1976). *Is alcoholism hereditary?* New York: Oxford University Press.

Goodwin, D. W. (1985). Alcoholism and genetics: The sins of the fathers. *Archives of General Psychiatry, 42,* 171–174.

Goyette, C. H., Conners, C. K., & Ulrich, R. F. (1978). Normative data on revised Conners Parent and Teacher Rating Scales. *Journal of Abnormal Child Psychology, 6*(2), 221–236.

Haberman, P. W. (1966). Childhood symptoms in children of alcoholics and comparison group parents. *Journal of Marriage and the Family, 28*(2), 152–154.

Hamburg, B. (1974). Early adolescence: A specific and stressful stage of the life cycle. In G. Coelho, D. A. Hamburg, & J. E. Adams (Eds.), *Coping and adaptation.* New York: Basic Books.

Harter, S. (1983). *The perceived competence scale for children.* Denver, CO: University of Denver.

Hess, R. D., & Holloway, S. D. (1984). Family and school as educational institutions. In R. D. Parke (Ed.), *The Family* (pp. 179–222). Chicago: University of Chicago Press.

Herjanic, B., & Reich, W. (1982). Development of a structured psychiatric interview for children: Agreement between child and parent on individual symptoms. *Journal of Abnormal Child Psychology, 10*(3), 307–324.

Herjanic, B., Herjanic, M., Wetzel, R., & Tomelleri, C. (1978). Substance abuse: Its effects on offspring. *Research Communications in Psychology, Psychiatry and Behavior, 3*(1), 65–75.

Hughes, J. M. (1977). Adolescent children of alcoholic parents and the relationship of Alateen to these children. *Journal of Consulting and Clinical Psychology, 45,* 946–947.

Jacob, T., & Leonard, K. (1986). Psychosocial functioning in children of alcoholic fathers, depressed fathers, and control fathers. *Journal of Studies on Alcohol, 47*(5), 373–380.

Jacob, T., Favorini, A., Meisel, S., & Anderson, C. (1978). The alcoholic's spouse, children, and family interactions: Substantive findings, and methodological issues. *Journal of Studies on Alcohol, 39,* 1231–1251.

Jastak, S., & Wilkinson, G. S. (1984). *The Wide Range Achievement Test—Revised.* Wilmington, DE: Jastak Associates.

Johnson, J. L. (1990). Forgotten no longer: An overview of research on children of chemically dependent parents. *Children of chemically dependent parents: Academic, clinical and public policy perspectives.* New York: Brunner/Mazel.

Johnson, J. L., & Bennett, L. A. (1988). *School aged children of alcoholics: Theory and research.* Center for Alcohol Studies, Rutgers University, New Brunswick, NJ: Alcohol Research Documentation, Inc.

Johnson, J. L., & Bennett, L. A. (1989). *Adult children of alcoholics: Theory and research.* Center for Alcohol Studies, Rutgers University, New Brunswick, NJ: Alcohol Research Documentation, Inc.

Johnson, J. L., & Rolf, J. E., (1988). Cognitive functioning in children from alcoholic and non-alcoholic families. *British Journal of Addictions, 83,* 849–857.

Jones, K. L., & Smith, D. W. (1973). Recognition of the fetal alcohol syndrome in early infancy. *Lancet, 2,* 999–1001.

Kaij, L. (1960). *Alcoholism in twins: Studies on the etiology and sequels of abuse of alcohol.* Stockholm: Almqvist & Wiksell.

Kammeier, Sister M. L. (1971). Adolescents from families with and without alcohol problems. *Quarterly Journal of Studies on Alcohol, 32,*(2), 364–372.

Kandel, E., & Mednick, S. A. (1988). IQ as a protective factor for subjects at high risk for antisocial behavior. *Journal of Consulting and Clinical Psychology, 56*(2), 224–226.

Kern, J., Hassett, C., Collipp, P., Bridges, C., Solomon, M., & Condren, R. (1981). Children of alcoholics: Locus of control, mental age, and zinc level. *Journal of Psychiatric Treatment and Evaluation, 3,* 169–173.

Knop, J., Teasdale, T., Schulsinger, F., & Goodwin, D. (1985). A prospective study of young men at high risk for alcoholism: School behavior and achievement, *Journal of Studies on Alcohol, 46,* 273–278.

Kosten, T. R., Rounsaville, B. J., & Kleber, H. B. (1985). Parental alcoholism in opioid addicts. *Journal of Nervous and Mental Disease, 173,*(8), 461–469.

Kovacs, M. (1983). The children's depression inventory: a self-rated depression scale for school-aged youngsters. (Unpublished manuscript, University of Pittsburgh School of Medicine.)

Kovacs, M., & Beck, A. T. (1977). An empirical clinical approach toward a definition of childhood depression. In J. G. Schulterbrandt & A. Raskin (Eds.), *Depression in childhood: Diagnosis, treatment, and conceptual models.* New York: Raven Press.

Kuhn, D. (1981). The role of self-directed activity in cognitive development. In I. E. Sigel, D. M. Brodzinsky, R. M. Golinkoff, & R. M. (Eds.), *New directions in Piagetian theory and practice* (pp. 353–358). Hillsdale, NJ: Erlbaum.

Lerner, R. M., & Foch, T. T. (1987). *Biological-psychosocial interactions in early adolescence.* Hillsdale, NJ: Erlbaum.

Lilienfeld, A. M., & Lillienfeld, D. E. (1980). *Foundations of epidemiology* (2nd ed.). New York: Oxford University Press.

Loeber, R. (1982). The stability of antisocial child behavior: A review. *Child Development, 53,* 1431–1446.

Maccoby, E. E., & Martin, J. A. (1983). Socialization in the context of the family: Parent-child interaction. In E. M. Hetherington (Ed.), P. H. Mussen (Series Ed.), *Handbook of child psychology: Vol. 4. Socialization, personality, and social development* (pp. 1–101). New York: Wiley.

MacDonald, K., & Parke, R. D. (1984). Bridging the gap: Parent-child play interaction and peer interactive competence. *Child Development, 55,* 1265–1277.

Masten, A. S., & Garmezy, N. (1987). Risk, vulnerability, and protective factors in developmental psychopathology. In B. B. Lahey & A. E. Kasdin (Eds.) *Advances in Clinical Child Psychology, Vol. 8,* New York: Plenum.

Mischel, W. (1968). *Personality and assessment.* New York: Wiley.

National Institute on Alcohol Abuse and Alcoholism (1985). *Alcoholism: An inherited disease,* DHHS Publication No. (ADM) 85–1426. Washington, DC: U.S. Department of Health and Human Services.

National Institute on Mental Health (1978). *Children at risk.* DHEW Pub. No. (ADM) 78–724. Washington, DC: Department of Health, Education and Welfare.

Neimark, E. D. (1985). Moderators of competence: Challenges to the universality of Piagetian theory. In E. D. Neimark, R. DeLisi, & J. L. Newman (Eds.), *Moderators of competence* (pp. 1–14). Hillsdale, NJ: Erlbaum.

Parsons, O. A. (1983). Cognitive dysfunction and recovery in alcoholics. *Substance and Alcohol Actions/Misuse, 4,* 175–190.

Parsons, O. A., & Farr, S. P., (1981). The neuropsychology of alcohol and drug use. In S. B. Filskov, & T. J. Boll, (Eds.), *Handbook of clinical neuropsychology* (pp. 320–365). New York: Wiley.

Patterson, G. R., & Stouthamer-Loeber, M. (1984). The correlation of family management practices and delinquency. *Child Development, 33,* 1299–1307.

Phillips, L. (1966). Social competence, the process-reactive distinction, and the nature of mental disorder. In P. H. Hoch & J. Zubin (Eds.), *Psychopathology of schizophrenia* (pp. 471–481). New York: Grune & Stratton.

Piaget, J. (1955). *The child's construction of reality.* New York: Routledge & Kegan Paul.

Piaget, J. (1963). *The origins of intelligence in children.* New York: Norton.

Piaget, J. (1970). *Genetic epistemology.* New York: Norton.

Piaget, J. (1971). *Biology and knowledge: An essay on the relations between organic regulations and cognitive processes.* Chicago: University of Chicago Press.

Reich, W., & Earls, F. J. (1982). *The home environment interview for children. Child and parent versions* (unpublished manuscript). St. Louis: Washington University.

Reich, W., Herjanic, B., Welner, Z., & Ghandy, P. R. (1982). Development of a structured psychiatric interview for children. Agreement on diagnosis comparing child and parent interviews. *Journal of Abnormal Child Psychology, 10,* 325–336.

Rimmer, J. (1982). The children of alcoholics: An exploratory study. *Children and Youth Services, Review, 4,* 365–373.

Rolf, J., Johnson, J. L., Israel, E., Baldwin, J., & Chandra, A. (1988). Depressive affect in school-aged children of alcoholics. *British Journal of Addiction, 83,* 841–848.

Rolf, J., & Read, P. B. (1984). Programs advancing developmental psychopathology. *Child Development, 55,* 8–16.

Roosa, M. W., Sandler, I. N., Beals, J., & Short, J. L. (1988). Risk status of adolescent children of problem-drinking parents. *American Journal of Community Psychology, 16(2),* 225–239.

Russell, M., Henderson, C., & Blume, S. (1985). *Children of alcoholics: A review of the literature.* New York: Children of Alcoholics Foundation, Inc.

Rutter, M., (1981). Parent–child separation: Psychological effects on the children. *Journal of Child Psychology and Psychiatry, 12,* 233–260.

Ryan, C., & Butters, N. (1983). Cognitive deficits in alcoholics. In B. Kissen & H. Begleiter (Eds.), *The pathogenesis of alcoholism: Vol. 7. Biological factors* (pp. 485–538). New York: Plenum.

Schaefer, E. S. (1965). Children's reports of parental behavior: An inventory. *Child Development, 36,* 413–324.

Schuckit, M. A., Goodwin, D. A., & Winokur, G. (1972). A study of alcoholism in half siblings. *The American Journal of Psychiatry, 128,* 1132–1136.

Shapiro, E. S. (1987). *Foreword.* In L. M. Montgomery, *Anne of Green Gables.* New York: Children's Classics.

Sher, K. J. (1987). What we know and do not know about CoAs: A research update. Paper presented at the MacArthur Foundation Meeting on Children of Alcoholics, Princeton, NJ, December 2, 1987.

Sigel, I. E., Brodzinsky, D. M., & Golinkoff, R. M. (1981). (Eds.) *New directions in Piagetian theory and practice.* Hillsdale, NJ: Erlbaum, 1981.

Spiker, C. C. (1966). The concept of development: Relevant and irrelevant issues. *Monographs of the Society for Research in Child Development,* Serial No. 107, *31*(5), 40–54.

Steinglass, P., Bennett, L. A., Wolin, S. J., & Reiss, D. (1987). *The alcoholic family.* New York: Basic Books.

Steinhausen, H., Gobel, D., & Nestler, V. (1984). Psychopathology in the offspring of alcoholic parents. *Journal of the American Academy of Child Psychiatry, 23,* 465–471.

Tarter, R. E. (1988). Are there inherited behavioral traits that predispose to substance abuse? *Journal of Consulting and Clinical Psychology, 56*(2), 189–196.

Tarter, R. E., Jacob, T., & Bremer, D. A. (1989). Cognitive status of sons of alcoholic men. *Alcoholism: Clinical and Experimental Research, 13*(2), 232–235.

Tarter, R. E., Hegedus, A., Goldstein, G., Shelly, C., & Alterman, A. (1984). Adolescent sons of alcoholics: Neuropsychological and personality characteristics. *Alcoholism: Clinical and Experimental Research, 8,* 216–222.

Ulleland, C. N. (1972). The offspring of alcoholic mothers. *Annals of the New York Academy of Sciences, 197,* 167–169.

Verhulst, F. C., Althaus, M. (1988). Persistence and change in behavioral/emotional problems reported by parents of children aged 4–14: An epidemiological study. *Acta Psychiatrica Scandinavica Suppl. No. 339*(77), 2–28.

Warner, R. H., & Rosett, H. L. (1975). The effects of drinking on offspring. *Journal of Studies on Alcohol, 36*(11), 1395–1420.

Watt, N. F., Anthony, E. J., Wynne, L. C., & Rolf, J. E. (1984). *Children at risk for schizophrenia: A longitudinal perspective.* New York: Cambridge University Press.

Watters, T. S., & Theimer, W. (1978). Children of alcoholics: A critical review of some literature. *Contemporary Drug Problems, Summer,* 195–201.

Werner, E. E. (1986). Resilient offspring of alcoholics: A longitudinal study from birth to age 18. *Journal of Studies on Alcohol, 47* 34–40.

West, M. O., & Prinz, R. J. (1987). Parental alcoholism and childhood psychopathology. *Psychological Bulletin, 102*(2), 204–218.

Wilson, C., & Orford, J. (1978). Children of alcoholics: Report of a preliminary study and comments on the literature. *Journal of Studies on Alcohol, 39,* 121–142.

Youman, J. R., Parsons, O. A., & Leber, W. R. (1985). Lack of recovery in male alcoholics' neuropsychological performance one year after treatment, *Alcoholism: Clinical and Experimental Research, 9,* 114–117.

7

Family Culture and Alcoholism Transmission

LINDA A. BENNETT and STEVEN J. WOLIN

In a suburban home outside Washington, DC, a couple in their late 50s recounts their family's experience with alcoholism. The Parkers, a working class family, have five grown children all living in the same community as the parents. Two of these children are married daughters who have children of their own. The father is critically ill due to excessively heavy drinking since adolescence. His drinking history is not so unusual, except perhaps for the phenomenal amount of alcohol he regularly consumed until a year ago. However, when we scrutinize the family context of Mr. Parker's drinking, some telling and not so predictable points emerge. These bits of evidence are helpful in formulating ideas about transmission of alcoholism.

QUESTION: *Mrs. Parker, how would you describe your drinking over the years?*

MOTHER: My husband and I went out and drank together from the time we first met. It was wartime and the places to meet were the bars. I didn't think much about it. It was the accepted thing: people met there, had a drink, played darts. It was like a social gathering.

Later on after we married, he would come home from work, get cleaned up, and off to the bar he'd go. And I got to thinking, well, the only way I am going to see anything of him is to go with him. I tell you that just about killed me. I mean sure it was fun. That first drink tasted horrible, the second one was a little better, and by the time I got to the third one, I didn't give a hang. But the next morning I would feel so sick. I just had to quit.*

FATHER: She never was a true alcoholic because a true alcoholic never has a hangover.

*In presenting family cases, we have drawn excerpts from the interviews, changing names and modifying some details to ensure anonymity of families.

talk openly in the family about your husband's drinking?

en the kids were growing up, his drinking was something
ived with. It gave us a lot of grief and misery so that when-
cv̵ ̱d, we pushed it away from us and did other things.

FATHER: And while they were trying to keep away from me, I was feeling
like I was being shut out of the whole goddamn mess, and I mean no-
body would talk to me. So I would just put on my jacket and go out
and get in my car and go on to one of the bars to drink.

QUESTION: *What was the impact of his drinking on family life?*

MOTHER: There was no social life. You couldn't have friends to the house,
and you couldn't get out and make friends. Family life was nothing but
turmoil. You couldn't talk with him because when we did, we got into a
heck of a lot of really bad sessions, but nothing was accomplished. We
just yelled and screamed at each other. And then the pressure would
build up slowly, slowly and then got to the point where you thought
you were going to blow your top.

QUESTION: *Were there times when Mr. Parker was intoxicated at dinner time?*

MOTHER: I am going to be very honest. Up until two years ago for quite a
long period of time I never saw him sober. He would wake up in the
middle of the night and get another drink. He just constantly kept it
going for five years at least. So, yes, he was intoxicated at dinner time.
He would sit here in the living room and eat and watch television while
the rest of us were at the table.

FATHER: She threw out my beer a lot of the time, but I recovered most of it.

QUESTION: *Mrs. Parker, how would you generally describe your reaction to the
alcoholism?*

MOTHER: With drinking, you get to the point of saturation where you can't
do anything about it, and it's affecting your life so much you try to push
it away. There is only so much you can take and you don't want any
more part of it. I've known for a few years that alcoholism is a disease,
but the thing is how long can you live with that disease and go along as
if it's all right. There's a point you get to and then the hell with it, I've
had enough and want no part of it because the disease is getting to you
then.

QUESTION: *Do any of your children have problems with alcohol?*

MOTHER: I don't think so. I hope not—up to this point. They are all social
drinkers, but I don't think any of them up to this point has a problem
with it.

FATHER: It depends on where you draw the line of problems.

MOTHER: Well, I don't think any of them are habitual drinkers.

The Parkers have been through the throes of alcoholism for close to 40 years. They have witnessed its deteriorating effects on the father's body, felt the social disintegration of family relationships, seen the disruption of family rituals, and weathered highly precarious financial circumstances throughout the years their children were growing up. *And alcoholism has already recurred in their children's generation.*

Mr. Parker no longer drinks, but he stopped only under conditions of dire medical necessity. The family tried all sorts of strategies to control his drinking. Mrs. Parker began by joining forces with him during their courting years and early marriage. When that didn't work and his drinking continued unabated, she and the children tried pushing him out of the rest of family life, giving him yet another excuse to go right back to the bars to drink and into the living room to eat dinner apart from the rest of the family. Intermittently they would scream, confront him, and throw out his liquor, but the results were all for naught. In the end, they just tried to make do. No strategy changed the bottom line fact that "the disease was getting to them."

Alcoholism pervades this family. All four of the father's brothers are alcoholic. While his parents were not drinkers, his grandfathers reportedly also abused alcohol, with one dying of alcohol-related causes. The really startling discovery, however, is that the mother is quite wrong about her children. Transmission of alcoholism has already recurred in the next generation. Based upon direct and extensive interview data with the two married daughters and their husbands, we determined that they do have alcohol problems. One daughter is a recovering alcoholic, and the other is married to an alcoholic and is a heavy drinker herself. Neither couple made any bones about these facts. It was not a family secret.

What might have the Parker family done to change the course of its intergenerational continuity of alcoholism? What went wrong with the mother's strategies for dealing with the father's drinking and intrusive behavior while intoxicated? And how can she possibly *not* be aware of her own children's alcoholism?

In an attempt to answer these sorts of questions, we have conducted two studies of family culture and alcoholism transmission (Bennett & Wolin, 1984; Bennett & Wolin, 1986; Bennett, Wolin, Reiss, & Teitelbaum, 1987; Wolin, Bennett, & Noonan, 1979; Wolin, Bennett, Noonan, & Teitelbaum, 1980). Drawing upon in-depth semistructured individual and couple interviews with multiple members of approximately one hundred families, we have identified certain family processes that serve as either precipitating or protective factors in the continuity of alcoholism. In this chapter, we review those studies and describe two family processes—distinctive family rituals and deliberate family heritage selection—which mediate between parental alcoholism and drinking problems in the next generation.

We present in some detail family case material that demonstrates differences among adult married siblings with respect to transmission and family culture.

ALCOHOLISM AS A FAMILY ILLNESS

Alcoholism is very much a family illness. More often than not, its presence alters the routines of daily life as well as the family's most special occasions. Furthermore, it has become a commonplace to note that alcoholism "follows in family lines." In other words, when alcoholism is diagnosed for one family member, the chances are very good that it has previously appeared in prior generations and that it will surface again in the next generation (Cotton, 1979; Hall, Hesselbrock, & Stabenau, 1983a,b; Hesselbrock, Stabenau, & Hall, 1985; Midanik, 1983). The recurrence of alcoholism in one or more children of an alcoholic parent is alarmingly frequent. Researchers and clinicians are not the only ones well acquainted with this pattern: the lay public has become highly aware of the familial nature of alcoholism. Many people are also very interested in looking for explanations for its recurrence, as well as preventive solutions.

In looking for explanations and solutions, we have taken a family culture approach (Bennett, 1989), rather than focusing on biological contributions. By acknowledging existing evidence that genetic predisposition is a contributing factor to familial transmission (e.g., Bohman, 1978; Cadoret, Cain, & Grove, 1980; Cadoret & Gath, 1978; Cloninger, Bohman, & Sigvardsson, 1981; Goodwin, Schulsinger, Hermansen, Guze, & Winokur, 1973; Goodwin, et al., 1974), we look to aspects of the family environment—which we call the family culture—for precipitating and protective factors which place offspring of alcoholics at increased or decreased risk to become alcoholic themselves.

Gomberg and Lisansky's (1984) depiction of alcoholism etiology voices our own perspective accurately and succinctly:

> It is our assumption that events leading to alcohol problems in adult life are myriad, that causation is indeed complex and interactional. Nonetheless, . . . it is not random selection or blind fate that determines problem drinking, but events in certain combinations and sequences that lead a person into problem drinking. (p. 234)

We have attempted to identify some of those combinations and sequences (or patterns) found within the realm of family culture that are significantly associated with transmission or nontransmission. Our focus has been on the overall context of growing up in intact families with an alcoholic parent. By family culture, we mean the patterns of behavior and the belief system of a family incorporating language, thought, action, and material objects and conveyed through the socialization of each new generation.

The concept of "family ritual" is central to the theoretical model and methodological approach of both studies. Family rituals are symbolic forms of communication between family members. Because of the satisfaction that family members experience through their repetition, rituals are performed in a systematic manner over time. Due to their special meaning and repetitive nature, rituals contribute to the establishment and preservation of a family's collective sense of itself, which we call the "family identity" (Bennett, Wolin, & McAvity, 1988; Wolin & Bennett, 1984; Wolin, Bennett, & Jacobs, 1988; Wolin et al., 1980). Family rituals offer an especially handy window through which to view the family and to assess the relative impact of chronic problems such as alcoholism upon family life.

RATIONALE FOR A FAMILY CULTURE MODEL

Several considerations favor studying familial alcoholism from a family culture perspective. To begin with, variation in drinking outcome among siblings having a common alcoholic parentage is a compelling argument. While some children of alcoholic parents grow up to become alcoholic themselves, other offspring from the same family do not always repeat the drinking problems of the prior generation. Unfortunately, scant information exists regarding epidemiological patterns for the *sons and daughters* of alcoholics, in comparison to much more extensive data on *fathers and mothers* and *siblings* of identified alcoholics. Most surveys on familial alcoholism examine family patterns by collecting data on parents and first and second degree relatives from children who are diagnosed as alcoholic. Thus, it is extremely difficult to accurately estimate the extent of transmission which moves *down* family lines from grandparents, to parents, and to children.

With respect to siblings, Hall et al. (1983b) have shown that risk for alcoholism when one sibling is already affected is very different for brothers and sisters. A substantial group of brothers of identified alcoholics are either heavy drinkers, probable alcoholics, or definite alcoholics (47.3% altogether), in comparison with 14.4% of the sisters. In this sample, considerable variability was found in drinking patterns among siblings even though at least one sibling was an identified alcoholic.

The frequent occurrence of sibling differences has several potential explanations, including purely genetic and penetrance factors, sex differences (e.g., Fillmore, 1975), birth order (e.g., Blane & Barry, 1973), differential identification with the alcoholic parent, and variable exposure to the parental alcohol behavior throughout childhood.

A second justification for a family culture approach is the "indirect" continuity of alcoholism over generations, such as happened in the Washington suburban family described earlier. For example, daughters of alcoholics reportedly often marry alcoholics without necessarily evidencing problems with alcohol themselves. Similarly, in the "skipped generation" situation, alcoholism appears in the grandparent generation, but does not reappear until the grandchild generation.

Studies of this phenomenon are not abundant, however. Hall and her colleagues (1983b) provide some useful data to support this observation. For example, among the proband group of 117 married alcoholic men, 62 had fathers who were problem drinkers. Of these, 34 (54.8%) were also married to an alcoholic. Among the 62 men in the study who had fathers who were also alcoholic, 28 were married to women whose fathers were either abstinent (16%) or social drinkers (29%). Unfortunately the drinking patterns of the wives are not specified.

In an unpublished survey by Kruzich in Texas of 405 male alcoholic servicemen, 40% had problem-drinking fathers, and 27% were married to women who also had problem-drinking fathers. Those men who evidenced both familial drinking patterns—problem drinking for their own fathers and for their wives' fathers—amounted to 54 individuals, or 13% of the sample. Information about the wives' drinking patterns is not available.

A third rationale has to do with the question of lifelong prognosis for young men and women who drink heavily or problematically. Children of alcoholics who in their youth show signs of impending alcoholism through heavy drinking periods do not always go on to become alcoholic. Fillmore (1975) has shown that while problem drinking in young adulthood (ages 16–25) is a significant predictor of drinking problems in middle age (early 40s) for both men and women, a substantial percentage of those young problem drinkers become moderate drinkers during their middle years. This is demonstrated more clearly for men than for women, since fewer men who were problem drinkers early in life are problem drinkers during middle age, while the incidence for women is very similar for both periods. Although a significant percentage of the variability among both men and women can be explained by correlations between problem drinking at time one and drinking problems twenty years later in life, Fillmore (1975) found that "Among both men and women there was a tendency to shift toward nonproblem drinking." She concludes that "the notion of irreversibility of problem drinking is open to question" (p. 827).

In short, we can state that heavy drinking or problem drinking in youth does not *always* lead to alcoholism and can be a precursor to moderate drinking in adulthood. The tendency toward potential alcohol problems early in the life of children of alcoholics—especially males—often later reverses itself with no long-term drinking problems developing.

To account for variation among siblings with alcoholic parentage, the incidence of indirect continuity of alcoholism through the generations of a family, and exceptions to a lifelong progression of chronic alcoholism, we have looked to differences both between families and within families.

THE TRANSMISSION STUDIES

The Alcoholism Transmission via Family Ritual Project

In an initial study of alcoholism recurrence and ritual disruption, we interviewed adult members from two generations of 25 families living in the Washington, DC area. All families had at least one parent who had been a chronic problem drinker or alcoholic during the now-grown children's childhood and adolescent years (following Goodwin et al., 1973, criteria for drinking levels). Two interview sessions were conducted individually with each family member. We focused upon the development and maintenance of six ritual areas of family life: dinner times, holidays, vacations, evenings, weekends, and having visitors in the home. In particular, we were interested in the extent to which each of these ritual areas had either remained stable or been disrupted through the progression of the parent's alcoholism.

In categorizing the extent of ritual change, a comparison was made between the ritual performance before the parental drinking became most severe and during the heaviest drinking years. These qualities were assessed: (1) consistency of roles for family members; (2) stability in family routines; (3) continued frequency of observance; (4) change in affect associated with the activity; (5) overall social and emotional atmosphere; (6) an alteration in attendance by family members; and (7) predictability of the ritual sequence.

We have discovered that families vary considerably with respect to the stability of their rituals as parental alcoholism grows more severe. The rituals may remain *distinctive,* in that the alcohol abuse behavior is kept distinct from the ritual itself, or they may become *subsumptive,* in that the alcohol abuse behavior subsumes the ritual.

Distinctive rituals are those that are minimally altered during the time of particularly severe parental drinking. Although exposed to alcoholic behavior, families with distinctive rituals kept them intact by resisting the disruptive influence of the drinking. Thus, the ritual's integrity and continuity were maintained.

In one family, the *son* reported that dinners remained the same over time:

> "Dinner was one of the most stable things. We always ate together, and my father was rarely late. It was the time of the day we saw the most of him. There were not many changes that I can remember."

His *sister* gave a similar account:

> "My dad sat at the head of the table, near the telephone, so that he could sidetrack calls. No chair was sacred, but we did take the same places. Everyone was together. We all took part in preparing whatever we were having. We sat around and talked after dinner about the day, school, things that had happened, world events. That's the way I always remember it."

The preservation of the dinnertime ritual in this family occurred despite the fact that the father was drinking alcoholically throughout the children's growing-up years.

In some alcoholic families, holiday celebrations are similarly resistant to alteration under the impact of alcohol abuse behavior. While dinners provide a measure of day-to-day stability around an ordinarily important event, holidays offer a view of how the family preserves an occasion that is special, as shown by this *son's* recountings:

> "Christmas was always an important time for us as a family unit. We did things that were very special and tried to use our imagination. We all went out shopping, but did not tell each other what we were buying. Everyone decorated the tree."

His *sister* reported a very similar theme:

> "Christmas was always a lot of fun. Even now, people come to watch us open our presents. Everyone was on their best behavior. And it has always been like that."

The alcoholic father in this family had been treated in an in-patient program and is an active participant in Alcoholics Anonymous. During his drinking years, he lost a job, often drove on the wrong side of the road, passed out early in the evenings, and was verbally abusive to members of the family. Although his wife wanted "to run," she lived through "four to five years of hell" before he stopped drinking. In short, the fact that the family kept its holiday rituals distinct was not a function of less severe alcoholism in the family.

Subsumptive rituals, in contrast, evidence gradual or an abrupt change as the parental drinking worsens. Eventually the ritual is subsumed by the alcohol abuse behavior. The difference between "normal" and "drinking" periods during dinnertimes is emphasized in this *son's* recollections of a subsumptive dinnertime in his family:

> "When my father was not really ripped, he held the floor and dominated all conversations. That was normal. He would make it very unpleasant for us. He would pick at us, put us down. It got increasingly frequent. Dad got a whole lot sloppier, disorganized. As he drank more, dinner got progressively worse, and he went through a gradual decline."

His *sister's* description includes observations about what was going on
with other family members at the time, as well as the dramatic change in
her father's demeanor:

> "Mom got slack on housework when Dad started drinking, and dinner-
> time stopped being formal and balanced. There were two different din-
> nertime periods, one where we were still kind of a family and hanging
> out with Dad. After his drinking got bad, he wouldn't even show up for
> dinner lots of times, but would be in bed sleeping. I was about sixteen."

Major intrusions by the drinking upon holiday celebrations are often recalled in stark terms. In one family where the mother was an alcoholic, the
daughter and son felt their disrupted Christmas to be a major loss and a
great disappointment. According to the *daughter:*

> "The family Christmas card was a big tradition: A photograph of each
> child and parent was pasted on a background drawn in. The grandmoth-
> ers just loved it. I was sorry to see the tradition go. Mother lost interest.
> The Christmas card tradition deteriorated when I was in high school.
> One year I did the cutting and pasting. At that point things were done
> haphazardly and with less care. One year we even had a plastic tree."

The mother's detachment from the holiday celebration was also a jolt for
her *brother:*

> "My Mother was less and less involved with the holiday as the years went
> by. It meant that it was less special because she was the one who had
> done all the work for the decorations and bought all the presents. One
> year when Mother was drinking, my Father realized that she wasn't go-
> ing to do anything. So he went out and did the shopping. He bought
> one present for each person and wrapped them in newspaper. We were
> all standing around for Mother to get up because that was the tradition.
> She finally came staggering in around 11:00. I felt a chill come over me,
> and I didn't want to be around."

Our results showed that those families whose rituals were most subsumed by the alcoholism ("subsumptive families") evidenced a greater incidence of intergenerational continuity of the alcoholism among the grown
children interviewed than those families which kept their rituals distinct
from the alcohol abuse behavior ("distinctive families") (Wolin et al., 1979,
1980).

Of the six families that had at least one offspring who was a problem
drinker or an alcoholic, four were subsumptive to the extent that all six
rituals had been disrupted as the parental drinking worsened. Two others
were moderately subsumptive in that some of their rituals had been altered.
Among the 12 families with no evidence of alcoholism, problem drinking,
or heavy drinking in the children's generation, five were distinctive in that
none of their rituals had been disrupted during the heaviest drinking pe-

TABLE 7.1. Ritual Change Type for Ten Families by Alcoholism Transmission Category[a]

Ritual change type	Alcoholism transmission	
	Transmitters ($n = 4$)	Nontransmitters ($n = 6$)
Subsumptive	4	1
Distinctive	0	5

$p<.025$ Fisher's Exact Test.
[a]Adapted from Wolin et al. (1979), p. 591.

riod, six were moderately subsumptive, and one was subsumptive. The seven families in which at least one of the children was a heavy drinker, but as yet had not evidenced problem drinking or alcoholism, were evenly divided between subsumptive, moderately subsumptive, or distinctive. Since there is no way to predict the eventual outcome of those children who are heavy drinkers, we conducted an analysis on those 10 families who were fully distinctive or subsumptive and who were clearly transmitter or nontransmitter families. (Of the four transmitter families, all were subsumptive; of the six nontransmitter families, five were distinctive, and one subsumptive.) In this analysis, we found a significant association between subsumptive family rituals and the transmission of problem drinking or alcoholism into the children's generation ($p<.025$, Fisher's Exact Test). (See Table 7.1.)

The Alcoholism and Family Heritage Project

With this initial finding—that those families that kept their rituals intact even during the heaviest drinking years evidenced less transmission of alcoholism to the next generation—we planned the second transmission study. A new theme emerged in this two-generational project, which has been subsequently demonstrated to exert, first, a significant influence on alcoholism transmission among adult children of alcoholics (Bennett, Wolin, Reiss, & Teitelbaum, 1987) and, second, on the level of behavior problems among school-aged children of alcoholics (Bennett, Wolin, & Reiss, 1988). This theme is the family's level of *deliberateness* in establishing and maintaining family rituals and other highly valued patterns of family life.

High deliberateness represents the successful execution of a newly-married couple's expectations for the formation of their own family ritual structure vis-à-vis their family of origin backgrounds. *Highly deliberate* couples plan early in marriage how they wish to be similar to or different from their families of origin and are able to follow through on those ideas. *Low deliberate* couples either never develop such a plan and instead take a fatalistic view of their future together, or they do have a plan that simply does not work out. Choice of a particular family heritage is not sufficient in and of itself to place a couple at greater or lesser risk for alcoholism transmission. Instead, we argue, the couple needs to be *deliberate* in its pursuit of a specific family heritage.

The alcoholism and family heritage project is a two-generation study of 68 married children from 30 alcoholic families of origin and their spouses. All 30 of these families of origin with an alcoholic parent/s were intact during the growing-up years of the now-married children. Within the 30 families of origin, 22 had fathers who were alcoholic; of the other eight, four were mother-alcoholic and four, both-parent alcoholic families. At least one parent was either alcoholic or a problem drinker, according to criteria of Goodwin et al. (1973). At least two grown, married children and their spouses from each of the 30 families of origin were interviewed. Of the 68 offspring couples from these 30 families, 27 included at least one problem drinker or alcoholic. Thirty-five were female and 33 were male. Their mean age was 33 years. Families came from the metropolitan areas of Washington, DC, Baltimore, Minneapolis, and Philadelphia, as well as rural areas and small towns located in Virginia, Delaware, Pennsylvania, and Tennessee. The study group was socially and demographically heterogeneous. Most family members were interviewed in their homes.

Each child and spouse took part, first, in an individual interview regarding family life when he or she was a child (the "family of origin interview"). Later, both husband and wife participated jointly in a session focusing on their present family life ("nuclear family interview"). A semistructured format was used for both sessions, and parallel questions were asked regarding individual and shared experiences of husband and wife. The family of origin sessions covered many aspects of family history over three generations, including demography, family alcohol and other drug history, interpersonal relationships in the nuclear and extended families, and the organization of family and household responsibilities.

Special attention was paid to dinnertime and holiday rituals. Basic descriptions of these two ritual areas were elicited, followed by details of stability and change over time as the parental drinking became more severe in the alcoholic families. The nuclear family interview paralleled the family of origin interview, but focused on the current generation as compared with the couple's two families of origin. An extensive history of drinking and other drug use of each spouse and their children was also taken during this interview.

In order to reliably code the interview data into theory-derived categories, the research team developed a coding manual and trained two coders who had not been previously involved in the research and who were not privy to the working hypotheses of the study. In coding data for a particular family, each coder read the entire data set for a given family of origin and then focused on the three interviews for each couple in the family. Thus, the coders began with an overview of all the data collected for the family.

The coding manual provided detailed instructions for locating and interpreting specific information in the large data set, a procedure often referred to as "holistic coding." Since it was not usually possible to specify that a particular code could be determined only on the basis of the answer to a particular question, it was necessary to direct the coders to a whole complex of material in their consideration of information relevant to the selection of a particular category. This required that the coding manual indicate those places in the transcribed interview data where the pertinent material was most likely to be found and to specify explicit guidelines for interpreting various types of responses of the couples.

Using this method, the coders coded each of the 68 couples for several theory-derived family process dimensions such as the distinctiveness or subsumptiveness of rituals in the family of origin, level of ritualization of dinnertimes and holidays in both families of origin, extent of contact between the couple and the alcoholic family of origin, and the level of deliberateness in the couple's family ritual heritage choice.

Fourteen predictor variables were selected on the basis of the theoretical model. Of the 14, nine referred to the family of origin background of the adult children of their spouses (family of origin variables), and five pertained to the nuclear family experience of the couple from the time of their courtship and marriage to the current period (nuclear family variables). Among the nine origin family variables, six were family process dimensions while three had to do with family demography and/or alcohol history: (1) the child being second born in birth order; (2) the child being the son of an alcoholic father; and (3) the spouse having an alcoholic parent. (See Table 7.2.) The single outcome variable was the couple's status as alcoholic or nonalcoholic. Those couples with one or two heavy drinking spouses were categorized as nonalcoholic.

The kappa statistic, a change-corrected measure of agreement, was used to determine whether the coder agreement was better than chance, no better than chance, or less than chance (Bartko & Carpenter, 1976). A two-tailed test of significance was performed for each kappa to determine whether the coder agreement was better than chance at the $<.05$ level of significance (Bennett et al., 1987, pp. 117–119).

Multiple regression analysis was applied in a two-step hierarchical method. Since the outcome may be due at least partly to shared family membership among those siblings taking part in the study, the first step in the analysis calculated the variance due to family membership. Next, the predictor variables were entered in order to determine whether the increment in variance beyond the variance accounted for by family membership

TABLE 7.2. Fourteen Predictor Variables[a]

Origin family variables
1. Dinner ritual level, child's family: highly ritualized or not
2. Holiday ritual level, child's family: highly ritualized or not
3. Dinner ritual level, spouse's family: highly ritualized or not
4. Holiday ritual level, spouse's family: highly ritualized or not
5. Ritual change in dinnertime, child's family: distinctive or not
6. Ritual change in holidays, child's family: distinctive or not
7. Child is second born: yes or no
8. Child is son of an alcoholic father: yes or no
9. Spouse has an alcoholic parent: yes or no

Nuclear family variables
10. Spouse family heritage maintained: yes or no
11. Level of family heritage from previous generation: low, moderate, or high
12. Novel elements evident in nuclear family identity: yes or no
13. Extent of contact with child's origin family: low, moderate, or high
14. Level of deliberateness in family heritage outcome: low, moderate, or high

[a]Adapted from Bennett et al. (1987), pp. 118–119.

alone was significant. Table 7.3 presents the results of the statistical analysis (Bennett et al., 1987, pp. 124–126). The fourteen predictor variables contributed significantly to the couples' alcoholism outcome ($p<.01$). This lends support to the overall model.

Looking at the specific predictors of nontransmission, we find, first, that it was protective *not* to be the son of an alcoholic father, a family membership status which very likely combines biological and environmental influences from the family heritage. The sons of alcoholic fathers group

TABLE 7.3. Hierarchical Multiple Regression Analysis ($N=68$)[a]

Predictor variables	R^2	Incremental F	Probability of increment	Overall F
Shared family membership	.467			1.15
Family membership plus 9 origin family variables and 5 nuclear family variables	.802	2.91	.01	2.26

[a]Adapted from Bennett et al. (1987), p. 125.

constituted the most transmitted-to sex–age category. Second in predictive importance, high deliberateness in family heritage selection was found to be protective. Additionally, we found that being second born, coming from a family with distinctive dinnertimes, marrying a spouse from a family with highly ritualized dinnertimes, and marrying a spouse from a non-alcoholic family were protective. In contrast, maintaining a high degree of contact with the child's alcoholic family of origin placed the couple at increased risk for alcoholism (Bennett et al., 1987). (See Table 7.4)

Distinctive dinnertimes in the child's family of origin are not significantly correlated with high deliberateness on the part of the couple (correlation coefficient −.018). as we might expect on the basis of our conceptual model. However, these two variables measure family processes in two different generations of the family. Furthermore, distinctiveness is based upon the individual child's perspective of his/her origin family, which might be different from that of the other siblings. In contrast, level of deliberateness reflects the couple's joint experience. We would expect to find greater congruence between distinctive family rituals and high deliberateness within the same generation, using a whole family approach to categorize the family.

TABLE 7.4. Predictor Variables Contributing Most Significantly to Outcome (N=68)[a]

Predictor variables	Direction	F	Probability of F
Child is son of an alcoholic father	Risk	10.63	<.002
High level of deliberateness in family heritage outcome	Protective	8.66	<.006
Spouse's family dinner ritual level high	Protective	5.30	<.02
Child's family dinner ritual distinctive	Protective	4.09	<.05
Spouse's family had an alcoholic parent	Risk	3.17	<.08
Contact high with child's origin family	Risk	2.62	<.115
Child is second born	Protective	2.56	<.12

[a]Adapted from Bennett et al. (1987), p. 125.

Since we found that highly deliberate couples were significantly more protected from alcoholism transmission and low deliberate couples were at considerably greater risk, we devote the remainder of the chapter to a discussion of the concept of deliberateness.

DELIBERATENESS IN FAMILY HERITAGE SELECTION AND TRANSMISSION

The importance of replicating or rejecting rituals and other family patterns from the prior generation figures centrally in our two-generation model. The newly-married couple begins with two possible legacies to draw upon in establishing its own family identity and family ritual traditions. Depending in part upon the alcohol legacy and upon the ritual focus of these families, the couple's adoption of a particular family heritage may be instrumental in the transmission process.

A child who has grown up in a family culture with chronic parental alcohol abuse may choose to break with this past by abrogating his or her family ritual traditions. Instead, that child may selectively carry over some of the family's more sound behaviors and values into the next generation. Whatever the particular decisions this offspring makes with regard to choice of a spouse and family ritual heritage, this critical juncture offers an opportunity to determine new directions that may be healthier than those practiced previously.

A couple has four options open to them in establishing a family heritage. They can replicate the child's ritual and interactional heritage; they can adopt the spouse's; they can develop a heritage that combines elements of both families of origin, with neither dominating; or they can develop an entirely new family heritage, drawing upon neither of their families of origin as potential models.

According to the results of our study, heritage choice in and of itself does not place a couple at greater or lesser risk for alcoholism transmission. Because an alcoholic family background produces a tenacious hold over children's lives, the alcoholism-free couple needs to establish a clear path for their future. In our terms, the couple must be deliberate in its pursuit of a specific heritage outcome.

Highly deliberate couples exhibit explicit expectations, communicated through statements in the interview session of intentions that were fulfilled. In such families, there was a plan early in marriage, and the couple has successfully followed through on that plan. Talk and ideas are transformed into action. Such couples evidence a thinking through and anticipate both the good and the problematic aspects of life that they are likely to encounter. Not only do they make the effort to anticipate and have a sense of what to expect; they also believe that they hold some measure of control over their future. They find ways to ensure these desired outcomes.

Of the 68 couples in the study, 12 were highly deliberate; of these, 75% were not alcoholic.

Low deliberate couples follow a very different course. Their heritage outcomes are not consciously designed. They either accept with little forethought developments that arise as they move through their marriage and rely on fate to determine their course or they struggle uselessly with the world and with each other in haphazard attempts to order their lives, but to no avail. Ideal plans fall by the wayside. Of the 31 couples who were low on deliberateness, 77% were alcoholic.

Of the 25 couples who were *moderately deliberate* in that they were somewhat successful in carrying out their early marital plans for establishing their family heritage, 11 were alcoholic and 14 were nonalcoholic. Thus, these couples did not fit a very clear pattern one way or the other with regard to transmission.

DELIBERATENESS AND TRANSMISSION: DIFFERENCES AMONG SIBLINGS

The following three siblings from the same alcoholic family of origin and their spouses illustrate the difference between level of deliberateness and alcoholism transmission. Like the Parkers, they come from a working class family with several adult children. Two sisters and one brother—all of whom are married to spouses from families where the parents were moderate drinkers—were interviewed. Sylvia, the older of the two sisters, had explicit notions early in marriage as to what she and her husband Jerry should emulate or change from her own family background.

> "Yes, I had very strong feelings about what we should do. When I was growing up, we always had our hands in alcohol and all sorts of people living with us. I was determined that that would not happen in our lives. And I don't mean that we would reject people."

Sylvia's husband Jerry was happy to have her take the lead in deciding upon the nature of their family life together. However, he did have some pretty clear ideas as to how they should celebrate their holidays.

> "I thought things would continue much as before. We did carry on things the way they had been when we were children, especially around holidays. We both had a lot of Christmas and Thanksgiving celebrations. That's what we have done too. We do her family's thing on Christmas and mine on Thanksgiving. Right?"

SYLVIA: Yes. And we started out with really very little materially, and we have been growing together, both of us, reaching various plateaus and heading toward goals. In the beginning since we didn't come from goal-oriented families, we really had not thought through everything so clearly. *Then I started to realize that I could have a lot more control over*

things that were happening to us. And we sought to gain some of that control.
We were kind of growing and developing and maturing and learning
how to get the best out of what was available to us.

Sylvia and Jerry have developed a family heritage that draws in part from
both families of origin and their own novel way of doing things. Early in
marriage, they charted a course that they have followed together and they
represent the most highly deliberate couple in this family. They are not
alcoholic.

Sylvia's younger sister Carolyn had high hopes for a certain type of family when she married, but these hopes have not be realized. While she expected to emulate her husband's family of origin in her own family, in fact
they have primarily drawn upon on her family of origin background for
patterning their own family. According to Carolyn:

> "What I was really drawn to was his family's traditions which were
> much stronger than mine, and I really enjoyed them and felt comfortable
> with them. And for the holidays, they had more family togetherness, the
> whole family being there. And I want to carry that on. I never really
> did. It hasn't worked out that way."

In addition to holidays not turning out as Carolyn had expected, aspects
about family organization and relationships are a far cry from what either
she or her husband Nick had in mind at the time of their wedding. In
discussing these developments, they talk in very fatalistic terms. They
explained that the absence of family assistance from either side had contributed to their lack of family cohesion and to difficulties they had encountered in their marriage and raising their children. At marriage, both
had expected that the togetherness of his family of origin would continue.
It has not. There are no family reunions. And they do not celebrate Christmas with either set of grandparents. This has been a particular disappointment to Carolyn, who had happily anticipated close holiday times with all
of Nick's relatives:

> "I would like the family to be a little closer together. I mean the whole
> family. I don't feel we are presenting a normal family life to our
> children. My husband isn't there at holidays, like his father was. He's
> working."

Neither Sylvia nor Carolyn have experienced alcoholism in their marriages; they and their husbands are moderate drinkers, with no signs of any
heavy drinking. But Carolyn and Nick, who are low on deliberateness on
family heritage formation, have experienced very serious marital problems.

Older brother Robert in this family, however, is alcoholic. He and his
wife Lydia are also low on deliberateness. When we asked them about any
changes they had hoped to make at the time they married, Lydia noted:

"Yes, I did want to make some changes. I think it has backfired, though. I don't think I wanted to be as dominant a person as my mother, but I don't know if I have made the right choice or not with my children, the way they treat me sometimes. Maybe I should have been more firm."

While Robert had hoped to move away from the way his family had been when he was growing up, their family has, in fact, adopted the heritage of his family of origin.

"I guess at the time when young people get married, they want to pick up where their families left off. Everything has to be just so, only the best of everything, things that had worked for your parents, those you want to continue. And at first it was more or less that way."

Over the years, however, family life has not persisted in a more optimistic vein. According to Lydia's account:

"No, I don't think things have worked out the way we had expected them to. I thought, for one thing, that we would have more money. That we would be further ahead. We had planned to live in this town for five years, and then of course it's been fifteen years almost. It seems like we were closer earlier than we are now really. I think that as much as you love your children, they tend to overpower you."

This feeling of powerlessness—due to one's own children, lack of family help, or whatever—is often characteristic of low deliberate families. They may have strong wishes as to what kind of family they would like to have created, but things got the best of them. After years together and life not going according to plan, they tend to communicate a fatalistic resignation about what is really possible in life. It is just such couples, we submit, that are most vulnerable to carrying forth the alcoholism legacy. In Robert's case, his alcoholism is every bit as severe as his father's was. Although he has tried various well-meaning strategies to get control of his drinking, he has been uniformly unable to do so.

Furthermore, their oldest son, at age 13, is already drinking heavily and has come home intoxicated several times. While this annoys Lydia to no end and concerns them both, they have not been able to gain control of that situation either. The tragedy of this couple is the strong possibility that the alcoholic legacy will continue into their children's generation, against their best intentions.

HIGH DELIBERATENESS AND NONTRANSMISSION: THE SON OF AN ALCOHOLIC FATHER

While being the son of an alcoholic father places a person at increased risk to become alcoholic, many examples of nontransmission to such offspring are found in the study. David and Lucy, one such couple, are in their early 30s and have a son Ricky who is 11. David grew up in a middle class family in Pennsylvania with an alcoholic father and a moderate drinking mother; Lucy's father was a moderate drinker, and her mother abstained from alcohol. Both David and Lucy drink very occasionally, and have never experienced any problems with alcohol.

Given David's family background of being the son of an alcoholic father, and the first-born, he was automatically at increased risk to become alcoholic himself. Furthermore, his dinnertime rituals were subsumed by his father's drinking. In marrying Lucy, he appeared to have moved in the direction of establishing a healthier family identity. Her family was not alcoholic, and her dinnertime rituals were highly ritualized. Furthermore, they both had some pretty clear ideas as to what kind of family life they would create together.

QUESTION: *When you got married, did you have any traditions which you wanted to carry over from when you grew up?*

LUCY: Holiday traditions. We wanted to carry them over, but as far as home life goes, we made our own. David was determined to do that.

DAVID: It never entered my mind to be determined. I just felt we should live the way we wanted to live.

QUESTION: *Would you give an overall description of dinnertime in your home and how it has changed over the years.*

DAVID: It's never really changed much.

LUCY: Only as far as our son being added to the family.

DAVID: We always make it . . . it's an important time of our lives. It is the only time we get together each day. Always was. And I like to cook. So I get involved with dinners.

LUCY: I love it when he cooks.

DAVID: And we always wait for each other to eat, even if it means eating at 8:00. Even Ricky waits. He's the type of kid that has a lot of self-control when it comes to something like that.

QUESTION: *Are there ever any hassles, unpleasantries, over dinner?*

LUCY: Ricky doesn't eat his vegetables (*laughter*). You know, just normal sorts of things like that.

DAVID: We do have our bad nights. We're under so much pressure in our work and the kind of schedule we lead. Every once in a while we will get into a heated discussion, which we try to avoid.

LUCY: I try to avoid it. When I first started going to David's family's house for dinner, they were constantly fighting at the table. David's mother would be screaming at his brother, and his brother would be screaming back.

DAVID: Yeah, but for us that was normal.

QUESTION: *Is your dinnertime now at all like it was in your home when you were growing up?*

LUCY: Yeah, the togetherness is and the calm. The food definitely is different. The type of atmosphere is very much like it was in my family. I like that kind of atmosphere. In my family we were always together for dinner. There were times when there was not a lot of food on the table. But our meal was always a family affair. I was completely happy with it. It was a very calm time.

Then when I first started dating David, dinner in his home was unbelievable. Arguments. Food would stick in my throat when I went there because we never had that at my house. And I could never live with that in our family.

DAVID: It was very different in my family. We ate as we came in the house, and that was it. As you got older, it got even worse. As my Dad got older and his drinking got worse, meals together got to be impossible. He was staying out all the time. It certainly wasn't a time for conversation.

In many aspects of family life this couple had charted a course very much in contrast to how it was in David's childhood. They have drawn considerably more upon the model of Lucy's family, especially in setting the tone of family interaction. They feel a strong need for tranquility in the home, to offset many of the demands of the outside world. This was not achieved without a struggle, however. In the first year of their marriage, they experienced frequent verbal outbursts before they were able to work out the differences in expectations for their own family together.

As things have turned out thus far, Lucy's family heritage predominates in their family together, and she was *not* crushed in the early decision-making of this couple. Lucy may have been shocked at the beginning by the way his family behaved around dinnertime, but her quiet persistence not to repeat this element of his family past and David's loud outbursts early on have provided a constructive blend. The resulting family life which they have established pleases them both, and by now, David has become a strong advocate and supporter of a more controlled and congenial family life.

CONCLUSION

Where does alcoholism come into this discussion? Many of these examples seem almost devoid of drinking concerns. The subject of alcoholism, for example, does not reappear in David and Lucy's case following the specification of their drinking status and that of their parents. But, then, there are *alcoholic families* and *families with alcoholism,* and they are not one and the same. "Alcoholic families are behavioral systems in which alcoholism and alcohol-related behaviors have become *central organizing principles* around which family life is structured" (Steinglass, Bennett, Wolin, & Reiss, 1987, p. 47). We propose that one avenue out of an alcoholic family circle can occur by emphasizing nonalcoholic family behavior as a central organizing principle of family life.

Looking at this process from an individual and family development perspective, we see some critical points that an offspring of an alcoholic encounters as he or she moves from childhood into adulthood, life junctures which we believe can make a difference in whether or not the alcoholism recurs or is rejected. While individual dimensions, such as the "ego strength," of particular family members may be an important element in this process, we believe that family culture is particularly critical in determining the extent to which the family takes a relatively healthy or unhealthy course, even when parental alcoholism is present. We find the idea of *selective disengagement* from an alcoholic family system to very aptly encompass the protective family processes that occur over three critical junctures: family of origin ritual protection; discriminating spouse selection; and the deliberate establishment of a family heritage in adult life.

Within the childhood and adolescent years, disengagement can occur at either an individual or a family level. It is not uncommon for "resilient" or "successful" adult children of alcoholics to describe themselves as having felt different from the rest of the family when they were growing up. They attempted to find ways out, rather than getting overly enmeshed within the alcoholic family system. This can serve as a survival tactic. When the family itself is able to keep its rituals distinct from the alcohol abuse behavior of the parent during the childhood and adolescent years, it is using another disengagement tactic.

A second crucial step in *spouse selection.* In choosing a spouse, these are important considerations for a child of an alcoholic: Does the prospective spouse also come from an alcoholic family? Does that family offer solid and meaningful ritual traditions? According to our findings, marrying someone who comes from a nonalcoholic family and one that is highly ritualized can be a positive step.

The third step in selective disengagement involves being *highly deliberate in establishing a family heritage* that suits the wants and needs of the couple. It is important that the newly-married couple (1) envision a course to their lives; (2) believe that it is possible to direct that course; and (3) follow through on their vision with a reasonable degree of success.

In short, we are suggesting that breaking the cycle of familial alcoholism may have less to do with addressing the alcoholism per se and more to do with focusing on other aspects of family life which are indeed possible to control.

To return to the Parker family introduced at the beginning of this chapter, perhaps we can now shed some light on the transmission of alcohol problems among the two married daughters. Eleanor, the first-born, and Kitty, the third-born in the family, grew up participating in subsumptive dinnertimes. Because of the intrusive behavior of the father under the influence of alcohol, the family found it impossible to maintain consistent routines from day to day. Thus, there was no evidence of selective disengagement on the part of the family.

More telling developments took place when each daughter married and attempted to set up a new household and begin a family of her own. Eleanor, the oldest and a recovering alcoholic, was married to Rodney, who did not have an alcoholic parentage, and who never drank to excess himself. At the time they married, however, they did not share the same expectations for their own family and for the birth of their child.

QUESTION: *When you married, did you have any ideas of how you wanted to do things in a similar way to your families growing up?*

ELEANOR: I don't think I consciously did because I didn't like the way my family was. That doesn't mean that I didn't do it, but I don't think I wanted to.

RODNEY: I can't consciously think of any family routines I wanted to continue except for our family gatherings.

QUESTION: *Were there any particular things that you wanted to be different?*

ELEANOR: I knew I didn't want a drinking husband. That was the one thing I knew and it probably attracted me to Rodney. I knew that if we had children I didn't want to raise my children the way I had been raised. That if we had children, for them to have a better sense of love and caring than I feel that I got.

RODNEY: At one time very early on you gave me an ultimatum that it was either that I could not bring any beer into the house or.... and I said, well, I am going to bring beer into the house if I want to.

ELEANOR: Yeah, I was totally irrational about it.

QUESTION: *How do you think your expectations for life together have worked out since you were married?*

RODNEY: Well, considering what we have been through, it's going very well now. For a while there Eleanor, with her illness, could do nothing. She could not carry out household responsibilities, and now she does that very nicely. And so my expectations have been fulfilled. She does what I want her to do and what I expect her to do. And that is . . .

ELEANOR: To take care of you.

RODNEY: Right. Feed, wash my clothes, keep the house clean.

ELEANOR: Mow the grass.

QUESTION: *And that's what you had intended when you were married?*

RODNEY: I guess so, without really thinking about it.

QUESTION: *What about your expectations, Eleanor?*

ELEANOR: Well, I think my expectations have changed. If you are talking about my expectations at the beginning of our marriage, I think that's what I wanted to do, as Rodney describes. To take care of him and iron his shirts. But that didn't last long.

RODNEY: I sort of expected Eleanor to work, to have a job, and she couldn't seem to hold a job real well, and that has disappointed me.

QUESTION: *How did you feel about your pregnancy?*

ELEANOR: I was totally bonkers the entire time I was pregnant. I was a totally unreasonable person. Although I was looking forward to the baby, when she arrived, I was totally lost, totally lost.

QUESTION: *Did you feel unprepared for parenthood?*

ELEANOR: Yes.

RODNEY: It was unplanned. So naturally I had some reservations about it, financially, but I was happily resigned to it. Of course once Angela was born, you love her more and more all the time. I was disappointed the way Eleanor couldn't seem to handle it at first.

QUESTION: *Would you comment on the best times and worst times in your marriage?*

ELEANOR: I think probably the roughest time for me was after Angela was born. I think I was projecting onto Rodney ideas I had about men that I had gathered from living with my father, expecting the worst, and being ready to fight.

Eleanor's younger sister Kitty married Skip, the son of an alcoholic father. Skip came from a family where dinnertime rituals were very unritualized. Like Eleanor and Rodney, they went into parenthood with minimal forethought or planning. They have three children.

QUESTION: *How did you feel about your first pregnancy?*

KITTY: So so. I didn't think Skip was ready for kids even at the second pregnancy. At that time we were still much more involved in ourselves than with the family and the children. We more or less missed those years.

SKIP: We kind of fell into marriage and having children. That's the way it's supposed to be done.

QUESTION: *So you didn't think about it a whole lot ahead of time?*

SKIP: No.

KITTY: It was just the thing that you had been taught to do. That is what you do and that's how it has worked out. So we really missed all those years. I can't tell you how I felt about the pregnancies. A lot of times I felt hostility. Here are kids coming along, and I am tied down.

Skip and Kitty describe their family as being out of control. Furthermore, he is a problem drinker, and she, a heavy drinker. Like Eleanor and Rodney, they had maintained considerable social and physical contact with Eleanor and Kitty's alcoholic family of origin, and have looked to that family for direction in many parts of their life. Thus far, the verdict is still out for both couples with regard to how well they can yet overcome their alcoholic family identity. By the time of the interview, Eleanor and Rodney had superimposed some measure of control on their family life, and Eleanor was no longer drinking. In contrast, Kitty and Skip were still struggling to redirect their family life into a healthier, nonalcoholic direction.

In summary, we find that neither of the Parker daughters had the benefit of selective disengagement from an alcoholic family as children. Their spouses did not provide advantageous alternatives with respect to family background. Furthermore, each couple embarked on a low deliberate course in establishing its own family heritage. This is most clearly evidenced in their lack of planning for the birth and upbringing of their children. On a more optimistic note, both couples were trying to add a measure of deliberateness in their working out of day-to-day routines and in addressing their drinking problem. Hopefully, they will successfully break the cycle of alcoholism in their family.

The concepts of distinctive rituals and deliberateness as protective family processes deserve further examination under a variety of family conditions. In a more recent study, we have found that school-aged children of alcoholic parents are significantly less likely to evidence behavior problems when the family is highly deliberate in its ritual development (Bennett et al., 1988). We believe that it would be valuable to study families with other types of problems or psychopathology, such as clinical depression, to see whether ritual protection and/or high deliberateness are related to relatively better outcomes for the children. Furthermore, we think that these ideas should be tested also in "normal" families in terms of the well-being of offspring. Finally, the relationship between distinctiveness and deliberateness and other measures of individual and family dynamics should be empirically explored in both normal and troubled families.

REFERENCES

Bartko, J. J. & Carptenter, W. T. (1976). On the methods and theory of reliability. *Journal of Nervous and Mental Disease, 163.* 307–317.

Bennett, L. A., & McAvity, K. (1985). Family research: A case for interviewing couples. In G. Handel (Ed.), *The psychosocial interior of the family* (3rd ed.). New York: Aldine.

Bennett, L. A., & Wolin, S. J. (1984). The cross-generational transmission of alcoholism in families: The alcoholism and family heritage study. *Anali Klinicke bolnice "Dr. M. Stojanovic", 33,* 207–214.

Bennett, L. A., & Wolin. S. J. (1986). Daughters and sons of alcoholics: Developmental paths. *Alcoholism, Journal on Alcoholism and Related Addictions, 22*(1), 3–15.

Bennett, L. A., Wolin, S. J., Reiss, D., & Teitelbaum, M. A. (1987). Couples at risk for transmission of alcoholism: Protective influences. *Family Process, 26,* 111–129.

Bennett, L. A., Wolin, S. J., & Reiss, D. (1988). Deliberate family process: A strategy for protecting children of alcoholics. *British Journal of Addiction, 83,* 821–829.

Bennett, L. A., Wolin, S. J., & McAvity, K. (1988). Family identity, ritual, and myth: A cultural perspective on life cycle transitions. In Celia J. Falicov (Ed.), *Family transitions* (pp. 221–234). New York: Guilford.

Bennett, L. A. (1989). Family, alcohol, and culture. In M. Galanter (Ed.), *Recent developments in alcoholism* (pp. 111–127). New York: Plenum.

Blane, H. T., & Barry, H, Jr. (1973). Birth order and alcoholism: A review. *Quarterly Journal of Studies on Alcohol, 34,* 837–952.

Bohman, M. (1978). Some genetic aspects of alcoholism and criminality: A population of adoptees. *Archives of General Psychiatry, 35,* 269–276.

Cadoret, R. J., Cain, C. A., & Grove, W. (1980). Development of adoptees in adoptees raised apart from alcoholic biologic relatives. *Archives of General Psychiatry 37,* 561–563.

Cadoret, R. J., & Gath, A. (1978). Inheritance of alcoholism in adoptees. *British Journal of Psychiatry, 132,* 252–258.

Cloninger, C. R., Bohman, M., & Sigvardsson, S. (1981). Inheritance of alcohol abuse: Cross-fostering analysis of adopted men. *Archives of General Psychiatry, 38,* 861–868.

Cotton, N. S. (1979). The familial incidence of alcoholism: A review. *Journal of Studies on Alcohol, 40,* 89–116.

Fillmore, K. M. (1975). Drinking and problem drinking in early adulthood and middle age: An exploratory 20-year follow-up. *Quarterly Journal of Studies on Alcohol, 35,* 819–840.

Fillmore, K. M., & Midanik, L. (1984). Chronicity of drinking problems among men: A longitudinal study. *Journal of Studies on Alcohol, 45,* 228–236.

Gomberg, E. S. L., & Lisansky, J. M. (1984). Antecedents of alcohol problems in women. In S. C. Wilsnack & L. J. Beckman (Eds.), *Alcohol problems in women* (pp. 233–239). New York: Guilford.

Goodwin, D. W., Schulsinger, F., Hermansen, L., Guze, S. B., & Winokur, G. (1973). Alcohol problems in adoptees raised apart from alcoholic biologic parents. *Archives of General Psychiatry, 28,* 238–243.

Goodwin, D. W., Schulsinger, F., Moller, N., Hermansen, L., Winokur, G., & Guze, S. B. (1974). Drinking problems in adopted and nonadopted sons of alcoholics. *Archives of General Psychiatry, 31,* 164–169.

Hall, R. L., Hesselbrock, V. M., & Stabenau, J. R. (1983a). Familial distribution of alcohol use: I. Assortative mating in the parents of alcoholics. *Behavior Genetics, 13,* 361–372.

Hall, R. L., Hesselbrock, V. M., & Stabenau, J. R. (1983b). Familial distribution of alcohol use: II. Assortative mating of alcoholic probands. *Behavior Genetics, 13,* 373–382.

Hesselbrock, V. M., Stabenau, J. R., & Hall, R. (1985). Drinking style of parents of alcoholic and control probands. *Alcohol, 2,* 525–528.

Midanik, L. (1983). Familial alcoholism and problem drinking in a national drinking practices survey. *Addictive Behaviors, 8,* 133–141.

Steinglass, P., Bennett, L. A., Wolin, S. J., & Reiss, D. (1987). *The alcoholic family.* New York: Basic Books.

Wolin, S. J., Bennett, L. A., & Noonan, D. L. (1979). Family rituals and the recurrence of alcoholism over generations. *American Journal of Psychiatry, 136*(4B), 589–593.

Wolin, S. J., Bennett, L. A., Noonan, D. L., & Teitelbaum, M. A. (1980). Disrupted family rituals: A factor in the intergenerational transmission of alcoholism. *Journal of Studies on Alcohol, 41,* 199–214.

Wolin, S. J., & Bennett, L. A. (1984). Family rituals. *Family Process, 23,* 401–420.

Wolin, S. J., & Bennett, L. A., & Jacobs, J. (1988). Assessing family rituals in alcoholic families. In *Rituals in families and family therapy.* New York: W. W. Norton.

8

Marital Functioning Among Episodic and Steady Alcoholics

KENNETH E. LEONARD

Alcoholism clearly exerts a detrimental impact on the marital and family functioning of families in which one member is an alcoholic. The litany of problems is well known and includes marital conflict and divorce, economic difficulties, child abuse and neglect, and domestic violence. Despite the tremendous stresses that accompany alcoholism and are dysfunctional for the family, there is a growing awareness that many families remain intact and achieve some degree of stability. The basic family tasks are somehow accomplished, though not necessarily in an optimal fashion, despite the continued burden of a member who contributes less to the functioning and more to problems than if he or she were not an alcoholic. The recognition that many alcoholics continue to drink within a family framework has spurred research focused on the marital and family processes that occur within alcoholic families.

Although there are numerous issues which have been examined concerning the marital/family functioning of alcoholics and their families, one of the more recent issues has been the exploration of marital/family processes which might serve to reinforce and, therefore, maintain heavy alcohol use. The clinical concept of "enabling"—family members behaving in such a way as to allow the alcoholic to engage in heavy drinking—describes one group of such processes. For example, assuming the responsibilities of the alcoholic or providing excuses to an employer when the alcoholic is intoxicated may be necessary for continued family functioning, but may also shield the alcoholic from the potential negative consequences of his or her behavior. In a different vein, the family's inability or unwillingness to interact with the alcoholic when drinking may provide him or her a respite from undesired family demands. In doing this, the other members of the family may be able to interact in a fairly normal way and accomplish a variety of familial tasks. As a consequence, the family may be unwilling to allow the alcoholic to participate in family tasks even when sober, thereby inadvertently or purposefully punishing the alcoholic for sobriety. Alternatively, the family may avoid arguments and confrontations with the alcoholic while he or she is drinking, perhaps because they believe it will be futile, or might result in an escalation of conflict or even a violent response. As a result, members of the family may wait until the alcoholic is sober to express their anger and frustration, again perhaps punishing the alcoholic for sobriety. These examples serve to illustrate the variety of different ways that family processes may encourage, or fail to discourage, heavy drinking. In these examples, the family's adaptation to the challenges posed by the behavior of the alcoholic may reinforce and maintain his or her drinking. Family tasks are accomplished *despite* the drinking of the alcoholic. However, most of the clinical, theoretical, and empirical considerations of the role of family processes in maintaining the alcoholic's drinking have focused on the adaptive functions of the alcoholic's drinking. That is, does the drinking of the alcoholic result in behaviors which have a positive impact on the family that would not occur in the absence of drinking? Are there certain family tasks that are accomplished as a result of the drinking of the alcoholic?

ALCOHOLISM PHASE AND MARITAL/FAMILY INTERACTIONS

The work of Steinglass and his associates has been the most influential in this regard (Steinglass, Bennett, Wolin, & Reiss, 1987; Steinglass & Robertson, 1983). From a family systems perspective, Steinglass has argued that among alcoholic families, alcohol consumption may have an adaptive value to the family by allowing the alcoholic and his family to interact in a way in which certain important tasks could be accomplished which otherwise might not be accomplished. As a result, alcohol consumption would be reinforced, and the family would come to rely on both sober and intoxicated interactions to maintain family functioning and to solve family problems.

Although this approach to alcoholism and the family has tremendously important treatment implications, few studies have examined this issue empirically. The "adaptive value" of drinking model was initially derived from clinical observations of conjointly hospitalized alcoholic "couples" during periods of intoxication and sobriety (Davis, Berenson, Steinglass, & Davis, 1974; Steinglass, Davis, & Berenson, 1977). For example, Steinglass et al. (1977) observed 10 married couples in which at least one member was alcoholic. These couples participated (three couples at a time) in a 7- to 10-day inpatient program. The facility provided a homelike atmosphere in which behaviors typical of the home environment could be observed. Alcohol was freely available to the couples over the first seven days. On the basis of clinical observations, these authors concluded that "interactional behavior during intoxication was first, exaggerated or amplified, and second, restricted in range" (p. 8).

Subsequently, studies of family interaction were conducted in which alcoholic couples were compared as a function of alcoholism phase; that is, whether the alcoholic had been drinking during the week preceding the study (wet) or had not been drinking (dry). Steinglass (1979) studied 17 alcoholic families consisting of a mother, father, and a child 12 years or older who participated in a problem solving task. This task consisted of family members sorting three separate decks of cards containing patterned sequences of letters and nonsense syllables. The first card sort was completed independently by each family member. The second sort was completed by each member in communication with the other members, and the third sort was again completed independently. Two variables were derived: configuration, which indicated the degree to which family members' interactions led to a subsequent improvement or deterioration in problem solving; and coordination, which indicated the degree to which the family, both while communicating and subsequently, produce similar versus dissimilar solutions.

Families were classified as either wet or dry on the basis of whether the alcoholic had been drinking or not in the week preceding the task. The results indicated that wet families were lower on coordination than were dry families. That is, while communicating among themselves, and in the sort that followed, wet families produced sorts less similar to each other than did dry families. Despite this lack of family coordination, the wet families benefited as much as the dry families from the communication period. The wets had higher configuration scores than did the drys, though the difference was not significant. Nonetheless, the scores of the wets suggested that the discussion improved problem solving abilities for the members. In subsequent analyses, it was found that families with the *most* alcohol-related consequences also achieved the best configuration scores.

Steinglass (1981) examined the family interactions of 31 alcoholic families who were observed in their homes over a six-month period. Two observers, each focusing on one member of the couple, charted a variety of characteristics including the presence and/or consumption of alcohol, the location in the home of the targeted member, the presence of other family members and their distance from the target, verbal interactions between the target and other family members, and the content and outcome of the interaction. Observations were made on nine different occasions, incuding both weekday evenings and weekend afternoons.

Alcoholic families were divided into stable wet (alcoholic was drinking throughout the six months of the study), stable dry (alcoholic was abstinent throughout study), and transitional. The results indicated that stable wet families scored higher on distance regulation (members dispersed around house, spent more time alone) than either the stable dry or the transitional families. Transitional families scored low on distance regulation (were close together) and low on content variability (narrow range of content, affect, and outcome of interactions). Stable dry families were intermediate on distance regulation but higher on content variability. The author's basic conclusion was that "the drinking phase of the alcoholic was associated with a stable . . . pattern of interactional behavior in the home" (p. 583).

Support for the conclusion that marital/family interactions are related to drinking phase is also provided by Roberts, Floyd, O'Farrell, and Cutter (1985). These investigators observed the behavior of 30 marital couples in which the husband was an alcoholic. These couples participated in a discussion to resolve disagreements identified through the use of the Revealed Difference Questionnaire. Couples in which the husband had been sober for two years or more were compared with couples in which the husband had been sober less than four months. Husbands with longer periods of sobriety talked more, but asked fewer questions, and expressed fewer disagreements and aggressive comments than did husbands with short periods of sobriety.

ALCOHOL CONSUMPTION AND MARITAL INTERACTION

Although the above studies suggest differential marital/family behavior as a function of whether the husband is in a drinking versus sober phase of alcoholism, they do not necessarily indicate that the altered interactions occur *while* the alcoholic is drinking nor that they are *adaptive* to the family. These studies are suggestive; however, studies involving empirically based observations of alcoholics while they were sober and while they were actually drinking are more pertinent.

The earliest study of the marital interactions of alcoholics while drinking and while not drinking was conducted by Billings, Kessler, Gomberg, and Weiner (1979). In this study, alcoholic, maritally distressed (but not alcoholic), and control couples were asked to role-play several standard scenarios that were designed to establish conflicting motives and goals for each member of the couple. The couples enacted these scenes twice, once with alcohol available and once with no alcohol available. Although alcoholics and their wives displayed more hostility and less friendliness than the normal control couples, they were not different from the maritally distressed couples. Furthermore, the presence of alcohol did not differentially influence the alcoholic couples in contrast to the distressed or normal couples. Unfortunately, however, the alcohol manipulation was quite weak, with approximately 50% of the subjects not consuming any alcohol. Among those who did consume some alcohol, most had only one or two drinks. Even the alcoholics did not drink an appreciable amount of alcohol, attaining a blood alcohol concentration of only .026.

Three studies have employed more effective alcohol administration manipulations. Frankenstein, Hay, and Nathan (1985) recruited eight alcoholics and their spouses who were interested in treatment. These couples discussed minor marital problems, major marital problems, and alcohol problems under a no-alcohol and an alcohol condition. The results indicated that alcoholics spoke more and engaged in more problem description statements while they were drinking than while they were sober. Alcoholics also engaged in more problem solving than did their spouses, irrespective of alcohol condition. In a subsequent study, Frankenstein, Nathan, Hay, Sullivan, and Cocco (1985) found that outside observers of these interactions, as well as the members of the couple, tended to view the nonalcoholic spouse as dominant during the no-alcohol session and the alcoholic as dominant during the alcohol session.

In contrast, Jacob, Ritchey, Cvitkovic, and Blane (1981) observed eight alcoholic and eight nonalcoholic couples who discussed major conflicts in their relationships with alcohol available and under a no-alcohol condition. These investigators reported that alcoholic couples expressed higher levels of negativity when drinking than when not drinking, while the nonalcoholic couples did not alter their negativity as a function of alcohol availability.

Recently, Jacob and Krahn (1988) replicated and extended this study with a larger sample and with the addition of a control group consisting of depressive men and their wives. As with the Jacob et al. (1981) study, alcoholic couples were more negative than depressive or normal couples on drink night but were indistinguishable from these two groups on no-drink night. As this study also assessed parent–child interactions, participating couples were accompanied by their oldest child between the ages of 10 and 18. Although these children were not in the room while the couples participated in the marital interaction, the sex of the child did exert an influence on the marital interaction. Alcoholic couples in which the participating child was a male slightly decreased their positivity and problem solving on drink relative to no-drink night, while couples with sons in the other two groups increased their positivity and problem solving. In contrast, alcoholic couples with daughters dramatically increased their positivity and problem solving on drink versus no-drink night, while other couples with daughters were unaffected by the drink condition.

Although family systems approaches have argued that alcohol intoxication may have an adaptive value relative to the problem solving in the family, it would be misleading to interpret this as suggesting that the adaptive value would necessarily or uniformly be reflected in increased problem solving activity under intoxication. Indeed, clinical examples cited by Steinglass and others imply considerable heterogeneity with regard to the precise role of intoxication in altering problem solving activities. As one example, Steinglass et al. (1987) describe one family in which intoxication was used to delay decision making, an improvement over the family's typical impulsive style of decision making, by inducing conflict and distracting the family from the specific decision of interest. In another case, the drinking of the alcoholic was viewed as a behavior that allowed the family to interact assertively with others and mobilize help in times of crisis. Thus, from one alcoholic family to another, the particular manner in which intoxication was "adaptive" might vary considerably.

The heterogeneity of alcohol's adaptive influence on family functioning could be the result of numerous factors. Different family structures might influence the character of the family's response to alcohol. For example, different strengths and weaknesses within the individuals in the family, cultural factors, and life stage factors as well might lead to different responses to alcohol. Steinglass et al. (1987) suggest that alcoholism may be more easily adapted to by certain types of families, depending on the energy level, interactional distance, and characteristic behavioral range of the family. Additionally, they argue that the manner in which the alcoholism is expressed may create differential demands on the family. Some families, when confronted with these demands and stresses, may be unable to adapt. For those families who are able to adapt to the alcoholism, the specific form of their adaptation will differ as a function of the different demands encountered and resources available. As a consequence, family behaviors during intoxication may differ considerably from one family to the next as a function of the specific manifestations of alcoholism in the family.

ALCOHOLISM SUBGROUPS: EPISODIC/STEADY DIMENSION

Over the past 10–15 years, there has been a growing interest on the part of researchers in the delineation of specific types of alcoholism, types which might differ from each other with respect to etiology, natural history, and response to treatment. For example, Cloninger, Bohman, and Sigvardson (1981) divide alcoholics into male-limited, which is characterized by an early onset and by alcoholism and criminality in the parents, and milieu-limited, which is characterized by a later onset and alcoholism, but not criminality, in the parents. Hesselbrock and colleagues (Hesselbrock, Hesselbrock, & Stabenau, 1985) have examined alcoholics with antisocial personalities, concomitant depressive disorders, or no other psychiatric diagnosis. Morey, Skinner, and Blashfield (1984) utilized cluster analysis and identified three subgroups of alcoholics: early stage problem drinkers, affiliative alcoholics, and schizoid alcoholics. Zucker (1986) has proposed four different types of alcoholism: antisocial, developmentally cumulative, developmentally limited, and negative affect. Other typologies which have been suggested include primary–secondary (MacAndrew, 1981), essential–reactive (Rudie & McGaughran, 1961), familial–nonfamilial (McKenna & Pickens, 1981; Penick, Read, Crowley, & Powell, 1978), and early onset–late onset (Abelsohn & van der Spuy, 1978; Lee & DiClimente, 1985).

In our own work, we have focused on subtypes of alcoholism which relate more directly to the impact that alcoholism might have on the family. The most important of these variables is whether the alcoholic describes himself as a steady drinker, who drinks about the same amount on a day-to-day basis, versus an episodic (periodic, binge) drinker, who has some days on which he consumes considerably more and some days on which he may not drink at all. In the case of the steady alcoholic, his drinking represents a continual, predictable source of stress to the family and, therefore, may be more easily accommodated to by the family. Drinking by the episodic alcoholic is more variable and therefore less predictable by the family. As a result, the family may have more difficulty accommodating the family processes and daily routines to the behavior of the episodic alcoholic. Furthermore, from a developmental perspective, it seems likely that a family that has "accepted" the drinking of the alcoholic and has accommodated itself to the behavior of the alcoholic may be conducive to the development of a steady pattern of drinking. In contrast, a family who does not accept the behavior, but excludes the alcoholic from family interactions when he is intoxicated, may be more conducive to a more episodic pattern of drinking.

Distinctions between alcoholics who used alcohol on an intermittent basis and those who used alcohol in a more continuous fashion have been drawn since the 1800s (Babor & Lauerman, 1986). However, there is very little empirical literature examining differences between these two types of alcoholics. Among male VA patients, binge alcoholics had lower levels of education, more serious alcohol problems, and more treatment contacts (Tomsovic, 1974). In contrast, Sanchez-Craig (1980) reported fewer neuropsychological deficits among halfway house bout drinkers relative to daily drinkers, after controlling for age, IQ, drug use, and years of problem drinking. Among a more middle-class sample, binge drinkers were more likely to report liver problems and parental alcoholism and tended to have more alcohol-related arrests and hospitalizations (Connors, Tarbox, & McLaughlin, 1986).

Over the past five years, we have had the opportunity to assess episodic and steady alcoholics in the course of a larger study comparing the marital and family interactions of families in which the husband was either alcoholic, depressed, or was not psychiatrically disturbed. Families for this study were recruited through the use of newspaper advertisements calling for subjects to participate in a paid study of drinking and family functioning. In the case of the alcoholics, advertisements seeking heavy drinking men who were residing in intact families for at least five years, and who had a child between the ages of 10 and 18, were used. For families in which the father was depressed, the advertisement sought depressed men who had experienced some of the typical symptoms of depression (e.g., feeling sad, trouble sleeping, trouble eating, etc.) who were also residing in an intact family for at least five years and had a child between the ages of 10 and 18. Control families were recruited with ads seeking social drinking men in intact families for at least five years and also having a child between the ages of 10 and 18. Families who responded to the ad were provided with a description of the study and were intensively screened, using both self-report questionnaires and interviews including the Schedule for Affective Disorders and Schizophrenia (Spitzer & Endicott, 1977). On the basis of these screening procedures, certain families were not considered eligible for the study. In addition to the basic requirements (i.e., husband meets appropriate diagnosis, family has been together for five years, and there is a child between the ages of 10 and 18 residing in the home), the families had to meet the following criteria: the husband did not meet criteria for any other diagnosis except for the diagnosis of interest (a small number of alcoholics reported a depression secondary to their alcoholism and were included in the study); the wife did not meet criteria for any current major diagnosis; no medications, medical conditions, or other condition prevented the husband and the wife from participating in an experimental drinking situation (obviously, if the husband or the wife were abstainers, they were not eligible); and neither the husband, the wife, nor the participating child was currently in treatment. The purpose of these strict inclusion and exclusion criteria was to form a relatively homogeneous group of families in which father's diagnosis of alcoholism (or depression) was uncomplicated by other psychopathologies and in which the family dynamics would not be influenced by any current treatment interventions.

Each member of the participating families completed a vast array of self-report questionnaires concerning himself/herself and his/her view of the family and of family problems. Specifically, the mother and father were assessed with the Marlatt Drinking Profile (Marlatt, 1976), the Locke–Wallace Marital Adjustment Test (Locke & Wallace, 1959), the Dyadic Adjustment Scale (Spanier, 1976), the Minnesota Multiphasic Personality Inventory (MMPI) (Dahlstrom & Welsh, 1960), the Michigan Alcoholism Screening Test (Selzer, 1971), the Beck Depression Inventory (BDI) (Beck, Ward, Mendelson, Mock, & Erbaugh, 1961), and a variety of other questionnaires tapping relevant elements of sociodemographic, alcohol consumption and problems, and individual difference factors. The child also completed a self-report questionnaire that assessed a variety of constructs viewed as relevant for this age group. Both the parents and the child completed the Revealed Difference Test (RDT) (Bodin, 1966) and the Area of

Change Questionnaire (ACQ) (Weiss, Hops, & Patterson, 1973) (modified for parent-child relationships when necessary) with respect to the other two members of the family who were participating in the study. Thus, for example, the father completed the RDT and ACQ on both his wife and his adolescent child.

In addition to completing these self-report instruments, each family participated in a laboratory study of drinking and problem solving. On the basis of the RDT and the ACQ, conflict topics were chosen for each family combination (mother–father, mother–child, father–child, and mother–father–child). Subsequently, each combination interacted and was videotaped for approximately 20 minutes (10 minutes resolving differences on the RDT and 10 minutes discussing a conflict area relevant for that specific family combination). Each family engaged in the conflict resolution interactions on two different nights. On one of those nights, the family was provided with snacks and nonalcoholic beverages. On the other night, the mother and father were provided with their typical alcoholic beverage. The order of these alcohol versus no alcohol sessions was counterbalanced.

The videotaped discussions were rated by trained raters with an abbreviated version of the Marital Interaction Coding System (MICS) (Weiss, Patterson, & Hops, 1976). The abbreviated system contains 16 unique behavioral codes and several combination codes that reflect verbal and nonverbal behaviors. The trained raters were blind to the group status of the family, to the alcohol administration condition, and to the specific nature of the project. Each interaction was rated by one primary rater, and 25% were rated by a second rater to assess reliability. Across the 16 codes, the average interrater reliability was 72%. Three summary codes were utilized for analyses (Jacob & Krahn, 1987): positivity, negativity, and problem solving.

CHARACTERISTICS OF EPISODIC AND STEADY ALCOHOLICS

Given the great wealth of data collected within this study, we have been able to examine a variety of aspects concerning the family functioning of episodic and steady alcoholics. Of considerable importance is the fact that episodic and steady alcoholics, while comparable in numerous respects, differ from each other in several important ways in addition to their reported pattern of consumption. Although many of the differences only approached conventional levels of significance, nonetheless, these differences should caution against the conclusion that differences in family processes are solely the result of the differences in the pattern of drinking.

In terms of sociodemographic characteristics, episodic and steady alcoholics were quite similar. On the average, the alcoholics were 42 years old, and the wives were 39 years old. Given the requirements of residing in an intact family and having a child between the ages of 10 and 18 in the home, it should not be surprising that most of the couples had been married for a considerable length of time. Nearly all (94%) reported being married for 10 years or more, with the average length of time being 17 years. Despite the longevity of these marital relationships, a sizable proportion of the families were reconstituted (i.e., one or both of the partners had a previous marriage or entered into the marriage with a child from a previous relationship). This tended to be more common among the episodic alcoholics and their spouses (33%) than among steady alcoholics and their spouses (16%), though the difference was not significant. For the most part, the couples were drawn from the lower to middle socioeconomic levels, with most of the alcoholics and their wives completing high school (76%) but few completing college (6% of husbands and 2% of wives).

The marital functioning of episodic and steady alcoholics, as measured by the Locke–Wallace Marital Adjustment Test and the Dyadic Adjustment Scale, tended to be comparable. The average Locke-Wallace score for the alcoholic husbands was 89, while the average for the wives was significantly lower, 73, scores which are clearly indicative of marital distress. The difference between husbands' and wives' scores is significant for both groups and replicates a recent finding by O'Farrell and Birchler (1987). Of interest, despite the observed difference, was a significant correlation between the Locke–Wallace scores of episodic alcoholics and their wives ($r = .51$). Among steady alcoholics, there was no relationship between the marital satisfaction scores of the husbands and wives ($r = .02$). This pattern of findings was also observable with respect to the total Dyadic Adjustment scores.

Similarly, there were few differences between episodic and steady alcoholics or between their wives with respect to scores on the MMPI or on the Beck Depression Inventory. The primary difference of note was that episodic alcoholics scored significantly higher on scale 9 (mania) than did steady alcoholics (73 vs. 63). High scorers on scale 9 have been described as impulsive individuals. Further, the average profile for the episodic alcoholics was a 4–9–8, with all three scales elevated above 70. In contrast, the steady alcoholics were characterized by a 4–2 profile, with only scale 4 elevated above 70. The profile manifested by the episodic alcoholic is suggestive of a hostile, alienated, and impulsive individual, while the average profile of the steady alcoholics is suggestive of a passive dependent or inadequate personality. However, these descriptions must be considered rather tentative in view of the absence of significant differences on many of the MMPI scales. None of the MMPI scales differentiated episodic and steady wives from each other, and few wives from either group manifested significant elevations on any of the MMPI scales. (It should be recalled, however, that families in which wives had a current major disorder were not eligible for the study.)

Despite the relatively few differences between steady and episodic alcoholics with respect to sociodemographic, marital, and personality characteristics, they could be distinguished from each other with respect to drinking-related variables. Episodic alcoholics reported a lower average daily consumption of alcohol than did steady alcoholics. This finding is not particularly surprising in that steady alcoholics were defined on the basis of drinking roughly the same amount daily or nearly every day, while episodics were defined as drinking considerably less or nothing at all several days out of the week. Nonetheless, in light of the determination of episodic/ steady group membership from a single, self-report item, this finding lends support to the validity of the group classification.

Overall, the two groups evidenced the same degree of severity with regard to alcohol problems, as indicated by the absence of any significant group differences on the Michigan Alcoholism Screening Test (MAST). The average MAST score for the alcoholics was 24 (SD = 10; range = 6–42). There were also no differences on the medical consequence or control problem items of the Feighner criteria. However, episodic alcoholics endorsed more of the social consequence items and fewer of the prior identification items than did steady alcoholics. These differences can be seen also in terms of the specific alcohol problems endorsed by episodic and steady alcoholics. Episodic alcoholics were more likely to be involved in a fight and to have had an argument with a friend as a result of drinking during the preceding year than were steady alcoholics. They were also more likely to report missing work and skipping meals than were steady alcoholics. The episodic alcoholics were more likely to report that their father or mother was an alcoholic than were steady alcoholics, and the episodic alcoholics tended to report an earlier age of first intoxication.

In summary, the episodic alcoholics in our sample, relative to the steady alcoholics, could be characterized as impulsive (on the basis of the MMPI scale 9 differences), family history positive, early onset, and having more social problems associated with drinking, in particular, problems with hostility (fights and arguments). This description of the episodic alcoholic overlaps with other types of alcoholics. Male-limited has been characterized by an early onset and by alcoholism and criminality in the parents, as well as frequent fighting and arrests and high levels of impulsivity. However, Cloninger (1987) associates these characteristics with the inability to abstain, which seems more relevant to steady alcoholics than to episodic alcoholics. Family history positive alcoholics have been characterized as having an earlier onset of alcohol problems, more social and personal problems due to drinking, and greater hostility and aggression (McKenna & Pickens,

1981; Penick et al., 1978); more antisocial behavior (Frances, Timm, & Bucky, 1980); and more arrests (McKenna & Pickens, 1981; Penick et al., 1978). Differences in alcohol consumption patterns, however, have not been reported.

Early onset alcoholics tend to have a positive family history for alcoholism, higher hostility and greater emotional disturbance, and gamma alcoholism (e.g., short spells of abstinence between bouts, periodic intoxication, and social disorganization; Abelsohn & van der Spuy, 1978). Lee and DeClimente (1985) found that early onset alcoholics reported higher scores on the social role maladaptation, loss of control while drinking, and negative consequences subscales of the Alcohol Use Inventory and somewhat lower scores on the sustained drinking pattern scales. However, no differences were found regarding the family history of early and late onset alcoholics (possibly because of the very high rate of family positives in the sample).

Studies of alcoholics with an additional diagnosis of antisocial personality suggest that antisocial alcoholism is associated with an earlier onset of drinking and drinking problems, a bilineal alcoholism pedigree (alcoholism both in the mother's and the father's family), and higher levels of psychosocial problems associated with alcohol misuse. Interestingly, Cadoret, Troughton, and Widmer (1984) reported that antisocial alcoholics, relative to alcoholics without additional psychiatric diagnoses, are more likely to report drinking heavily in one day, blackouts, and binge drinking; an early age of first intoxication and first alcoholism symptom; more fighting while drinking; job problems; more symptoms of depression; and more *manic* symptoms (recall that our episodic alcoholics scored high on scale 9 of the MMPI, the Mania Scale).

Despite the minor inconsistencies which might be attributable to different sample characteristics, the studies considered together suggest that the episodic alcoholics whom we describe represent a more socially disruptive, impulsive, and hostile type of alcoholic, prone to instances of very heavy consumption and periods of relatively little consumption, and characterized by a family history of alcoholism and an early onset of drinking and drinking problems.

Although the characteristics of the episodic alcoholics correspond closely to other types of alcoholics described in the literature, the characteristics of steady alcoholics do not clearly correspond to other types. As noted above, these alcoholics manifested an average 4–2 MMPI profile, suggestive of a passive dependent or inadequate personality. They have a later onset of alcohol problems, few aggressive problems, relatively fewer social problems, and are less likely to report parental alcohol problems. In many regards, these alcoholics appear similar to the Type I or milieu-limited alcoholics described by Cloninger (1987). It is of interest that he too ascribes a passive dependent or anxious personality to this group of alcoholics.

ALCOHOL CONSUMPTION AND
MARITAL SATISFACTION

The possibility of different family processes among episodic and steady alcoholics was first suggested in a series of analyses conducted by Jacob, Dunn, and Leonard (1983). These analyses were based on 27 alcoholics who, at that time, had completed their participation in the family interaction study described above. The primary focus guiding these analyses was to explore the relationship between individual and family functioning, on the one hand, and different characteristics of alcoholism, on the other. Specifically, in this study and a second one (Jacob, Dunn, Leonard, & Davis, 1985), correlations were computed between husband's and wives' reports of individual functioning (MMPI and BDI) and marital functioning (Locke–Wallace MAT and Dyadic Adjustment Scale) and different parameters of drinking and drinking problems. In the Jacob et al. (1983) paper, the drinking variable of interest was the average daily alcohol consumption reported over the past 30 days. Several findings emerged from these analyses. First, husbands who reported drinking more in the preceding 30 days also reported better marital functioning and received marginally lower scores on several MMPI scales. Of considerably greater importance, a similar relationship was observed between the wife's individual and marital functioning and the husband's alcohol consumption. That is, husbands who reported higher levels of alcohol consumption had wives who reported somewhat better marital functioning, lower levels of depression, and received lower scores on several MMPI scales.

Although these findings were significant for the sample as a whole, the relationship between heavy alcohol consumption on the part of the husband and relatively better individual and marital functioning on the part of the wife was noticeably stronger and more pervasive among steady drinking alcoholics than among episodic alcoholics. Furthermore, for steady alcoholics, the correlation between the husband's drinking and the wife's functioning is considerably stronger than the relationship between the husband's drinking and his own functioning. As a result, it is difficult to make the argument that heavy drinking among the steady alcoholics enhanced their own individual functioning, and thereby enhanced the functioning of their spouses.

ALCOHOL CONSUMPTION AND THE MARITAL
INTERACTIONS OF EPISODIC
AND STEADY ALCOHOLICS

Although the observed relationship between alcohol consumption and spouse functioning did not appear to be mediated through the husband's functioning, it would be misleading to conclude that increases in alcohol consumption caused improved functioning on the part of the spouse. Given the cross-sectional nature of these results, it is plausible that wives who were less distressed by their husband's drinking were less likely to attempt to apply controls over his drinking. Additionally, it is possible that a variety of selective factors resulted in a large sample of steady and heavy drinking alcoholics with adaptive and healthy wives. Despite these cautions, the interesting interpretation is that for steady drinkers, alcohol consumption may be a stabilizing factor in the family. Thus, when the husband is drinking more, the functioning of the spouse is improved.

A key element of this hypothesis is that alcohol consumption, in contrast to the absence of alcohol, alters the marital and/or family interactions of steady alcoholics in such a way as to improve family functioning, but that the interactions of episodic alcoholics are altered in a different way, a way that would not be functional for the family. In our research, we have been able to address this issue by examining the impact of alcohol consumption on couples attempting to work toward resolution with respect to one of their reported areas of marital conflict. While this paradigm is clearly relevant to the assessment of improved marital interactions, it does not exhaust the possible ways in which alcohol could improve marital and family functioning. For example, an alcoholic who retreats to his bedroom when drinking, but is uncommunicative, depressive, or hostile when not drinking, might create a very dramatic improvement in family functioning while he is drinking by virtue of his absence from the family interactions. Clearly, these kinds of improvements will not be assessed by the problem solving interaction tasks. However, enhanced problem solving can be observed within this paradigm, and thus it represents an important tool in determining whether alcohol consumption improves marital interactions among steady alcoholics and their wives.

As noted earlier, couples in which the husband was an alcoholic, a depressive, or a normal control participated in two sets of family discussions, one with alcohol available and one with only nonalcoholic beverages available. Since the occurrence of these two conditions was counterbalanced, differences between drink and no-drink conditions could not be attributed to order effects. Each set of family discussions consisted of a husband–wife (father–mother), father–child, mother–child, and a father–mother–child combination. The order of these discussions was randomly assigned and counterbalanced across the alcoholic, depressed, and control groups, with the constraint that the father–mother–child interaction always occurred either first or last. In order to analyze these data for differences between episodic and steady alcoholics, Jacob and Leonard (1988) conducted analyses of variance for one between-group factor (episodic/steady) and two within-group factors (alcohol: drink vs. no-drink and member: husband vs. wife).

Several findings were of interest. First, since the alcoholics were allowed relatively free access to alcohol, it is of importance to determine whether episodic and steady alcoholics consumed comparable amounts of alcohol and achieved similar blood alcohol levels. Over the entire evening, the alcoholics consumed an average of 3.4 oz of ethanol, the equivalent of roughly seven standard size drinks, with no difference between episodic and steady alcoholics. The final blood alcohol level of the alcoholics was .075, with again no differences between episodic and steady alcoholics. Thus, any differences that we observe cannot be attributed to different amounts of alcohol or degrees of intoxication.

With regard to marital interaction behaviors, there was a significant interaction between group membership and alcohol consumption with respect to problem solving. Although tests for simple effects were not significant, the interaction appeared to indicate that episodic alcoholics decreased their problem solving from no-drink to drink night, while steady alcoholics increased their problem solving.

Additionally, there was a significant group-by-member interaction. This interaction suggested that among steady alcoholics, wives were more negative than husbands, while among episodic alcoholics, husbands were more negative than wives. This interaction should be considered in light of the group-by-condition-by-member interaction that approached significance. Two simple effects were significant; steady alcoholics were less negative than their wives on drink night and episodic alcoholics were more negative than their wives on drink night. Among steady alcoholics, both husbands and wives displayed a nonsignificant increase in negativity on drink night. Among episodic alcoholics, husbands also evidenced a nonsignificant increase, while wives actually decreased in negativity on drink night (Figure 8.1).

The differential patterns of responsiveness to alcohol on the part of the steady and episodic alcoholics suggested somewhat different processes. Among the episodic alcoholics, the presence of alcohol in the interaction led to an increase in negativity on the part of the husband and an overall decline in the problem solving behaviors of the couple. This suggested a coercive control process, whereby the husband's negativity may have prevented active problem solving. In contrast, steady alcoholics and their wives both increased their negativity and increased their problem solving, suggesting that the negativity may have emerged from a more intense problem solving style.

In order to more fully describe these interactional differences, the behaviors comprising negativity were examined more closely. Although three of the behaviors, criticize, put-down, and negative response, were strongly suggestive of negativity, one behavior, disagree, did not seem particularly negative. In fact, Jacob and Krahn (1987) indicate that not all coding systems view disagree as negative. Furthermore, at least in males, the disagree

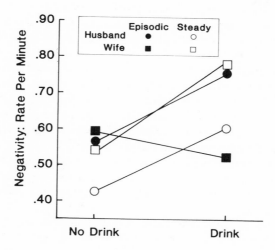

FIGURE 8.1. Negativity as a function of episodic/steady group, condition, and member. From Jacob and Leonard (1988). Copyright 1988 by the American Psychological Association. Reprinted by permission.

code loaded on several different factors, including negativity, positivity, and problem solving. Further evidence for the differentiation of hostility and disagree codes can be seen by examining the intercorrelations of these codes within the control, steady alcoholic, and episodic alcoholic samples. Among control and steady alcoholic couples, the husband's level of hostility was unrelated to his rate of disagree on no-drink night, while this relationship was marginally significant among episodic alcoholics ($r = .36$). On drink night husband hostility was unrelated to husband disagree for steady alcoholic couples ($r = .04$), was moderately correlated for control men ($r = .39$), and was strongly associated among episodic men ($r = .63$). Among wives, there tended to be a significant correlation between her hostility and disagree for both drink and no-drink night. However, as with the husbands, the association between wife hostility and wife disagree was much stronger among episodic wives on drink night ($r = .86$). When the correlations between husband and wife behaviors are examined, the distinction between disagree and hostility is further supported. Except for episodic alcoholics on drink night, husband hostility and wife disagree tended to be unrelated, as did husband disagree and wife hostility. In contrast, there tended to be uniformly strong correlations between husband hostility and wife hostility and between husband disagree and wife disagree. Preliminary sequential analyses using log-linear procedures suggested that couples tended to reciprocate hostility with hostility and disagree with disagree. Hostility, however, was not more likely to follow a disagree than would be expected on the basis of base rate behavior, nor was disagree more likely to follow hostility.

Reanalyses of the episodic and steady alcoholic interactions were conducted on the hostility codes. According to these analyses, there was a significant group-by-condition-by-member interaction. This interaction was largely comparable to the interaction described above for negativity. That is, episodic husbands increased their hostility from no-drink to drink night, while their wives tended to decrease their hostility. Among steady alcoholic couples, both husbands and wives tended to increase their hostility from no-drink to drink night. As a result of these analyses, hostility, independent of disagreement, was viewed as a potentially important code to investigate in further analyses.

The above analyses are suggestive of differential problem solving processes as a function of the episodic/steady dimension and alcohol administration. Since the analyses focus on the frequencies of different behaviors, we can conclude only that episodic and steady couples behave differently when drinking than when sober. Whether the sequential structure of marital interactions differs between episodic and steady alcoholics or is influenced by the alcohol administration is not addressed in these analyses. Log-linear analyses examining the sequences of behavior in marital interactions are currently in progress, and some preliminary results concerning the episodic/steady dimension, alcohol administration, and sequential interactions are available.

Log-linear modeling techniques predict the natural logs of cell frequencies of multiway contingency tables from the classification variables that were utilized to construct the table. Cell frequencies may be predictable from main effects in a classification variable (e.g., differential proportions for the various levels of the variable) or from interactions between two or more variables. Two-way interactions indicate that the cell frequencies are predicted by the joint influence of two variables, after controlling for the marginal frequencies of the two variables. In the present set of analyses, two multiway tables were constructed, one representing only husband $\longrightarrow$ wife sequences of behavior, and the other representing wife $\longrightarrow$ husband sequences. At present, we have examined only one specific sequence, hostile reciprocity. Variables utilized to construct the multiway tables were: antecedent behavior (hostility, other behavior), consequent behavior (hostility, other behavior), condition (no-drink night, drink night), group (episodic, steady, control), and which half of the interaction (first or second).

For both tables, assessment of effects proceeded in a hierarchical fashion, with the assessment of an interaction controlling for all of the main effects and lower order interactions implicit in that interaction. These preliminary analyses contrasted episodic with control couples and steady with control

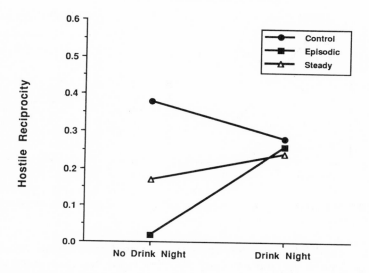

FIGURE 8.2. Husband hostile reciprocity as a function of group and condition.

couples. Finally, although there are numerous effects which are tested in log-linear models, our current presentation will be restricted to those indicating a sequential structure, which differs as a function of episodic/steady group membership.

In the wife–husband sequences, after controlling for the main effects and two-way associations, there was a significant four-way interaction, indicating that the antecedent–consequence structure was different as a function of drink condition and group membership.

The parameters indicating the strength of husbands' hostile reciprocity are displayed as a function of group and drink condition in Figure 8.2. As can be seen in this figure, control husbands were less likely to reciprocate hostility on drink night than on no-drink night. In contrast, episodic husbands dramatically increased their hostile reciprocity on drink night. Steady alcoholic husbands only slightly increased their hostile reciprocity on drink night.

In the analysis of wife ⟶ husband sequences, there was a highly significant five-way interaction involving antecedent, consequence, group, drink condition, and interaction half. This interaction indicates that wives' hostile reciprocity differed as a function of group, drink, and the interaction half. Control wives exhibited a moderate level of reciprocity and did not alter their hostile reciprocity as a function of drink condition or interaction half. As displayed in Figure 8.3, among episodic wives, hostile reciprocity increased over the interaction on no-drink night and decreased over the in-

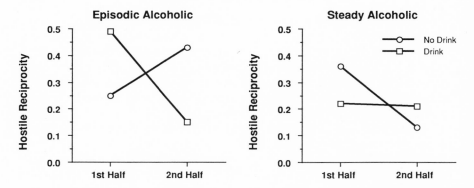

FIGURE 8.3. Wife hostile reciprocity as a function of group, condition, and interaction half.

teraction on drink night. Steady wives decreased their hostile reciprocity over the time of the interaction on no-drink night, but maintained a similar level of reciprocity over the interaction on drink night.

DISCUSSION

Overall marital adjustment, as reflected in self-report scales, did not differentiate between episodic and steady alcoholics or their spouses. However, more detailed analysis of episodic and steady alcoholics reveals a variety of differences in marital processes. Importantly, these processes also appear to be influenced by alcohol consumption and, therefore, may have implications for the continuation versus cessation of abusive drinking in these couples.

Among episodic alcoholics, there is evidence of a shift in the power in the relationship when drinking occurs. This shift may be brought about by the increased hostility on the part of the alcoholic husband and may reflect a coercive control process. There are several different lines of evidence which support this model. First, in the Jacob and Leonard (1988) study, episodic alcoholics increased their negativity from no-drink to drink night. Wives of these men slightly decreased their negativity on drink night. Concurrently, the episodic couples reduced their attempts at problem solving on drink versus no-drink night. Although these analyses are not sequential, the results are suggestive of a process whereby husband negativity on drink night suppresses wife negativity and suppresses both husband and wife problem solving. Initial sequential analyses have explored the first aspect of this issue, the relationship between husband and wife hostility. In the absence of alcohol, episodic alcoholics manifested no hostile reciprocity. Over the course of the no-drink interaction, wives of episodic alcoholics increased the level of their hostile reciprocity. This could be interpreted to suggest that as the wives realized that their husbands were not reciprocating their hostility, they felt safe to reciprocate his hostility. On drink night, episodic alcoholics increased their level of hostile reciprocity, although the level did not differ from steady alcoholic or control husbands on drink night. Wives of episodic alcoholics again altered their hostile reciprocity over the course of the interaction. However, they decreased their reciprocity dramatically, suggesting that as their husbands began to reciprocate, the wives inhibited their hostile reciprocity.

Among steady alcoholics, the findings suggest a somewhat different picture. The cross-sectional relationship between husband's drinking and wife's marital satisfaction and depression suggested that the more the husband was drinking, the more maritally satisfied and less depressed was the wife. In the analysis of frequencies of behavior, both husbands and wives increased their negativity and their hostility from no-drink to drink night. However, steady wives were more negative than their husbands on both drink night and no-drink night. Moreover, this increased negativity was accompanied by increased problem solving behaviors. The sequential analyses suggested that the husband's hostile reciprocity was moderate and did not change from no-drink to drink night. Wives of steady alcoholics decreased their hostile reciprocity over the course of the interaction on no-drink night. There are a variety of potential explanations for this. Given the low level of husband negativity and moderate level of hostile reciprocity on no-drink night, it does not seem likely that his hostility inhibited his wife's hostile reciprocity as the interaction proceeded. Perhaps her initial level of hostile reciprocity represented an attempt to get him more involved in the problem solving task. Her reduction in hostile reciprocity may have been a response to the failure of the reciprocity to get her husband involved. On drink night, when there was an increase in negativity and problem solving, the wives of the steady drinking alcoholics manifested a moderate level of hostile reciprocity and did not change over the interaction. Although this is somewhat speculative at this point, one possible interpretation is that problem solving activities in these couples are energized when the husband has been drinking. Given this activation, it may not have been necessary for the wife to utilize hostile reciprocity to involve her husband.

As noted previously, there is some overlap between the episodic/steady dimension and other alcoholism subtypes. Specifically, episodic alcoholics appear to be more socially disruptive, impulsive, and hostile, and are more likely to have a positive family history of alcoholism. The characteristics of the steady alcoholics were less clear, though there is the suggestion of a passive dependent or inadequate individual. As a result, there may be different kinds of alcoholics manifesting different drinking patterns and different marital processes while drinking. At this point, the chain of causality is unclear. Our original hypothesis was that the drinking patterns, by virtue of the differential ease with which they could be incorporated into family life, would lead to differential marital processes. However, it is possible that differential responses to alcohol by different types of alcoholics could lead to different marital processes, and that families in which the drinking style of the alcoholic and the family reaction to the drinking "fit" are more likely to remain intact than families in which there is a lack of "fit." For example, a marriage in which the husband's response to alcohol consumption is heightened hostility and coercion may be unlikely to survive if the husband drinks steadily. However, if he drinks on occasion, the family may be better able to compartmentalize his hostile behavior. Similarly, a passive-dependent alcoholic who is able to effectively interact with his spouse only while drinking may develop a steady drinking pattern, and his family may be able to adapt to this pattern. Longitudinal studies of alcohol use in developing families are necessary to address these issues.

Aside from the development of these marital interaction differences, it is of importance to determine whether these processes are adaptive to the family and whether they have an impact on the continued drinking of the alcoholic. Among the episodic alcoholics, drinking may be adaptive for the family by allowing the alcoholic to express relationship dissatisfactions that otherwise might not be expressed. Alternatively, this process may not be adaptive to the family at all, but may serve a positive function for the alcoholic—the suppression of problem solving attempts by his spouse. Among steady alcoholics, drinking may energize the alcoholic's problem solving attempts, and, despite the accompanying negativity, this may be of considerable importance to the continued marital functioning. Further research tying these marital processes to marital and drinking outcomes is currently under way and will hopefully begin to address the ways in which alcohol consumption is adaptive as opposed to destructive to the marriage and family.

Acknowledgment. Portions of this work were supported by Grant No. R01AA03037 to Theodore Jacob from the National Institute on Alcohol Abuse and Alcoholism.

REFERENCES

Abelsohn, D. S., & Van der Spuy, H. I. J. (1978). The age variable in alcoholism. *Journal of Studies on Alcohol, 39,* 800–808.

Babor, T. F., & Lauerman, R. J. (1986). Classification and forms of inebriety historical antecedents of alcoholic typologies. In M. Galanter (Ed.), *Recent developments in alcoholism,* Vol. 4 (pp. 113–144). New York: Plenum.

Beck, A., Ward, C., Mendelson, M., Mock, J., & Erbaugh, J. (1961). An inventory for measuring depression. *Archives of General Psychiatry, 4,* 53–63.

Billings, A. G., Kessler, M., Gomberg, C. A., & Weiner, S. (1979). Marital conflict resolution of alcoholic and nonalcoholic couples during sobriety and experimental drinking. *Journal of Studies on Alcohol, 40,* 183–195.

Bodin, A. (1966). Family interaction, coalitions, disagreement, and compromise in problem, normal and synthetic family triads. Unpublished doctoral dissertation, State University of New York at Buffalo. (University Microfilms No. 66-7960)

Cadoret, R., Troughton, E., & Widmer, R. (1984). Clinical differences between antisocial and primary alcoholics. *Comprehensive Psychiatry, 25,* 1–8.

Cloninger, C., Bohman, M., & Sigvardson, S. (1981). Inheritance of alcohol abuse: Cross-fostering analysis of adopted men. *Archives of General Psychiatry, 38,* 861–868.

Cloninger, C. R. (1987). A systematic method for clinical description and classification of personality variants. *Archives of General Psychiatry, 44,* 573–588.

Connors, G. J., Tarbox, A. R., & McLaughlin, E. J. (1986). Contrasting binge and continuous alcoholic drinkers using demographic and drinking history variables. *Alcohol and Alcoholism, 21,* 105–110.

Dahlstrom, W. G., & Welsh, G. S. (1960). *An MMPI handbook.* Minneapolis: University of Minnesota Press.

Davis, D. I., Berenson, D., Steinglass, P., & Davis, S. (1974). The adaptive consequences of drinking. *Psychiatry, 37,* 209–215.

Frances, R. J., Timm, S., & Bucky, S. (1980). Studies of familial and nonfamilial alcoholism. I. Demographic studies. *Archives of General Psychiatry, 37,* 564–566.

Frankenstein, W., Hay, W. M., & Nathan, P. E. (1985). Effects of intoxication on alcoholics' marital communication and problem solving. *Journal of Studies on Alcohol, 46,* 1–6.

Frankenstein, W., Nathan, P. E., Hay, W. M., Sullivan, R. F., & Cocco, K. (1985). A symmetry of influence in alcoholics' marital communication: Alcohol's effects on interaction dominance. *Journal of Marital and Family Therapy, 11,* 399–410.

Hesselbrock, V. M., Hesselbrock, M. W., & Stabenau, J. R. (1985). Alcoholism in men patients subtyped by family history and antisocial personality. *Journal of Studies on Alcohol, 46,* 59–64.

Jacob, T., Dunn, N., & Leonard, K. (1983). Patterns of alcohol abuse and family stability. *Alcoholism: Clinical and Experimental Research, 7,* 382–385.

Jacob, T., Dunn, N. J., Leonard, K. E., & Davis, P. (1985). Relationship between alcoholism and psychiatric symptoms of spouse: An attempt to replicate. *American Journal of Drug and Alcohol Abuse, 11,* 55–67.

Jacob, T., & Krahn, G. (1987). The classification of behavioral observation codes in studies of family interaction. *Journal of Marriage and the Family, 49,* 677–687.

Jacob, T., & Krahn, G. L. (1988). Marital interaction of alcoholic couples: Comparison with depressed and nondistressed couples. *Journal of Consulting and Clinical Psychology, 56,* 73–79.

Jacob, T., & Leonard, K. E. (1988). Alcoholic-spouse interaction as a function of alcoholism subtype and alcohol consumption interaction. *Journal of Abnormal Psychology, 97,* 232–237.

Jacob, T., Ritchey, D., Cvitkovic, J. F., & Blane, H. T. (1981). Communication styles of alcoholic and nonalcoholic families when drinking and not drinking. *Journal of Studies on Alcohol, 42,* 466–482.

Lee, G. P., & DiClimente, C. C. (1985). Age of onset versus duration of problem drinking on the Alcohol Use Inventory. *Journal of Studies on Alcohol, 46,* 398–402.

Locke, H., & Wallace, K. (1959). Short marital adjustment and prediction tests: Their reliability and validity. *Marriage and Family Living, 21,* 251–255.

MacAndrew, C. (1981). What the MAC scale tells us about men alcoholics. *Journal of Studies on Alcohol, 42,* 604–625.

Marlatt, A. (1976). The drinking profile: A questionnaire for the behavorial assessment of alcoholism. In E. Mash & L. Terdal (Eds.), *Behavior therapy assessment: Diagnosis, design and evaluation* (pp. 121–137). New York: Springer Publishing Co.

McKenna, T., & Pickens, R. (1981). Alcoholic children of alcoholics. *Journal of Studies on Alcohol, 42,* 1021–1029.

Morey, L. C., Skinner, H. A., & Blashfield, R. K. (1984). A typology of alcohol abusers: Correlates and implications. *Journal of Abnormal Psychology, 93,* 408–417.

O'Farrell, T. J., & Birchler, G. R. (1987). Marital relationships of alcoholic, conflicted, and nonconflicted couples. *Journal of Marital and Family Therapy, 13,* 259–274.

Penick, E., Read, M., Crowley, P., & Powell, B. (1978). Differentiation of alcoholics by family history. *Journal of Studies on Alcohol, 39,* 1944–1948.

Roberts, M. C., Floyd, F. J., O'Farrell, T. J., & Cutter, H. S. G. (1985). Marital interactions and the duration of alcoholic husbands' sobriety. *American Journal of Drug and Alcohol Abuse, 11,* 303–313.

Rudie, R. R., & McGaughran, L. S. (1961). Differences in developmental experience defensiveness, and personality organization between two classes of problem drinkers. *Journal of Abnormal Psychology, 62,* 659–665.

Sanchez-Craig, M. (1980). Drinking pattern as a determinant of alcoholics' performance on the trail-making test. *Journal of Studies on Alcohol, 41,* 1082–1090.

Selzer, M. (1971). Michigan Alcoholism Screening Test: The quest for a new diagnostic instrument. *American Journal of Psychiatry, 127,* 1653–1658.

Spanier, G. (1976). Measuring dyadic adjustment: New scales for assessing the quality of marriage and similar dyads. *Journal of Marriage and the Family, 38,* 15–30.

Spitzer, R. L. & Endicott, J. (1977). Schedule for Affective Disorders and Schizophrenia—Lifetime version. New York: New York State Psychiatric Institute, Biometrics Research.

Steinglass, P. (1979). The alcoholic family in the interaction laboratory. *The Journal of Nervous and Mental Disease, 167,* 428–436.

Steinglass, P. (1981). The alcoholic family at home: Patterns of interaction in dry, wet and transitional stages of alcoholism. *Archives of General Psychiatry, 38,* 578–584.

Steinglass, P., Bennett, L., Wolin, S., & Reiss, D. (1987). *The alcoholic family.* New York: Basic Books.

Steinglass, P., Davis, D. I., & Berenson, D. (1977). Observations of conjointly hospitalized "alcoholic couples" during sobriety and intoxication: Implications for theory and therapy. *Family Process, 16,* 1–16.

Steinglass, P., & Robertson, A. (1983). The alcoholic family. In B. Kissin & H. Begleiter (Eds.), *The biology of alcoholism: Vol. 6. The pathogenesis of alcoholism: Psychosocial factors* (pp. 243–307). New York: Plenum.

Tomsovic, M. (1974). 'Binge' and continuous drinkers: Characteristics and treatment follow-up. *Quarterly Journal of Studies on Alcohol, 35,* 558–564.

Weiss, R., Hops, H., & Patterson, G. (1973). A framework for conceptualizing marital conflict, a technology for altering it, some data for evaluating it. In R. W. Clark & L. A. Hamerlynck (Eds.), *Critical issues in research and practice: Proceedings of the Fourth Banff International Conference on Behavior Modification* (pp. 309–342). Champaign, IL: Research Press.

Weiss, R., Patterson, G., & Hops, H. (1976). Marital interaction coding system. Unpublished manuscript. University of Oregon.

Zucker, R. A. (1986). The four alcoholisms: A developmental account of the etiologic process. In P. C. Rivers (Ed.), *Nebraska symposium on motivation, 34, Alcohol and addictive behavior.* Lincoln, NE: University of Nebraska Press.

9

Sexual Functioning of Male Alcoholics

TIMOTHY J. O'FARRELL

Historically, Shakespeare summarized our knowledge about the behavioral effects of alcohol, presumably for both alcoholic and nonalcoholic males, with the statement in *Macbeth* that "drink . . . provokes the desire but mars the performance." Silvestrini (1926) summarized some of the physiological effects of prolonged alcohol abuse when he described the frequent occurrences of impotence, testicular atrophy, and gynecomastia in patients with alcoholic cirrhosis and speculated that these symptoms resulted from changes in the metabolism of sex hormones.

Literature on the relationship between alcohol and human sexual behavior has grown considerably in recent years (O'Farrell, Thompson, & Weyand, 1986) and a number of compilations and reviews of this literature have appeared (e.g., O'Farrell, Weyand, & Logan, 1983; Wilson, 1977). As a result of this growing interest, some preliminary information about the nature and extent, possible causes, and course over time of male alcoholics' sexual problems has begun to appear in the literature. This chapter provides a detailed review of the literature on *male* alcoholics' sexual adjustment problems with the goal of summarizing current knowledge and suggesting needed future research.

NATURE AND EXTENT OF MALE ALCOHOLICS' SEXUAL ADJUSTMENT PROBLEMS

Over 20 reports from 10 countries have indicated that a substantial proportion of male alcoholics seen in treatment settings have sexual adjustment problems. Averaging together the results of the various studies indicates that nearly 60% of alcoholics experience at least one sexual dysfunction, with lowered libido and erection difficulties, both of which average a 40%

prevalence rate, being the most frequently reported problems.* Although these average figures should be interpreted cautiously since definitions, criteria, and prevalence vary considerably across studies, they are much higher than the 2% general population prevalence rate for impotence (at age 40) reported by Kinsey, Pomeroy, Martin, and Gebhard (1948).

Studies that included comparison group data strengthen the conclusion of a heightened prevalence of sexual adjustment problems among alcoholics (e.g., Jensen, 1984; Tan, Johnson, Lambie, Vijayasenan, & Whiteside, 1984; Whalley, 1978). Most studies compare alcoholics to normal controls without major medical, psychiatric, or marital problems. Such studies find that alcoholics uniformly show greater prevalence of dysfunctions, greater impotence as determined both by self-report and by nocturnal erection studies, lower frequency of sexual intercourse, and less sexual satisfaction. Lowered libido is greater among alcoholics than in normals in some but not all studies depending on sample characteristics (e.g., age, partner available or not) and on how lessened sexual desire is defined (e.g. intercourse vs. masturbation frequency).

POSSIBLE CAUSES OF ALCOHOLICS' SEXUAL PROBLEMS

Although many alcoholics have sexual problems—some of them serious enough to be classified as sexual dysfunctions—not all alcoholics have such problems. Relatively little is known about what factors differentiate alcoholics who have sexual difficulties from those who do not. A variety of plausible explanations for alcoholics' sexual difficulties have been proposed. These explanations are presented and evaluated in this section.

Physical Causes of Alcoholics' Sexual Problems

Pharmacological Effects

A large body of literature in both human and animal experiments (see Wilson, 1977, 1981 for reviews) shows that acute alcohol intake beyond very low doses decreases potency and increases time to ejaculation in direct relation to the amount of alcohol consumed. The precise relationship of these laboratory findings to clinical samples of alcoholics is unclear. One question has to do with individual differences in tolerance for alcohol and in particular the acquisition of increased behavioral tolerance that is often

---

*A table is available on request from the author that summarizes these 22 studies including sample description; percentage of sample experiencing lowered libido, erection difficulties, premature ejaculation, retarded ejaculation, and at least one dysfunction; and criteria and definitions of dysfunction used.

considered diagnostic of alcoholism. Perhaps alcoholics and those developing an alcoholism problem do not suffer the same impairment in sexual function as nonalcoholics at similar dose levels of alcohol consumption. Such basic research questions have not been studied. Alcoholics in clinical settings report retrospectively an association between higher amounts of alcohol consumed and greater extent of sexual dysfunction, generally impotence and delayed or impaired ejaculation (e.g., Fahrner, 1987; Jensen, 1979; Mandell & Miller, 1983). These reports are consistent with experimental studies of alcohol's acute negative effects on sexual functioning. However, the fact that sizable subgroups of patients in these and other studies (e.g., Van Thiel, Gavaler, & Sanghir, 1982) reported that dysfunction was independent of amount consumed and continued despite reduced consumption makes it clear that factors in addition to alcohol's acute pharmacological effects are responsible for the maintenance of alcoholics' sexual dysfunctions. Finally, in such retrospective clinical investigations, alcohol's acute negative effects on sexual functioning cannot be evaluated separately from chronic effects due to other physical factors such as neurological and hormonal consequences and/or to psychosocial factors.

Neurological Effects

Human penile erection involves the peripheral and central nervous systems. According to Wagner and Jensen (1981), alcoholic polyneuropathy is a well-known complication in chronic alcoholics, mainly affecting the somatic peripheral nerves. They further state that disturbances of erection as well as ejaculation are to be expected, and that studies (presumably of patients in their clinical practice) of the reflexes necessary for erection such as bulbocavernosus reflex have shown these to be affected. Others (Duncan, Johnson, Lambie, & Whiteside, 1980; Tan et al, 1984) have indicated that alcoholics who had damage to the brain and to peripheral nerves also showed autonomic nervous system abnormalities, specifically with the vagal nerve. They speculated that sacral nerves, also part of the autonomic nervous system and necessary for erection, might be impaired and contribute to impotence in alcoholics. Alcoholic dementia, caused by diffuse central nervous system impairment, also may contribute to sexual problems. Alcoholic dementia even in its milder manifestations may reduce the alcoholic's ability to understand the fine nuances in the dyadic relationship and possibly in the sexual relationship also, thus creating emotional consequences that decrease the likelihood of satisfactory sex (Jensen, Gluud, & Copenhagen Study Group, 1985).

What evidence supports the often cited (e.g., Lemere & Smith, 1973; Snyder & Karacan, 1981; Wagner & Jensen, 1981) connection of neurological damage with alcoholics' potency problems? Only two studies located by this reviewer present data on this question. The first study by Tan et al. (1984) found more evidence of neurological damage including CNS damage, peripheral neuropathy, and evidence of damage to the parasympathetic nervous system among six impotent alcoholics whose nocturnal penile tumescence (NPT) results indicated a likely organic etiology for their impotence than did seven alcoholics with NPT-diagnosed psychogenic impotence. Tan et al. recommended that further studies to compare the frequencies of neurological abnormalities in alcoholic patients with and without impotence are required to determine whether these abnormalities may have a causal role in alcoholic impotence. The second study by Jensen et al. (1985) of 18 men with alcoholic cirrhosis found the sexually dysfunctional men did not experience significantly more neurological abnormalities than those without dysfunction. As Jensen cautions, the small sample may have precluded detecting significant effects. In addition, the sexually dysfunctional group was not homogeneous with respect to type or likely cause (psychogenic vs. organic) of dysfunction since it contained both erectile and other dysfunctions and the impotence cases had not been screened by NPT or other methods into those likely to have an organic etiology.

Vascular Effects

Adequate blood supply to the penis is necessary for erection. Wincze (1988) indicates that epidemiological studies show alcoholics to have a higher prevalence of hypertension, and hypertensives are a group with increased impotence. In these studies, however, no relationship was found between alcoholism and atherosclerosis of the aorta or peripheral vessels. Vascular impairment as a factor affecting alcoholics' impotence has not been studied systematically, and few would argue a vascular basis as a primary etiology for alcoholics' impotence. Nonetheless, it seems plausible that vascular causes may contribute to some cases of impotence in alcoholics and that this should be evaluated clinically with alcoholics who complain of impotence, as is done with other impotent patients.

Hormonal and Endocrine Effects

Alcohol-induced changes in sex hormone levels have been well studied. Acute and chronic alcohol ingestion reduces the level of serum testosterone in men. A great deal of clinical and laboratory investigation has shed light on the biochemical mechanisms involved in the alcohol-induced reductions in testosterone. Cicero (1983) sees the acute and chronic depression of testosterone levels of males as resulting from direct effects of alcohol on the pituitary gland and the testes as well as from degradation of male sex hormones in the liver. Thus, as Van Thiel and Chaiao (1983) have noted, alcohol affects testosterone levels through actions at three sites: the brain, the testes, and the liver. First, alcohol seems to damage areas of the hypothalamus and pituitary that control the function of the testes. The hypothalamus produces a series of hormones, or peptides, that stimulate the pituitary which, in turn, releases two hormones (LH, luteinizing hormone, and FSH, follicle-stimulating hormone). In males, these two hormones stimulate the testes to produce testosterone and sperm. Second, alcohol directly damages testicular tissue. Histologic examination showed that the seminiferous tubules were diminished in diameter. Furthermore, the Leydig cells, which are necessary for secretion of testosterone, the principal male hormone, appear to suffer direct damage (Gavaler & Van Thiel, 1982; Van Thiel, 1985). Third, alcohol-induced liver dysfunction compounds the hormonal decrements produced by alcohol to the hypothalamic–pituitary–gonadal axis and to the testes. Alcohol intake contributes to a greater rate of testosterone catabolism in the liver and in cirrhosis the level of female sex hormone increases. Thus cirrhosis patients show the most severe "feminizing" effects including enlargement of mammary glands (gynecomastia), reduction in muscle and increase in fat, reduction in size of testicles (testicular atrophy/hypogonadism), and changes in the pattern of pubic hair to a female distribution.

Hormonal changes caused by excessive alcohol consumption have been well-studied as described above. However, as Wincze (1988) has noted, the correlation between measured hormonal levels and sexual problems of alcoholics has been less well-studied. Tan et al. (1984) found higher elevated plasma concentrations of FSH and LH among 6 organically (NPT) impotent alcoholics than among 7 psychogenically (NPT) impotent alcoholics but did not find differences in prolactin and testosterone levels. Van Thiel et al. (1982) reported that among 60 impotent alcoholics, those who spontaneously recovered potency after 9–12 months' abstinence showed normal gonadotropin responses to LH releasing factor, or clomiphene, or both and normal testicle size (i.e., not abnormally decreased in size). Further, large doses of hormone replacement produced improved potency in many of those who did not show a spontaneous recovery. Cornely, Schade, Van Thiel, and Gavaler (1984) found both greater hormonal abnormalities and greater prevalence, duration, frequency, and severity of impotence in alcoholics as compared to nonalcoholic cirrhotic patients. Finally, two studies found no correlation between hormone levels and dysfunction. Fahrner (1987) reported that chronic alcoholics with a high prevalence of sexual dysfunction had normal levels of testosterone and Jensen et al. (1985) found no differences in testosterone levels between alcoholic cirrhosis cases with and without sexual dysfunction. However, these two studies failed to evaluate hormones other than testosterone and they included a variety of sexual dysfunctions, not just impotence.

Medical Diseases

The presence among alcoholics of medical diseases that may cause sexual problems is another physical factor to be considered. Wincze (1988) indicates that epidemiological studies show alcoholics to have a higher prevalence of hypertension, and hypertensives are a group with increased impotence. Diabetics also have increased prevalence of alcoholism and of impotence (Renshaw, 1975). Liver disease including alcoholic cirrhosis has been the disease most widely studied in relation to alcoholics' sexual dysfunction. Silvestrini (1926) was among the first to describe the frequent occurrence of impotence in patients with alcoholic cirrhosis. Until fairly recently the impotence was presumed to be caused by changes in the metabolism of sex hormones secondary to the liver disease. Currently, the findings of a number of studies question the primary role of the liver disease and ascribe greater importance to the direct effects of the chronic excessive drinking as the cause of both the cirrhosis and the hormonal abnormalities related to the impotence. Van Thiel et al. (1982) found no correlation between the severity of liver disease and the chance of a spontaneous recovery of adequate sexual functioning among impotent alcoholics. Cornely et al. (1984) found greater prevalence and severity of impotence as well as more severe sex hormone abnormalities in alcoholic cirrhosis patients than in patients with cirrhosis without an alcoholic basis. Jensen et al. (1985) found a similar extent of sexual dysfunction in alcoholics with and without cirrhosis. Further, alcoholic cirrhosis patients with sexual dysfunction did not differ in severity of liver disease from those without dysfunction in the Jensen et al. (1985) study.

To understand better the role of physical factors, both cross-sectional and longitudinal studies with larger samples are needed. Cross-sectional studies should include careful quantitative measurements of alcohol consumption, neurological, hormonal, and vascular parameters, as well as the extent of liver disease. Potent and impotent alcoholics could be compared with the latter further subdivided by NPT into presumed organic and psychogenic cases. Longitudinal studies could measure the same variables periodically and track these same subgroups of patients over time to provide a better understanding of the relationships among the physical parameters and changes in the alcoholic's sexual functioning.

Psychosocial Causes of Alcoholics' Sexual Problems

Psychological Factors

Sexual function is highly influenced by intrapsychic factors. *Performance anxiety* in males is a strong distractor of sexual concentration and can interfere with sexual behavior. Persons who have experienced erectile failures in the past may precipitate additional episodes of impotence by worrying about their potency (Masters & Johnson, 1966, 1970). Masters and Johnson (1970) reported that secondary impotence developing in a male in his late forties or early fifties has a higher incidence of direct association with excessive alcohol consumption than with any other single factor. When a man is traumatized by the inability to achieve or to maintain an erection while under the influence of alcohol he frequently develops major concerns for sexual performance and rarely associates his initial disability with its direct cause. They further (Masters & Johnson, 1970) indicated that alcohol is the second most frequent cause of impotence. For alcoholics who have been impotent when drinking heavily, sobriety may result in performance anxiety about the possible recurrence of impotence. This anxiety may lead to avoidance of and loss of desire for sex and, if they attempt sexual intercourse, may produce the impotence they fear. Alcoholics who after starting sobriety try to "have a few drinks" to reduce their performance anxiety often are unable to limit their alcohol intake and suffer alcohol-induced impotence as a recurring phenomenon. Social anxiety or phobia may interfere with sexual arousal or performance as well. Hence, persons who lack a basic sense of sexual or interpersonal self-confidence in relation to their partners may experience episodes of sexual dysfunction that are induced by anxiety. Persons who drink heavily during sexual episodes may experience a pharmacologically induced impotence. For alcoholic males who drink to assuage the social anxiety of their interpersonal relations (or their performance anxiety induced by prior erective failure), this pharmacologically induced impotence may be a recurring phenomenon.

No data beyond clinical observation exist to directly support performance anxiety as a contributor to alcoholics' sexual difficulties because research has not focused on this factor. However, indirect support comes from one study in which psychologically based sex therapy targeted at least in part to reducing sexual anxiety improved alcoholics' sexual dysfunctions more than a minimal treatment control (Fahrner, 1987).

The belief or expectancy that alcohol will improve sexual activities may play a role in the development of alcoholics' sexual difficulties. The alcoholic who strongly believes that alcohol is helpful or necessary for satisfactory sex and has avoided serious sexual dysfunction during drinking generally has used alcohol to accompany most or all sexual activities, and may find that entering alcoholism treatment and sobriety lead to diminished sexual activity and desire. In this regard, McCarthy (1984), a well-known sex therapist, described "a syndrome observed in clinical practice but which has received little research attention in either alcoholism or sex therapy literature" (p. 33). The pattern involves men who have maintained sexual functioning while drinking and begin experiencing erection difficulties when they stop drinking and start an alcoholism recovery program. Such a male can come to believe he has a choice of being a "potent drunk" or an "impotent abstainer" and often chooses the former. McCarthy (1984) sees a psychogenic origin in such cases in which the alcoholic has learned to use alcohol to facilitate sexual activities and must relearn comfortable sexuality in a sober state. Anxiety over any initial sexual failures in sobriety can cause recurring impotence and sexual avoidance based on sexual performance anxiety.

The belief or expectancy effects of alcohol on sexual response have been studied extensively via questionnaire and experimental drinking studies. Questionnaire studies of respondents' expected effects from drinking alcohol have found a strong tendency for subjects to endorse the belief that drinking enhances sexual pleasure and sexual performance among a variety of nonclinical samples, including college students (Brown, Goldman, Inn, & Anderson, 1980; Rohsenow, 1983; Southwick, Steele, Marlatt, & Lindell, 1981), young adolescents (Christiansen, Goldman, & Inn, 1982), executives (Johnson, 1974), and working-class middle-aged males (Connors, O'Farrell, Cutter, & Logan, 1986). The strength of this belief was greater in heavier than lighter drinkers (Brown et al., 1980; Rohsenow, 1983; Southwick et al., 1981) and in alcoholics than in problem and nonproblem drinkers (Connors et al., 1986). Experimental social psychological studies of sexuality among male college student social drinkers (see Lang, 1985, and Wilson, 1981, for comprehensive reviews) manipulate independently both the belief that alcohol has/has not been consumed and the alcohol dose (i.e., actual beverage content being alcohol or no alcohol). These studies indicate that, when relatively low alcohol doses (BAL $\leq$ .04%) are used, subjects who believed they had consumed alcohol, whether or not they actually had done so, indicated greater sexual arousal measured by self-report and/or physiological (i.e., penile tumescence via plethysmograph) methods in response to erotic stimuli (Briddell & Wilson, 1976; Lang, Searles, Lauerman, & Adesso, 1980; Wilson & Lawson, 1976). Belief or expectancy of alcohol consumption produced increased arousal even though actual alcohol consumption did not.

The direct relevance of these survey and experimental studies of alcohol expectancy effects to sexual problems of clinical samples of alcoholics remains to be demonstrated. However, Mandell and Miller (1983) present data consistent with the expectancy studies. They indicated that retrospective life history interviews with alcoholics suggested a developmental course for sexual dysfunction in at least some alcoholics. Initially alcohol had been used to overcome anxiety and facilitate sexual performance but as consumption increased over time so did dysfunction. Longitudinal research is needed to understand what role alcoholics' greater beliefs in the aphrodisiac properties of alcohol (which laboratory studies have shown to be placebo effects operating at low doses) play in the development of alcoholics' sexual problems. One can speculate that these greater beliefs may be perpetuated by the effects of acquired behavioral tolerance in which greater amounts of alcohol can be consumed without behavioral impairment and the pairing of alcohol consumption with sexual pleasure may thus occur repeatedly over long time periods. Researchers conducting longitudinal studies of populations at risk for alcoholism could contribute greatly to our

knowledge of the development of alcohol-related sexual problems if they
included alcohol expectancy and sexual behavior measures in their data sets.

Social, Interpersonal, and Relationship Factors

Among the more chronic and socially disabled alcoholics are a large number of single or divorced men with low social resources (e.g., jobs, income,
residence) and problems with establishing long-standing relationships for
whom sexual problems seem secondary to their social and interpersonal
deficits (Wagner & Jensen, 1981). For such men, lack of a consistent partner and preoccupation with social and other difficulties may preclude a satisfactory sexual adjustment.

Lack of a sexual partner may play an important role in alcoholics' sexual
problems, as Whalley (1978) and others (e.g. Levine, 1955) have speculated, but only Jensen (1979) specifically examined possible differences
between alcoholics with and without a steady sexual partner. Jensen's findings showed that single alcoholics, when compared with those having a
steady sexual partner: (1) did not differ on type or frequency of sexual
dysfunction experienced or on masturbation frequency; (2) had less frequent sexual intercourse, a finding that was most pronounced in those over
40 for whom no intercourse was the modal frequency at the time of the
study. For men 35 or younger, single alcoholics had more sexual problems.
Finally, for those who reported they became sexually aroused by alcohol,
single patients were more likely to have sexual problems than were those
with steady partners.

Anger and discord between the alcoholic and his partner can be an important
factor in producing sexual dissatisfaction and dysfunction in married alcoholics. Wiseman (1985) indicates that the wife's anger and disgust with her
alcoholic husband when he is actively drinking arise from two sources. The
first is that she is so angry with him in general over alcohol-related and
other negative events in the marriage that she is too upset to have intercourse. The second is that the wife is repelled by being intimate with a
drunken man. Therefore the wife refuses or passively endures intercourse
often leading to a marked reduction in sexual frequency and satisfaction.
Sex also can become part of the couple's power struggle over the alcoholic's
drinking when the wife withdraws from sexual activity in an attempt to
control the alcoholic's drinking. Once the alcoholic stops drinking and begins sobriety, the relationship tension and sexual avoidance do not necessarily change quickly (especially in the more chronic, severe cases) and may
contribute to maintenance of the couple's sexual maladjustment and mal-
aise. Very often one or both partners, more often the nonalcoholic spouse,
will hold onto her anger well into sobriety as a way of protecting herself
from further hurt and disappointment. The wife fears that if she opens up

her heart again the alcoholic will return to drinking. For some couples, resuming regular sexual activity represents recommitting themselves to a relationship from which they had psychologically removed themselves over a number of years.

Relationship discord as a cause of alcoholics' sexual difficulties has been described eloquently and in rich clinical detail in the exploratory interview study in Wiseman (1985) as described above. Further empirical support for Wiseman's (1985) theorizing comes from two studies by O'Farrell and colleagues which indicate the marital conflict is related to sexual dissatisfction and dysfunction among alcoholics. To examine the role of marital conflict in alcoholics' sexual adjustment, two recent studies by O'Farrell and colleagues compared alcoholics and their wives in a spouse-involved alcoholism treatment program with two groups of nonalcoholic couples, those seeking counseling for serious marital conflicts and a group who were satisfied with their marital relationships.

The first study (O'Farrell, Choquette, & Birchler, 1989), which was part of a larger project on alcoholics' marital relationships (O'Farrell & Birchler, 1987), examined sexual satisfactions and dissatisfactions among these three groups of couples. Results showed that alcoholic and maritally conflicted couples did not differ and that both groups reported less frequent intercourse, more disagreement over sex, and more desires for change in their sexual relationships than did nonalcoholic, nonconflicted couples. O'Farrell et al. interpreted these results as meaning that the marital conflict shared in common by the alcoholic and maritally conflicted couples led to less sexual satisfaction than among the nonconflicted couples. They also suggested that the sexual dissatisfaction experienced by alcoholics was not a unique concomitant of alcoholism but, rather, secondary to the alcoholics' distressed marital relationships. The O'Farrell et al. study used only couples married and living together; used accepted objective measures to establish the level of marital satisfaction in the nonalcoholic couples and to screen the nonalcoholic couples for both alcohol and major psychiatric disorders; ensured that the groups were equivalent on demographic and other variables likely to affect the results; and examined sexual satisfaction measures rather than only dysfunction. However, sources of the couples differed geographically in that the conflicted nonalcoholic couples were from a San Diego marital therapy clinic while the other two groups of couples were drawn from the Boston area. In addition, a comprehensive evaluation of sexual adjustment was not conducted since no measures of sexual dysfunction were included and the only sexual satisfaction measures assessed were those that could be drawn from the marital relationship questionnaires used in the larger study from which these results were drawn.

In the second study by O'Farrell and colleagues (O'Farrell, Choquette, Cutter, & Stoykovich, 1989), 26 married couples with an alcoholic (ALC) husband were compared with 26 maritally conflicted (MC) and 26 non-conflicted (NC) couples without alcohol problems (all couples from the Boston area) on *both* sexual dysfunction and a wide range of sexual satisfaction variables. On the basis of the marital conflict presumed to be shared by the ALC and MC couples, it was predicted that ALC would resemble MC and both would score lower than NC couples on measures of sexual satisfaction. The results supported this prediction indicating that the alcoholic and conflicted couples experienced less sexual satisfaction than the nonconflicted couples on a variety of measures including satisfaction with frequency of intercourse, privacy and context of sex, ease of refusing a sexual request, wives' overall sexual satisfaction, and husbands' satisfaction with specific aspects of sex. A second prediction in the O'Farrell, Choquette, et al. (1989) study was that marital conflict and the physical effects of prolonged alcohol abuse would combine to make ALCs greater than both NCs and MCs on sexual dysfunction, particularly impotence, diminished sexual interest, and retarded ejaculation. For impotence, a trend toward significance provided the only support for the hypothesis, with ALCs reporting more impotence than NCs or MCs which did not differ. The level of the ALC husband's interest in sex did not differ from MC husbands and both ALC and MC husbands showed diminished interest in sex compared to NC husbands. Similar findings occurred for premature ejaculation. Groups did not differ on retarded ejaculation.

The O'Farrell, Choquette, et al. (1989) results indicate that both male alcoholics and their wives and MC nonalcoholic couples experience less sexual satisfaction across a range of measures and more sexual dysfunction (specifically husbands' diminished sexual interest and premature ejaculation) than NC couples. However, impotence was the only aspect on which alcoholics reported more difficulties than did MC couples. On the basis of these results, O'Farrell et al. suggest that, with the possible exception of impotence, most of the sexual adjustment problems which married male alcoholics suffer may be a function of the marital unhappiness they experience. They suggest further that the physical effects of alcohol may account for the increased impotence over and above what can be explained on the basis of marital conflict. Certain limitations to interpretation of the O'Farrell et al. studies should be noted. Similar levels of sexual dissatisfaction and dysfunction in the ALC and MC couples do not necessarily arise from the same processes in the two groups, namely, marital conflict and unhappiness, as interpreted by O'Farrell et al. Possibly different or additional factors are at work in the ALC than in the MC group. For example, both acute and chronic physical effects of alcohol ingestion may lead to greater impotence which may produce other dysfunctions as well as sexual avoidance and dissatisfaction. Unfortunately, measures of variables that might implicate physical factors in alcoholics' sexual problems were not included in the O'Farrell et al. or other psychosocial studies. Similarly, measures implicating psychosocial factors have not been included in studies conducted by investigators examining physical factors.

Other Factors Related to Alcoholics' Sexual Problems

Age, duration of the alcoholism problem, and severity of the alcoholism are other factors that do not fall conveniently into psychosocial or physical causes but that have been studied in relationship to alcoholics' sexual problems.

Age has received the most attention. Jensen's (1984) study of 30 married alcoholics and 30 married medical practice controls found that alcoholics over age 40 had lower sexual frequency and more sexual problems than those aged 40 and under. O'Farrell, Choquette, et al. (1989) examined the relationship of age and sexual adjustment in their study of ALC, MC, and NC couples. The O'Farrell et al. study produced three main findings with regard to age. First, the older the husband the more dissatisfied was the

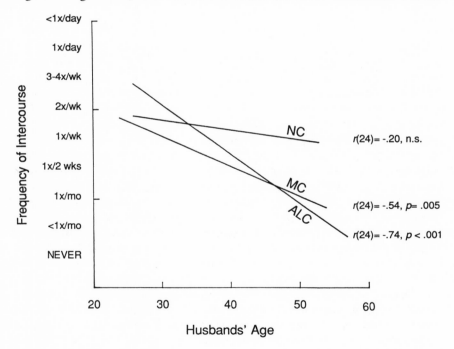

FIGURE 9.1. Regression lines for frequency of intercourse predicted by husbands' age for three groups of couples. ALC = couples with an alcoholic husband; MC = conflicted couples without alcohol problems; NC = nonconflicted couples without alcohol problems. From O'Farrell, Choquette, Cutter, and Stoykovich (1989).

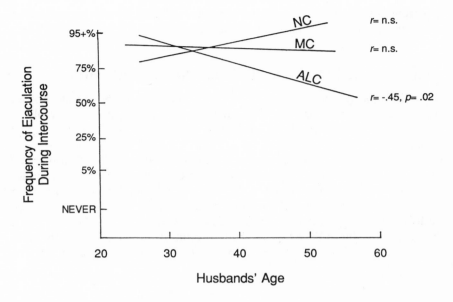

FIGURE 9.2. Regression lines for frequency of husband's ejaculation during intercourse predicted by husband's age for three groups of couples. ALC = couples with an alcoholic husband; MC = conflicted couples without alcohol problems; NC = nonconflicted couples without alcohol problems. From O'Farrell, Choquette, Cutter, and Stoykovich (1989).

couple with their frequency of intercourse and the greater was the frequency of impotence experienced. These results are *not* unique to alcoholics but occurred irrespective of the type of couple. Second, less frequent intercourse among older husbands occurred in both the ALC and MC couples but age was *not* related to intercourse frequency among the NC couples. Figure 9.1 shows that age was more strongly related to intercourse frequency among the ALC than among either the MC or NC couples. Third, more frequent retarded ejaculation in older husbands occurred *only* in the alcoholic couples since age was not related to ejaculation frequency in the other couples (see Figure 9.2).

Duration of alcoholism also has been studied in relation to alcoholics' sexual problems with mixed results. Two studies (Akhtar, 1977; Mandell & Miller, 1983) report greater sexual dysfunction with greater duration of heavy drinking. However, as Akhtar notes, the effects of age in determining the severity of dysfunction cannot be ruled out with certainty since age and length of problem drinking tend to be highly correlated. However, other studies found no relationship between the duration of the alcoholism and the occurrence of sexual dysfunction (Jensen, 1979) or the chance of a spontaneous recovery to adequate sexual functioning among impotent alcoholics (Van Thiel et al, 1982).

Alcoholism severity also has been studied. Holosko (1979) found a positive relationship between alcoholics' drinking problem severity measured by summing five unitary measures—number of years' drinking, teenage drinking, social and behavioral problems due to drinking, previous alcohol treatment, and present alcohol consumption—and the extent of sexual dysfunction and dissatisfaction. The relationship prevailed when the effect of other factors (e.g., age, physical health problems) was controlled statistically.

LONGITUDINAL STUDIES OF ALCOHOLICS' SEXUAL PROBLEMS

Given the extent of sexual dissatisfaction and dysfunction among clinical samples of alcoholics, it is a matter of some clinical and scientific importance to know the course over time of these problems. Clinically we wish to answer the patient's question "If I discontinue drinking will my sex life improve?" Scientifically, longitudinal studies have the potential for casting light on questions of etiology. Given that the physical effects of prolonged heavy drinking and the relationship distress noted in alcoholics' marriages are both plausible determinants of alcoholics' sexual adjustment problems, what happens when attempts are made to decrease the drinking through alcoholism treatment, improve the marriage relationship with marital therapy, or directly treat the sexual problems through sex therapy or hormone replacement therapy?

Course of Alcoholics' Sexual Problems after Alcoholism Treatment

The few clinical reports and alcoholism treatment outcome studies that present incidental data on recovery of sexual function (e.g., Bruning, 1986; Gross, Carpenter, & Adler, 1971; Jensen 1979; Lemere & Smith, 1973) generally suggest that sexual adjustment does not improve during and soon after alcoholism treatment—a conclusion also reached by the most extensive longitudinal study of the course of male alcoholics' sexual adjustment problems after alcoholism treatment to date conducted in Munich, Germany. Fahrner (1987) studied 116 alcoholic patients using a questionnaire about sexual functioning. Seventy-five percent of the patients reported at least one sexual dysfunction, mostly erectile dysfunction and loss of libido, but also premature or delayed ejaculation. Questionnaires mailed at 9 months after the hospital discharge showed no significant differences in prevalence of sexual dysfunction between treatment and follow-up assessments. Furthermore, at follow-up, abstinent and relapsed alcoholics did not differ in the extent of sexual dysfunction experienced. Fahrner concluded that alcoholics' sexual problems have psychological causes and need sex therapy since testosterone levels were normal and abstinence from alcohol did not significantly reduce the overall prevalence of sexual dysfunction.

Fahrner's (1987) report is extremely important but not without problems. Subject attrition at follow-up was high with only a 69% completion rate. No information was gathered from the alcoholics' spouses/partners, and, since 42% were not married, lack of a sexual partner may have influenced the results (Whalley, 1978). Although prevalence rates of all dysfunctions combined for the sample as a whole were unchanged, it is unclear from Fahrner's report whether individual patients who were dysfunctional initially were still dysfunctional at follow-up. Similarly, the pattern of individual patient change for specific dysfunctions (e.g., impotence) is not presented. Possibly some patients improved while others got worse and/or some dysfunctions got worse while others got better. Some clinical reports have described a subgroup of patients who became dysfunctional when they get sober after having been relatively functional during their drinking career. This could account for the lack of differences between the relapsed and abstinent groups. Finally, confidence in the reports of both drinking and sexual adjustment would have been increased if patient reports of their drinking had been confirmed by collateral informants and if evidence had been presented that the alcoholic was abstinent when completing the mailed questionnaire.

Sexual Adjustment Changes after Marital Therapy Plus Alcoholism Treatment

A few marital therapy outcome studies present incidental data on recovery of sexual function. Steinglass (1979) reported data from 10 alcoholic couples showing no change or a decrease in sexual satisfaction immediately and 6 months after participation in a 6 week course of multiple-couples group therapy. It was suggested that improved marital communication resulting from the therapy was associated with perceptions of increased marital difficulties and decreased satisfaction. Cohen and Krause (1971) compared the results after at least 6 months follow-up of treatment based on the disease concept of alcoholism with treatment based on alcoholism as a symptom of family problems. The disease-oriented treatment was most successful in reducing the husband's drinking while the family-oriented treatment was most successful in improving marital and sexual satisfaction. These results led Cohen and Krause to speculate that improvement occurred in the areas focused on in treatment and that changes in drinking and in marital/sexual satisfaction were relatively independent. McCrady, Noel, Abrams, Stout, and Nelson (1986) randomly assigned 53 alcoholics and their spouses to one of three outpatient spouse-involved behavioral treatments. This study, which showed significant decreases in the alcoholics' drinking and improvements in marital satisfaction from pretreatment to

6-month follow-up for all three types of spouse-involved treatment, also showed concomitant increased frequency of sexual intercourse but no increased satisfaction with sex (as rated on a 1–7 scale).

O'Farrell, Kleinke, and Cutter (1989) are conducting an ongoing longitudinal study that remedies problems of prior investigations by studying only married alcoholics, using both alcoholic and spouse reports of sexual adjustment and drinking, examining change after initial assessment for each individual not just for group data, getting at least 90% completion of follow-up, and including a matched sample of community controls against which to compare the alcoholics' follow-up functioning results. The study examined the impact on alcoholics' sexual adjustment of receiving alcoholism counseling with and without behavioral marital therapy (BMT). Using data currently available on results from before and after treatment, a series of predictions were tested.

The first prediction—that if alcoholism counseling reduced the drinking, then impotence should improve—was supported. Figure 9.3 shows fre-

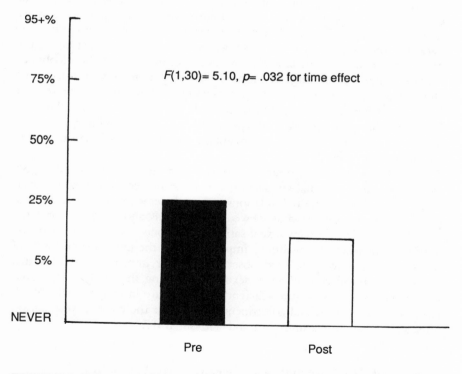

FIGURE 9.3. Mean frequency of husbands' difficulty maintaining erection before and after alcoholism counseling with or without marital therapy. From O'Farrell, Kleinke, and Cutter (1989).

TABLE 9.1. Impotence in Alcoholics Before and After Treatment and in Maritally Conflicted and Nonconflicted Couples Without Alcohol Problems[a]

Frequency of impotence	Alcoholics		Maritally conflicted	Nonconflicted
	Pre	Post		
Never	27.2%	39.4%	65.4%	61.5%
At least 5% of the time	72.8%	60.6%	34.6%	38.5%
At least 25% of the time	54.5%	36.4%	15.4%	15.4%

[a]These data are from O'Farrell, Kleinke, and Cutter (1989).

quency of difficulty maintaining erection (as reported by wives) decreased significantly over a 3- to 5-month period from before to after alcoholism counseling. Despite these improvements, alcoholics still experienced significantly more and over twice the rate of serious impotence reported by demographically similar nonalcoholic couples (see Table 9.1). Thus, the clinical significance of the short-term improvements in impotence is questionable but further improvements may occur later in the 2-year follow-up period. Other aspects of marital, family, and psychosocial functioning improve to the level of matched community controls when the alcoholic's drinking improves (Billings & Moos, 1983), so perhaps sexual functioning also will improve during later months of recovery. On the other hand, once a sexual dysfunction is established, possibly psychological (e.g., the alcoholics' performance anxiety), interpersonal (e.g., spouse withdrawal of affection), or organic factors may maintain the sexual dysfunction despite alcoholism recovery.

The second prediction, that if marital therapy improved marital adjustment then gains in sexual satisfaction should occur, received some support. BMT produced substantial relationship improvements but only modest gains in sexual satisfaction as viewed by husbands and no gains from the wives' perspective. Perhaps sexual satisfaction is one of the last areas of the alcoholics' marital relationship to improve. Thus, the limited time frame of the study may have precluded observing further improvements in sexual satisfaction and in recovering of sexual functioning that will emerge later, during the 2-year follow-up. Currently, analyses are in progress which will examine changes in sexual adjustment throughout the entire 2-year period after alcoholism counseling with and without BMT.

Results of Psychosexual Sex Therapy with Alcoholics

Two early reports examine the use of sex therapy to ameliorate alcoholics' sexual adjustment problems. Renshaw (1978) reported three case histories describing successful sex therapy with alcohol-abusing diabetics and their wives. She describes very brief interventions consisting of education and specific instructions that were successful in resolving the complaints of impotence but how durable the improvements were is unknown since follow-up data are not presented. Focusing directly on therapy to change sexual dissatisfaction, Gad-Luther and Dickman (1979) conducted a pilot study in which five alcoholic couples (in which the alcoholic had achieved considerable abstinence) showed improved scores on several scales of the LoPiccolo and Steger (1974) Sexual Interaction Inventory after receiving ten 3-hour sessions of a structured group therapy using specific behavioral techniques, exercises, and homework assignments. As Gad-Luther and Dickman note, their pilot study suggests a need for further research that includes a control group and targets both sexual dissatisfactions and dysfunctions.

Fahrner (1987) conducted the first comparative, controlled outcome study of sex therapy with dysfunctional alcoholics. Fahrner (1987) evaluated a short-term psychologically based behavioral sex therapy program during inpatient alcoholism treatment for 16 sexually dysfunctional patients by comparing pre, post, and 5-month follow-up (3 months after hospital discharge) questionnaire results with those of 11 demographically and symptomatically similar control patients who received 1 hour of "nonspecific counseling." The sex therapy program consisted of 10 session, each lasting 90 minutes. The goals of the behavioral treatment were sex instructions, change of negative attitudes toward sex, increase of skills in sociosexual behavior, and improvement of sexual dysfunction. Female partners of the treated patients were not involved in treatment because of the distance between the clinic and home. Role-playing was used to practice new social behavior, and masturbation training was used to rebuild effective and satisfying sexual functioning. Instructions by the therapists, group discussion, and homework assignments were also considered important elements of the therapy.

Results showed significant improvement from pre- to posttreatment among the sex therapy patients but not the controls on sexual knowledge, sexual attitudes, and social assertiveness in sexual situations—all areas in which both groups of patients had shown similar deficits at first assessment. Similar significant improvements, from pre to follow-up, in sexual dysfunction occurred in the treatment but not the controls group. Specifically, before sex therapy 88% (14) indicated sexual dysfunction and 12% (2) never had sexual contacts. Sexual dysfunctions decreased significantly: only 33% (5) of the sex therapy patients had dysfunctions at follow-up. In the control group there was no significant change in the number of sexual dysfunctions: 75% continued to suffer from sexual dysfunction. Differences between the two groups in the number of relapses were not found. No one in the control group or in the experimental group relapsed in the 3 months after clinic discharge. In addition, dysfunctions had lasted an average of 6 years in both sex therapy and control groups and the frequency overall and of specific types of dysfunction (i.e., loss of libido, erectile dysfunction, and premature ejaculation) did not differ between the two groups.

Fahrner's (1987) report is the first controlled outcome study of psychologically based behavioral sex therapy with sexually dysfunctional male alcoholics. Care was taken to insure that treatment and control groups were similar on demographics and sexual problem severity, although comparisons on alcoholism variables were not described. Still, the sample appears to have serious alcohol problems and significant sexual difficulties. Notably, a follow-up assessment was included also. The value of this study would have been increased considerably by two additional features. First, if results had been presented separately for different types of dysfunction and for each individual patient we could have learned much more. For example, were alcoholics with serious impotence cured by 3 months of abstinence and 10 sessions of individual (non-partner-involved) sex therapy? Who were the third of treated patients whose dysfunctions persisted at follow-up? Second, corroborating data from the patients' partners would have increased confidence in the results since, given the essentially no treatment control group, sex therapy patients' responses may have been due in part to demand effects to please the therapist.

Hormone Replacement Therapy and Spontaneous Improvement of Impotent Alcoholics

Van Thiel et al. (1982) looked at the reversibility of sexual dysfunction in 60 chronic alcoholic men with at least 3 months' abstinence at study entry who complained of impotence and/or loss of libido. During a follow-up period of regular monitoring for 2 years, 25% ($n = 15$) of the patients reported a spontaneous return of normal sexual functioning. Spontaneous recovery occurred only during the first year of observation. Indicators at study entry associated with this spontaneous recovery of sexual functioning were: (1) absence of testicular atrophy, (2) normal gonadotropin response to LH releasing factor and/or clomiphene administration, and (3) normal spermatozoa concentrations in ejaculates. Interestingly, no correlation was evident between the severity of the liver disease present, years of alcohol abuse, or amount of alcohol ingested and the chance of a spontaneous recovery to adequate sexual functioning. The 45 patients not recovering spontaneously in the first 2 years of the study were treated sequentially with clomiphene and human chorionic gonadotropin to no effect. Finally, an oral exogenous androgen, fluoxymesterone, produced a return to potency in 32 out of 45 cases. A side effect of reduced spermatozoal concentrations in ejaculates (which implies decreased infertility) was noted at the unusually high doses of androgen required to attain potency. However, more common side effects of very large doses of exogenous androgen (e.g., prostatic hypertrophy, gynecomastia, acne, hirsutism, priapism, hypercalcemia, and jaundice) were not observed.

The Van Thiel et al. (1982) study is one of the few reported studies which deals directly with the reversibility of sexual dysfunctioning in chronic alcoholics. Replication of these results in a study that corrected some of the problems with this study would certainly add to our knowledge in this important area. Unfortunately, the study is greatly weakened by the absence of more detailed and objective measures of sexual functioning. Objections could also be raised concerning experimenter bias since there were no attempts to keep results of hormonal data blind from sexual functioning data. Further objective information is essential to better delineate the important interplay between hormones and sexual functioning in chronic alcoholics. The criteria of return to "normal sexual function," at which time the subject was no longer followed in the study, included all of the following: occasional morning erections, ability to obtain and maintain an erection for at least 50% of attempts during the preceding 3 months, and ability to obtain an ejaculate. Both the criteria and the lack of follow-up data are open to question, the former because they designate recovered many who meet customary criteria (e.g., Masters & Johnson, 1970) for dysfunction, and the latter because the durability of the results presented in the study cannot be assessed. The Van Thiel et al. results for hormone replacement therapy as a treatment for impotence in alcoholics require replication in a controlled outcome study.

Conclusions re Longitudinal Studies of Alcoholics' Sexual Adjustment Problems

Our knowledge in this area is probably more limited than in any other aspect of alcoholics' sexual adjustment problems. The few descriptive studies of the course over time of alcoholics' sexual adjustment problems after alcoholism and/or marital therapy show modest improvements at best. Sexual adjustment data were limited in scope at least in part because they were collected incidentally as part of studies conducted for some other purpose. Data were collected during early stages of the recovery period with follow-up periods longer than 6 months rare or nonexistent.

The one study which examined prospectively a large series of unselected cases treated for alcoholism concluded that recovery from sexual dysfunction did not occur in spite of abstinence up to 1 year after entering impatient alcoholism treatment (Fahrner, 1987). Further, the only study of a sizable sample of dysfunctional alcoholics found only 25% spontaneous recovery after 12–18 months of abstinence and only among those without testicular atrophy or abnormal endocrine functioning (Van Thiel et al., 1982). Given the paucity of data and the limitations in these two pioneering studies noted above, we badly need long-term prospective studies both of a large number of cases entering alcoholism treatment programs and of samples of dysfunctional alcoholics, especially those suffering from impotence. The following recommendations apply to both of these types of studies. Multifaceted measurement of sexual adjustment should include self-reported and partner-reported sexual satisfaction and dysfunction, including a detailed description of the development and current status of any dysfunction experienced, and objective assessment of sexual responding to visual stimuli using penile plethysmography (Barlow, Becker, Leitenberg, & Agras, 1970) and NPT (Karacan et al., 1978; Karacan, Snyder, Salis, Williams, & Derman, 1980). Investigators should use state-of-the-art methods to assess carefully the neurological, endocrine, alcohol intake, and marital adjustment factors thought to contribute to alcoholics' sexual adjustment problems. Subjects should be followed with repeated measurements taken throughout a period of at least 2 years.

Studies of intervention although extremely limited show promise of psychologically based sex therapy and for hormone replacement therapy for cases of impotence that do not recover aftr 12–18 months abstinence. Controlled outcome studies of both types of treatment are needed and should include the same careful, comprehensive, multifaceted assessment procedures recommended for prospective descriptive studies above along with follow-up data to assess durability of results. Ideally, large enough samples could be used to randomly assign to treatment and control methods and to sequentially examine less to more intrusive methods (e.g., sexual enhancement therapy, direct sex therapy, and hormone replacement). Research is needed to find methods to correct sex hormone imbalance without reducing fertility.

OVERALL SUMMARY AND CONCLUSIONS

Extent and Causes of Alcoholics' Sexual Problems

Over 20 reports from 10 countries have indicated that a substantial proportion of male alcoholics seen in treatment settings have sexual adjustment problems. Studies which included comparison group data strengthen the conclusion of a heightened prevalence of sexual adjustment problems among alcoholics. Such studies find that alcoholics uniformly show greater prevalence of dysfunctions, greater impotence as determined by both self-report and nocturnal erection studies, lower frequency of sexual intercourse, and less sexual satisfaction. Lowered libido is greater among alcoholics than in normals in some but not all studies depending on sample characteristics (e.g., age, partner available or not) and on how lessened sexual desire is defined (e.g., intercourse vs. masturbation frequency).

Although many alcoholics have sexual problems, studies of alcoholics' sexual problems have not provided a definitive or singular explanation of the etiology of these problems. Generally causation is considered most likely to be multifactorial with factors generally grouped broadly into psychosocial and organic or physical categories.

Among psychosocial factors, relationship discord secondary to alcohol-related stressors for men with partners has the strongest support as an influence on sexual dissatisfaction. Partner unavailability has been implicated also for both sexual dissatisfaction and dysfunction. Expectations that alcohol will facilitate sexual experiences, which have been found to be stronger in alcoholics than normal drinkers, have not been studied in relation to the development or maintenance of alcoholics' sexual problems despite speculation that these beliefs predispose alcoholics to sexual problems. Finally, sexual performance anxiety based on past sexual failures or predisposing personal characeristics has been the subject of considerable clinical theorizing but no research among alcoholics.

Among organic or physical factors, sex hormone changes due to the effects of chronic excessive alcohol intake on the liver, testicles, and the hypothalamic–pituitary–testicular axis have the strongest support among physical factors as causes of alcoholics' impotence problems. Alcoholic liver disease (cirrhosis) had until recently been thought to be the primary cause of sex hormone metabolism changes that produced impotence but recent studies ascribe greater importance to direct effects of the chronic excessive drinking as the cause of both the cirrhosis and the hormonal abnormalities associated with impotence. Studies showing that alcoholics retrospectively report a relationship between amount consumed and extent of sexual problems are consistent with the extensive body of experimental studies which shows a negative dose-related effect of acute alcohol intake on erection and ejaculation latency. Drinking-related neurological damage to neural pathways involved in producing erection, frequently mentioned as a cause of alcoholic impotence, has been investigated in only one study, which found greater neurological damage among NPT-diagnosed organically impotent than among psychogenically impotent alcoholics.

Age and duration and severity of the alcoholism are factors which do not fit neatly into either psychosocial or physical causes. Older, more chronic and more severe alcoholics have more sexual problems.

Course of Alcoholics' Sexual Problems

Knowledge of the course of alcoholics' sexual problems over time is very limited. We do not have an adequate knowledge base to guide clinicians who must deal with patients' and families' concerns about the likelihood of recovery of sexual functioning and satisfaction. Two pioneering but methodologically flawed prospective studies indicated, respectively, that alcoholics' sexual dysfunctions did not recover in spite of abstinence up to 1 year after inpatient alcoholism treatment, and only 25% of impotent alcoholics, namely, those without testicular atrophy and abnormal sex hormone levels, recovered potency after 12–18 months of abstinence. Studies of intervention methods consist of one study each of psychologically based sex therapy and of sex hormone replacement therapy and results for both methods were sufficiently positive to recommend further research on both.

Critical Appraisal and Recommendations for Research

A number of methodological and conceptual shortcomings can be identified in the literature reviewed in this chapter. The measurement, definition, and criteria for sexual problems have varied considerably from study to study and have not been described in sufficient detail in most studies. Individual studies have suffered from a narrowness of perspective in the aspects of sexual behavior studied, the type(s) of etiological factor(s) considered, the sophistication of measurement procedures used, and the samples investigated. One is reminded of the story of how the blind men each perceived the elephant differently based on their own limited and narrow experience of the elephant.

Studies have emphasized dysfunction, especially impotence, often to the exclusion of other aspects of alcoholics' sexual behavior. With few exceptions studies have not provided an extensive and multifaceted measurement of alcoholics' sexual behavior that includes both a wide range of sexual satisfaction variables (e.g., overall satisfaction, initiation and refusal patterns, frequency, communication about sex, affection expressed during sex) and sexual dysfunctions. Further, the sexual adjustment of the partner of the alcoholic is rarely assessed. Studies also tend to focus on one class (e.g., psychosocial vs. physical) or type (e.g., hormonal, relationship) of etiological factor. This is unfortunate since a multifactorial etiology seems most likely, with different factors having relatively greater importance for different aspects of sexual adjustment (e.g., dissatisfaction vs. dysfunction) and different patients with the same problem (e.g., psychogenic vs. organic impotence). The narrowness of perspective extends to the measurement of variables within a given study. Frequently one factor will be measured with state-of-the-art methods when other factors are measured crudely or not at all. For example, a study with a psychosocial orientation may have excellent questionnaire and interview measures of sexual behavior but little or no data on hormonal or other physical factors, while the reverse may be true in a study of organic factors in alcoholic impotence. Finally, the samples investigated also have been limited since they have consisted almost entirely of clinical samples primarily of men in treatment for alcoholism but also those being seen for liver dysfunction or complaints of impotence.

The most detailed investigations have been conducted with impotent alcoholics being evaluated for this sexual complaint, which points up the difficulty of conducting detailed and explicit inquiries and extensive and sometimes intrusive testing related to sexual behavior unless the person is seeking help.

Recommendations for research including both suggested methodological requirements and types of studies needed flow directly from the appraisal of the literature just completed. Many of the methodological suggestions pertain to the measurement and presentation of data on sexual adjustment and related factors. Multifaceted measurement of sexual adjustment is recommended and should include a wide range of sexual satisfaction/dissatisfaction variables as well as indices of the various sexual dysfunctions. Questionnaire measures should be followed by interviews in order to determine the history and symptom pattern including onset, frequency, intensity, and duration of any problems reported. Similar data should be gathered from partners when they are available. Self-report data should be supplemented by objective measures of sexual behavior including nocturnal erection studies and penile plethysmography in response to viewing erotic stimuli whenever possible. Presentation of sexual adjustment data in research reports should be as detailed as possible given our limited knowledge. Individual subject's data should be presented. Specific dysfunctions should be examined separately and not aggregated into an overall dysfunction index or into groupings of related dysfunctins. The definition and criteria for each dysfunction should be clearly described. Finally, investigators should use state-of-the-art methods to assess the neurological, endocrine, vascular, alcohol intake, relationship, and other factors thought to contribute to alcoholics' sexual adjustment problems. Such multidimensional measurement requires a multidisciplinary research team with sophisticated psychological, sexological, medical, and alcoholism expertise. Realistically, not all studies will be able to reach this ideal.

Among the types of studies needed, prospective longitudinal investigations could provide the most important information. Descriptive longitudinal studies of large samples of cases entering alcoholism treatment and of dysfunctional alcoholics, especially those suffering from impotence, would provide needed information. We need to know what happens to alcoholics' sexual adjustment problems with abstinence. Simple descriptive studies could provide this information. Of even greater value would be longitudinal studies that measure both sexual adjustment and factors thought to affect it since the hypothesized etiological links could be examined in such studies. Treatment intervention studies using a randomized controlled outcome study design also are badly needed. Psychologically oriented sex therapy and hormone replacement therapy should be studied further for dysfunctional cases. Marital and sex relationship enhancement therapy should be evaluated for those with sexual dissatisfaction but not dysfunction. Ideally, subjects would be assessed to determine the nature of (e.g., dissatisfaction and/or dysfunction) and the likely cause of their problems (e.g., psychogenic, organic, mixed) so that differential predictions based on patient–treatment matching could be tested.

Cross-sectional studies providing only descriptive prevalence data in clinical samples of alcoholics or in comparison group studies are not likely to contribute a great deal of new knowledge since many similar studies have already been done. However, such studies could be valuable if they went beyond descriptive prevalence data. For example, studies of alcoholic samples that examined differences among alcoholics with and without specific sexual problems would be valuable. Comparison group studies designed to explicate etiological factors also are needed. Studies of alcohol use and sexual behavior in a representative national sample of men would contribute greatly to our knowledge. Klassen and Wilsnack (1986) have provided such data for women.

In conclusion, we have noted that sexual adjustment is an area of alcoholics' behavior and relationships that often has been neglected in both treatment and research. This chapter has summarized the slowly accumulating body of knowledge about sexual functioning of alcoholics. Hopefully, it will contribute to further needed research in this area.

Acknowledgments. Preparation of this chapter was supported by the Veterans Administration.

REFERENCES

Akhtar, M. J. (1977). Sexual disorders in male alcoholics. In J. S. Madden, R. Walker, & W. H. Kenyon (Eds.), *Alcoholism and drug dependence* (pp. 3–13). New York: Plenum.

Barlow, D. H., Becker, R., Leitenberg, H., & Agras, W. S. (1970). A mechanical strain gauge for recording penile circumference changes. *Journal of Applied Behavioral Analysis, 3,* 73–76.

Billings, A., & Moos, R. (1983). Psychosocial processes of recovery among alcoholics and their families: Implications for clinicians and program evaluators. *Addictive Behaviors, 8,* 205–218.

Briddell, D. W., & Wilson, G. T. (1976). The effects of alcohol and exectancy set on male sexual arousal. *Journal of Abnormal Psychology, 85,* 225–234.

Brown, S., Goldman, M., Inn, A., & Anderson, L. (1980). Expectations of reinforcement from alcohol: their domain and relation to drinking patterns. *Journal of Consulting and Clinical Psychology, 48,* 419–426.

Bruning, G. R. (1986). Phenomenological study of the experiences of the alcoholic and non-alcoholic spouse during the first three years of the recovery process. (Doctoral dissertation University of Southern California, 1986. *Dissertaion Abstracts International, 47,* 429B.

Christiansen, B., Goldman, M., Inn, A. (1982). Development of alcohol-related expectancies in adolescents: Separating pharmacological from social-learning influences. *Journal of Consulting and Clinical Psychology, 50,* 336–344.

Cicero, T. J. (1983). Alcohol effects on the endoctrine system. In: National Institute on Alcohol Abuse and Alcoholism. Biomedical processes and consequences of alcohol use, (pp. 53–91). Alcohol and Health Monograph No. 2. DHHS Pub. No. (ADM)82–1191. Washington, D.C.: Government Printing Office.

Cohen, D. C., & Krause, M. S. (1971). *Casework with the wives of alcoholics.* New York: Family Service Association of America.

Connors, G. J., O'Farrell, T. J., Cutter, H. S. G., & Logan, D. (1986). Alcohol expectancies among alcoholics, problem drinkers, and nonproblem drinkers. *Alcoholism: Clinical and Experimental Research, 10,* 667–671.

Cornely, C. M., Schade, R. R., Van Thiel, D. H., & Gavaler, J. S. (1984). Chronic advanced liver disease and impotence: Cause and effect. *Hepatology, 4,* 1227–1230.

Duncan, G., Johnson, R. H., Lambie, D. G., Whiteside, E. A. (1980). Evidence of vagal neuropathy in chronic alcoholics. *Lancet, 2,* 1053–1057.

Fahrner, E. M. (1987). Sexual dysfunctions in male alcohol addicts: Prevalence and treatment. *Archives of Sexual Behavior, 16,* 247–257.

Gad-Luther, I., & Dickman, D. (1979). Psychosexual therapy with recovering alcoholics, a pilot study. *Journal of Sex Education and Therapy, 1,* 11–16.

Gavalier, J. S., & Van Thiel, D. H. (1982). Adverse effects of ethanol upon hypothalamic-pituitary-gonadal function in males and females compared and contrasted. *Alcoholism: Clinical and Experimental Research, 6,* 179–185.

Gross, W. F., Carpenter, L. L., & Adler, L. O. (1971). Problems of adjustment reported by alcoholics prior to leaving a hospital treatment program. *Quarterly Journal of Studies on Alcohol, 32,* 454–456.

Holosko, M. J. (1979). *Sexual dysfunctioning of males undergoing treatment for alcoholism.* Unpublished doctoral dissertation. University of Pittsburgh.

Jensen, S. B. (1979). Sexual customs and dysfunction in alcoholics: *British Journal of Sexual Medicine, 6,* 29–32, 30–34.

Jensen, S. B. (1981). Sexual dysfunction in male diabetics and alcoholics: A comparative study. *Sexuality and Disability, 4,* 215–219.

Jensen, S. B. (1984). Sexual function and dysfunction in younger married alcoholics. *Acta Psychiatrica Scandinavica, 69,* 543–549.

Jensen, S. B., Gluud, C., and the Copenhagen Study Group for Liver Diseases. (1985). Sexual dysfunction in men with alcoholic liver cirrhosis: A comparative study. *Liver, 5,* 94–100.

Johnson, H. (1974). *Executive life-styles.* New York: Crowell.

Karacan, I., Wave, J. C., Dervent, B., Altinel, A., Thronby, J. I., Williams, R. L., Kaya, N., & Scott, F. B. (1978). Impotence and blood pressure in the flacid penis: Relationship to nocturnal penile tumescence. *Sleep, 1,* 125–132.

Karacan, I., Snyder, S., Salis, P. J., Williams, R. L., & Derman, S. (1980). Sexual dysfunction in male alcoholics and its objective evaluation. In W. E. Fann, I. Karacan, A. D. Pokorney, & R. L. Williams (Eds.), *Phenomenology and treatment of alcoholism* (pp. 259–268). New York: Spectrum.

Klassen, A. D., & Wilsnack, S. C. (1986). Sexual experiences and drinking among women in a U.S. national survey. *Archives of Sexual Behavior, 15,* 363–392.

Kinsey, A. W., Pomeroy, W., Martin, C., & Gebhard, P. (1948). *Sexual behavior in the human male.* Philadelphia: W. B. Saunders.

Lang, A. R. (1985). Social psychology of drinking and human sexuality. *Journal of Drug Issues, 15,* 273–289.

Lang, A., Searles, J., Lauerman, R., & Adesso, V. (1980). Expectancy, alcohol, and sex guilt as determinants of interest in and reaction to sexual stimuli. *Journal of Abnormal Psychology, 89,* 644–653.

Lemere, F., & Smith, J. W. (1973). Alcohol-induced sexual impotence. *American Journal of Psychiatry, 130,* 212–213.

LoPiccolo, J., & Steger, J. C. (1974). The sexual interaction inventory: A new instrument for assessment of sexual dysfunction. *Archives of Sexual Behavior, 3,* 585–595.

Levine, J. (1955). The sexual adjustment of alcoholics: A clinical study of a selected sample. *Quarterly Journal of Studies on Alcohol, 16,* 675–680.

Mandell, W., & Miller, C. M. (1983). Male sexual dysfunction as related to alcohol consumption: A pilot study. *Alcoholism: Clinical and Experimental Research, 7,* 65–69.

Masters, W. H., & Johnson, V. E. (1966). *Human sexual response* (pp. 267–269). Boston: Little, Brown.

Masters, W. H., & Johnson, V. E. (1970). *Human sexual inadequacy* (pp. 160, 163–169, 183–185). Boston: Little, Brown.

McCarthy, B. W. (1984). Returning to drinking as a result of erectile dysfunction. In D. J. Powell (Ed.), *Alcoholism and sexual dysfunction: Issues in clinical management* (pp. 33–34). New York: Haworth.

McCrady, B. S., Noel, N. E., Abrams, D. B., Stout, R. L., & Nelson, H. F. (1986). Comparative effectiveness of three types of spouse involvement in outpatient behavioral alcoholism treatment. *Journal of Studies on Alcohol, 47,* 459–460.

O'Farrell, T. J., & Birchler, G. R. (1987). Marital relationships of alcoholic, conflicted, and nonconflicted couples. *Journal of Marital and Family Therapy, 13,* 259–274.

O'Farrell, T. J., Choquette, K., & Birchler, G. R. (1989). *Sexual satisfaction in marriages of male alcoholics.* Manuscript submitted for publication.

O'Farrell, T. J., Weyand, C. A., & Logan, D. (1983). *Alcohol and sexuality: An annotated bibliography on alcohol use, alcoholism, and human sexual behavior.* Phoenix, AZ: Oryx.

O'Farrell, T. J., Thompson, D. L., & Weyand, C. A. (1986). Growing interest in alcohol and human sexuality revealed in the literature from 1941–1980. *Sexuality and Disability, 7,* 51–63.

O'Farrell, T. J., Kleinke, C., & Cutter, H. S. G. (1989). Sexual adjustment of male alcoholics: Changes from before to after receiving alcoholism counseling with and without marital therapy. Unpublished manuscript. Alcohol and Family Studies Laboratory, VA Medical Center and Harvard Medical School, Brockton, MA.

O'Farrell, T. J., Choquette, K., Cutter, H. S. G., & Stoykovich, C. A. (1989). Sexual satisfaction and dysfunction among alcoholic, maritally conflicted and nonconflicted couples. Unpublished manuscript. Alcohol and Family Studies Laboratory, VA Medical Center and Harvard Medical School, Brockton, MA.

Renshaw, D. C. (1975). Sexual problems of alcoholics. *Chicago Medicine, 78,* 433–436.

Renshaw, D. C. (1978). Impotence in diabetics. In J. LoPiccolo & L. LoPiccolo (Eds.), *Handbook of sex therapy.* New York: Plenum.

Rohsenow, D. (1983). Drinking habits and expectancies about alcohol's effect for self versus others. *Journal of Consulting and Clinical Psychology, 51,* 752–756.

Silvestrini, R. (1926). La reviviscenza mammaria nell'uomo affetto da cirrosi del Laennec. [Gynecomastia in men with Laennec's cirrhosis.] *La Riforma Medica, 42,* 701–704.

Snyder, S., & Karacan, I. (1981). Effects of chronic alcoholism on nocturnal penile tumescence. *Psychosomatic Medicine, 43,* 423–429.

Southwick, L., Steele, C., Marlatt, A., & Lindell, M. (1981). Alcohol-related expectancies: Defined by phase of intoxication and drinking experience. *Journal of Consulting and Clinical Psychology, 49,* 713–721.

Steinglass, P. (1979). An experimental treatment program for alcoholic couples. *Journal of Studies on Alcohol, 40,* 159–182.

Tan, E. T. H., Johnson, R. H., Lambie, D. G., Vijayasenan, M. E., & Whiteside, E. A. (1984). Erectile impotence in chronic alcoholics. *Alcoholism: Clinical and Experimental Research, 8,* 297–301.

Van Thiel, D. H. (1985). Ethyl alcohol and gonadal function. *Hospital Practice, 19,* 152–158.

Van Thiel, D. H., & Chaiao, Y. -B. (1983). Biochemical mechanisms that contribute to alcohol-induced hypogonadism in the male. *Alcoholism: Clinical and Experimental Research, 7,* 131–134.

Van Thiel, D. H., Gavaler, J. S., & Sanghir, A. (1982). Recovery of sexual function in abstinent alcoholic men. *Gastroenterology, 84,* 677–682.

Wagner, G. & Jensen, S. B. (1981). Alcohol and erectile failure. In G. Wagner & R. Green (Eds.), *Impotence: Physiological, psychological, surgical diagnosis and treatment* (pp. 81–87). New York: Plenum.

Whalley, L. J. (1978). Sexual adjustment of male alcoholics. *Acta Psychiatrica Scandinavica, 58,* 281–298.

Wilson, G. T. (1977). Alcohol and human sexual behavior. *Behavior Research and Therapy, 15,* 239–252.

Wilson, G. T. (1981). The effects of alcohol on human sexual behavior. *Advances in Substance Abuse, 2,* 1–40.

Wilson, G., & Lawson, D. (1976). Expectancies, alcohol and sexual arousal in male social drinkers. *Journal of Abnormal Psychology, 85,* 587–594.

Wincze, J. P. (1988). Recovery of sexual function in impotent male alcoholics. Unpublished manuscript. VA Medical Center and Brown University, Providence, RI.

Wiseman, J. P. (1985). Alcohol, eroticism and sexual performance: A social interactionist perspective. *Journal of Drug Issues, 15,* 291–308.

10

Summary: Family Processes and Alcoholism

KENNETH E. LEONARD

The impact of alcoholism on the lives of those who are intimately involved with the alcoholic has been recognized for some time. Temperance tracts of the 1830s, for example, describe the many negative effects experienced by the wives and children of inebriates. In the view of these writers, the excessive use of spirits in the father was strongly linked to subsequent alcohol problems in his children. Although the mechanism ascribed to this linkage, a Lamarckian notion that the alcohol had pharmacological properties which altered a man in such a way that he fathered inebriates (Levine, 1978), is not held today, descriptively, the temperance writers appear to be correct. Children of alcoholics, particularly sons, are at a heightened risk for the development of alcoholism. Of course, the transmission of inebriety was of concern to the Temperance Movement largely because the use of spirits was seen as the direct or indirect cause of a number of social ills, most notably, detrimental influences on family members. Throughout early temperance tracts are numerous references to the economic and social hardships suffered by the wives and children of drunkards. The tales of immorality included neglect of the needs of the family, as well as instances of extreme violence against family members. The culprit in all of these family problems was less the character of the habitual drunkard than the direct influence of the alcohol. In sum, the concern was that alcohol use had a very detrimental impact on the family functioning and would lead to alcoholism in the offspring.

Current research efforts concerning alcohol and the family that are described in this section roughly correspond to these concerns. One set of studies focuses on family processes that relate to the development of alcohol and other problems in the offspring, both of alcoholics and of nonalcoholics. Barnes's chapter describes parenting practices in families, whether the parents are alcoholic or not, that relate to adolescent drinking. Johnson's chapter focuses on the psychosocial deficits among children of alcoholics that occur, perhaps, because of parenting practices, or because of the specific challenges encountered as a child of an alcoholic, or as a result of an inherited temperament or cognitive characteristics that are associated with the risk for alcoholism. Even given these risks, being a child of an alcoholic does not necessarily lead to psychosocial dysfunction or to later alcohol problems. Bennett and Wolin's chapter establishes a link between family processes and whether alcohol problems are seen in the adult offspring of alcoholics.

A second set of studies concerns the relationship between alcohol consumption and marital functioning in alcoholics. In Bennett and Wolin's chapter, the manner in which the couple establishes family rituals and a family identity is linked to the development of alcohol problems in the offspring of alcoholics. Leonard's chapter examines differences in marital functioning and problem solving interaction between episodic and steady alcoholics and nonalcoholic spouses. O'Farrell's chapter calls attention to an important and neglected element of alcoholic marriages, sexual functioning, and its relationship to aspects of alcoholism and the marital relationship.

Integration of these chapters is rendered difficult by the considerable diversity exhibited among the different chapters. One is struck with the fact that although the authors are uniformly concerned with family processes, the concepts and methodologies are quite diverse. This diversity arises in part from the fact that different family processes are to be expected to operate relative to the different aspects of alcoholism. The diversity also can be partially attributed to the multidisciplinary roots of family studies (Jacob, 1987). Against this backdrop of diversity, a variety of methodological and conceptual issues stand out as important areas for future consideration. These do not exhaust the methodological issues relevant to the study of the family (see Larzelere & Klein, 1987, for a full discussion), but only the most pertinent to the alcohol and family area. They include: measurement of family processes, sampling of alcoholic families, and alcoholism as a general versus specific influence.

MEASUREMENT OF FAMILY PROCESSES

Across the five chapters, it is evident that family processes and outcomes are often measured quite differently. On the one hand, self-report of family processes is the most commonly utilized method. Studies of parenting practices and adolescent alcohol use described by Barnes assessed parenting practices by asking adolescents to report on their parents' behavior or by asking parents about their own behavior. In contrast to the use of these self-report scales, the work of Bennett and Wolin utilizes a semistructured interview with family members to elicit information concerning family rituals. This information is then coded by blind raters into the family process variables of interest. At the other extreme, the research reviewed by Leonard utilized direct observation of families, either in the home, going about their usual business (Steinglass, 1981), or in the laboratory, focused on a problem solving task. Each of these methods has strengths and weaknesses.

Self-report of family processes, like other self-reports, has the advantage of economy. Further, it allows the accumulation of experiences to be aggregated into a general pattern of family processes. Whether these reports are veridical with actual family processes is unclear. Given the private nature of the family, socially desirable distortions may be particularly apt to occur. Self-reports of family processes may also be influenced by factors which influence the *perception* of processes independent of the processes themselves.

Direct observations of laboratory tasks allow for the objective assessment of specific processes. However, the degree to which these processes generalize to actual family processes is a major question. Even when the task has a great degree of similarity to actual family tasks (i.e., discussion of family problems), the necessities of a laboratory study place constraints on the performance of the task. For example, family members are required to remain seated, remain in the laboratory, work toward a resolution of the problem for 10 to 15 minutes, and stay focused on the task. As a result, the processes identified in this structured setting may not correspond to actual processes that occur when the family attempts to solve a problem at home.

Home observations of actual behavior may be less problematic with respect to generalizability. However, the vast majority of actual family interactions may be irrelevant to the problem at hand. Important family process events may occur at such a low base rate that direct observation in the home may be impractical. Further, a certain amount of communication in a family occurs at a symbolic level or in a family dialect that is not necessarily accessible to an independent observer, whether that communication occurs in the home or in the laboratory. At present, the interrelationships among family processes as measured by these different procedures are not known and are a major issue for further research.

Not only do researchers measure family processes differently, family processes of interest encompass both molar and molecular behaviors. At the molecular level, the steady stream of family behavior is compartmentalized to the smallest understandable behavior, the thought unit. Family processes are viewed as the sequential structure of these individual behaviors. At the molar level, behavior-by-behavior associations are not of interest. Instead, molecular behavior is agglomerated, either explicitly or implicitly, and coded accordingly. Broad processes are of interest, such as support and control (Barnes, Chapter 5, this volume) and distinctive/subsumptive processes (Bennett & Wolin, Chapter 7, this volume). This issue relates in part to the choice of measures. Self-report inventories are most useful for molar processes. Molecular processes may not be easily observable by the relevant participants. Direct observations have most typically focused on molecular processes, though some observational studies have been concerned with molar processes (Steinglass, 1981). Studies of marital dysfunction and of aggressive children suggest strength in molecular approaches (Levenson & Gottman, 1985; Patterson, 1982). However, Bennett and Wolin's chapter demonstrates that molar processes, which are not always observable in molecular analyses, may be of considerable importance in understanding family functioning.

Differences in measurement also lie in whether processes are viewed as located within the individual, the interaction, or the family system. For example, the parental processes relevant to the development of adolescent drinking are most often seen as located within the parent. That is, the studies focus on whether the parent is warm or whether the parent exerts control. Sexual functioning also is typically seen as a process located in the alcoholic. Studies of marital processes often conceptualize these processes as the interaction of two or more individuals. The study of the family culture and family rituals, as well as some interaction studies, implicitly view the processes as residing in the family. It is unclear whether these represent alternative paradigms for describing marital and family processes or whether one approach is more valid or useful than the others. It is certainly the case that individual level characteristics can influence dyadic interactions and the family system and that dyadic interactions can influence the family system. However, in the causal chain of a specific outcome, which is the most useful manner of thinking about family processes? For example, a highly functional mother (individual level) may be able to display warmth and appropriate discipline to her children (individual and interactive level) and to interact with her husband in an appropriate way around his alcohol use (interactive) and thereby reduces his drinking within the family context (individual). Her coping ability (individual) and her relationship with her husband (interactive) may enable the formation of a distinctive family style (family systems) in which important family rituals are not disrupted by intoxication. When it is observed that the children from such a family are not socially debilitated and do not form alcoholic families, do we attribute this to the individual level (high mother functioning, father's drinking lower in family), the interactive level (effective maternal discipline, lessened parental conflict, lessened father-child conflict), the family systems level (distinctive family style), or to some combination of these levels. From an intervention perspective, this attribution would be of importance relative to who gets treated for what.

SAMPLING ISSUES

A second methodological issue raised in the studies of alcoholism and family processes is the sampling of alcoholic families for study. First, and perhaps most importantly, studies of family processes require the existence of a family. As simpleminded as this may sound, it has important consequences, particularly in the study of families of alcoholics. Many of the studies described in this section require, either explicitly in the protocol or implicitly in the topic, an intact family. It makes little sense to examine marital processes in a divorced couple or the alcoholic father's disciplinary interactions with the children in a family in which there is a nonalcoholic stepfather who is responsible for discipline. Thus, in many studies of alcoholic families, there is a strong likelihood that we are more likely to observe families in which alcoholism has been more or less accepted into the family. We do not tend to see families in which a problem drinker has ceased or moderated his drinking. Nor do we usually see families in which the alcoholic and his spouse have divorced, though some of the families will eventually reach this solution. As a result, generalizations of findings from these studies must be done very cautiously. Additionally, this points to the necessity of tracking alcohol and marital functioning longitudinally to determine the factors which lead to successful resolution of a heavy drinking pattern versus incorporation of the pattern into the family versus disintegration of the family unit.

A second sampling issue concerns the use of alcoholics and their families from clinical settings or from population samples. Many studies identify alcoholic families through clinical settings where the alcoholic or the spouse has presented for treatment (e.g., Herson, Miller, & Eisler, 1973; O'Farrell & Birchler, 1987; Steinglass, Davis, & Berenson, 1977). At present, little is known about the factors which differentiate alcoholics who seek treatment from alcoholics who do not. On a marital or family process level, there have been no studies that address the processes by which an alcoholic and/or his family might present for treatment, despite our knowledge that marital/family pressures are often reported to play a significant role in getting the alcoholic to treatment. As a result, it is probable that the marital and family processes of alcoholic families who present for treatment would be quite different from the processes of families who do not present for treatment. In an attempt to avoid the bias inherent in a treatment sample, some investigators have utilized newspaper advertisements to recruit alcoholics and their families for research (Jacob & Krahn, 1987; Steinglass, 1979). As with the clinical population, it is likely that alcoholics identified in this manner differ from the general population is some unknown way. Relatively few studies have attempted to utilize epidemiological approaches to identify alcoholics and their families for study. Some of the research described in the chapter by Barnes illustrates the usefulness of an epidemiologic approach to the study of parenting and alcohol use in adolescents. Application of this approach to other studies of alcohol and the family would be of considerable value.

A third sampling issue is related indirectly to both of the sampling issues described above. Since couples do not usually resort to treatment at the first sign of an alcohol problem, and, in particular, those that divorce relatively quickly may not ever present as an intact family, studies that rely on clinical samples of intact families tend to tap into a very selective time frame in the development of the family. As a result, many of the results from studies are most generalizable to those between the ages of 35 and 50 who have adolescent children. In particular, young alcohol abusers in their early 20s, in the early years of their first marriage, and having infants and young children are not typically sampled as part of research protocols. Thus, with the obvious exception of fetal alcohol effects, the impact of heavy alcohol consumption on infants and young children is virtually unstudied. To the extent that alcohol and marital processes manifest different relationships over the life span, research needs to examine the relationship across a broader age range than has been typically the case.

ALCOHOLISM AS A GENERAL VERSUS SPECIFIC INFLUENCE

Alcoholism may be viewed as exerting an influence on family processes, either through properties which it shares with other family disruptions or through more specific properties which are unique to this condition. For example, alcoholism is often viewed as a form of psychopathology. In many instances, other psychopathology accompanies the alcoholism, usually antisocial personality or depression (Hesselbrock, Hesselbrock, & Workman-Daniels, 1986). Differentiating between the general impact of psychopathology and the more specific impact of alcoholism is fraught with difficulties, particularly since other psychopathologies may have their own specific impact. Similarly, alcoholism is often accompanied by marital and family conflict, health problems, economic problems, and social problems. Some of these may be caused by the alcoholism, but others may simply be concomitants. These problems, too, have an influence on family processes.

Despite the general similarity that alcoholism shares with other conditions that influence the family, it also has specific aspects which are not shared. The presence of two different cognitive states, intoxicated and sober, is relatively unique. Although some psychopathologies cycle between two states (e.g., episodes of depression vs. normal functioning in depressives), the frequency of changes within alcoholics tends to be higher, and the characteristics of the states are quite different. Among other disturbances to the family, it is usually, but not always, possible to ascribe a clear causal attribution, either to the factors internal to the individual or to external factors. For example, in the case of a chronic disease, the causes are frequently assumed to be outside of the individual's control. With respect to marital conflict, the causes are often seen to reside in the individual. However, with alcoholism, there is often ambiguity in ascribing causality. Although alcoholism can be seen as having some of the features of a disease, it also can be seen as stemming from a moral failing in the individual. This particular configuration of attitudes about alcoholism may place the alcoholic's family in the confusing position of feeling angry (a reaction to an attribution of internal causality) about something over which they believe the alcoholic has no control (an attribution of external causality).

From a methodological standpoint, this issue will have a major impact on the selection of comparison groups, particularly among studies that seek to compare alcoholics to nonalcoholics. Studies seeking to understand the impact of alcoholism as a specific disorder should choose comparison samples designed to control for the general features of alcoholism which are deemed relevant. By implication, the conclusions of such studies must be carefully qualified in accordance with the aspects of alcoholism that have been controlled. The importance of this is most clearly illustrated in O'Farrell's chapter. Alcoholism has an impact on marital conflict, endocrine functioning, general health, and liver functioning, and all of these factors may play a role in sexual impairment. Throughout the studies reviewed in this chapter, a variety of specific comparison groups are utilized, each adding something different to our understanding of alcohol, alcoholism, and sexual functioning.

In sum, alcoholism may have a variety of impacts on family functioning. Some of these arise from the features that alcoholism shares with other disorders; some of these arise from disturbances caused by the alcoholism (but which can also be caused by other factors), and some arise from the unique elements involved in alcoholism. Disentangling these different influences will require a variety of methodological approaches and may have important implications for appropriate treatment interventions.

FUTURE RESEARCH DIRECTIONS

Although each of the authors has identified areas of needed research with respect to the specific issues discussed in their respective chapters, a variety of additional research directions can be identified. At the most basic level, methodological research addressing the comparability of self-report, quasi-observational, and observational measures of family processes is of tremendous importance. Issues concerning the level of analysis, both molar versus molecular and individually based versus interactively based versus systemically based, also require further work. Aside from the level of family processes, the content of family processes is of considerable importance. Most of the family interaction research thus far has focused either on family interaction broadly or on one specific family process, resolving conflict. This reflects as much about the historical roots of family interaction research as it does about the ascribed importance of this process to the family. O'Farrell's chapter, focusing on sexual functioning, addresses an important and neglected area of marital relationships. Other aspects of marital relationships need to be investigated. For example, how do alcoholics and their spouses regulate intimacy, and how is this influenced by alcohol consumption? How does alcoholism influence the couple's interaction with other social and family networks, and does this have implications for their own interactions? In short, the study of alcohol and family processes has started at the most obvious point of interest, conflict resolution, but should now proceed to other processes which are theoretically meaningful in the context of alcoholism and the family.

In addition to these needed methodological refinements, there is a vital need for research to address the interrelationship between alcohol and family functioning from a family developmental perspective. This perspective is similar to the position of Zucker (1979) and of Johnson (Chapter 6, this volume), but focuses on family development rather than individual development. A family developmental perspective suggests a variety of novel research possibilities. The influence of alcohol on family functioning, as well as the influence of family functioning on the development of alcohol problems, may differ across different phases of family development. In particular, the early years of marriage, in which many young men moderate their drinking behavior and in which marital patterns may be established, is one particularly important area for future research. The hypothesis of Bennett and Wolin concerning the transmission of alcoholism among offspring of alcoholics being a function of contact with the alcoholic family of origin and of a distinct decision to develop different family rituals than the alcoholic family of origin is one specific issue which could be addressed within such a longitudinal framework.

The impact of family social controls on drinking is also an important area of future research. Research by Holmila (1987) in Finland has pointed to a variety of informal controls which wives and husbands use in attempts to control excessive drinking by the spouse. In addition, families are confronted with a variety of normative developmental crises (birth of a child, child starts school, etc.) as well as more unexpected crises (loss of a job, death of a family member). Adjustment to these crises may very well be influenced by the presence of a heavy drinker or alcoholic in the family. As the family develops, a variety of specific studies becomes possible. Currently, there is considerable research concerning infant attachment within the framework of parent–infant interactions. Indeed, one study has examined parent–infant interaction among alcoholic women (O'Connor, Sigman, & Brill, 1987). How does alcoholism affect father–child interactions? Does alcoholism in the father influence mother–infant attachment? What impact do father–child and mother–child relationships have on the development of later psychosocial problems among children of alcoholics? Does a positive mother–child relationship protect the child of an alcoholic from the negative impact of the alcoholic father? These questions represent only some of the important areas for future research that arise from a family developmental perspective.

Finally, research progress concerning alcoholism and family processes will require shedding the implicit assumption of homogeneity among alcoholics. Within the alcoholism field, there has been a growing recognition that there are different subtypes of alcoholism within the heterogeneous alcoholic population. At present, there is not a consensus concerning the precise number and nature of different subtypes, but it is clear that research is attempting to devise more homogeneous subgroups of alcoholics and regularly includes these subgroups in substantive investigations. With the exception of the wet-transitional-dry distinction used by Steinglass and his colleagues (e.g., Steinglass, 1979) and the episodic/steady dimension described by Jacob and his colleagues (e.g., Jacob & Leonard, 1988), it is not certain whether any of the current subtypes will prove useful in studying the relationship between alcohol and family processes. Nonetheless, it is clear that alcoholism develops differently from one family to the next. The specific family challenges that arise from chronic heavy drinking differ from family to family, as does the reaction of the family. These parameters may come to define important subgroups of alcoholic families for which the relationship between alcohol use and family functioning are quite different. Importantly, such research may have implications for whether marital or family treatment would be useful, or detrimental, to the alcoholic and to the family.

REFERENCES

Herson, M., Miller, P. M., & Eisler, R. M. (1973). Interactions between alcoholics and their wives: A descriptive analysis of verbal and nonverbal behavior. *Quarterly Journal of Studies on Alcohol, 34,* 516–520.

Hesselbrock, V. M., Hesselbrock, M. N., & Workman-Daniels, K. L. (1986). Effect of major depression and antisocial personalilty on alcoholism: Course and motivational patterns. *Journal of Studies on Alcohol, 47,* 207–212.

Holmila, M. (1987). Young families and alcohol use in Finland and the Soviet Union. *Contemporary Drug Problems, 14,* 649–672.

Jacob, T. (1987). Family interaction and psychopathology: Historical overview. In T. Jacob (Ed.), *Family interaction and psychopathology: Theories, methods, and findings* (pp. 3–22). New York: Plenum Press.

Jacob, T. & Krahn, G. L. (1987). The classification of behavorial observation codes in studies of family interaction. *Journal of Marriage and the Family, 49,* 677–687.

Jacob, T. & Leonard, K. E. (1988). Alcoholic-spouse interactions as a function of alcoholism subtype and alcohol consumption interaction. *Journal of Abnormal Psychology, 97,* 231–237.

Larzelere, R. E. & Klein, D. M. (1987). Methodology. In M. B. Sussman & S. K. Steinmetz (Eds.), *Handbook of marriage and the family* (pp. 125–155). New York: Plenum Press.

Levenson, R. W. & Gottman, J. M. (1985). Physiological and affective predictors of change in relationship satisfaction. *Journal of Personality and Social Psychology, 49,* 85–94.

Levine, H. G. (1978). The discovery of addiction. Changing conceptions of habitual drunkenness in America. *Journal of Studies on Alcohol, 39,* 143–174.

O'Connor, M. J., Sigman, M., & Brill, N. (1987). Disorganization of attachment in relation to maternal alcohol consumption. *Journal of Consulting and Clinical Psychology, 55,* 831–836.

O'Farrell, T. J. & Birchler, G. R. (1987). Marital relationships of alcoholic, conflicted, and nonconflicted couples. *Journal of Marital and Family Therapy, 13,* 259–274.

Patterson, G. R. (1982). *Coercive family processes.* Eugene, OR: Castalia Publishing Company.

Steinglass, P. (1979). The alcoholic family in the interaction laboratory. *Journal of Nervous and Mental Disease, 167,* 428–436.

Steinglass, P. (1981). The alcoholic family at home. Patterns of interaction in dry, wet and transitional stages of alcoholism. *Archives of General Psychiatry, 38,* 578–584.

Steinglass, P., Davis, D. I., & Berenson, D. (1977). Observations of conjointly hospitalized "alcoholic couples" during sobriety and intoxication: Implications for theory and therapy. *Family Process, 16,* 1–16.

Zucker, R. A. (1979). Developmental aspects of drinking through the young adult years. In H. T. Blane & M. E. Chafetz (Eds.), *Youth, alcohol and social policy* (pp. 91–146). New York: Plenum Press.

PART III

FAMILY-ORIENTED TREATMENT

11

Family Treatment of Alcohol Abuse: Behavioral and Systems Perspectives

R. LORRAINE COLLINS

The topic of family treatment for alcohol abuse raises a variety of issues not all of which will be addressed here. This review will be limited to a description and evaluation of the two major approaches to family treatment of alcohol abuse: behavioral and family systems. Al-Anon, a self-help group for spouses and other relatives of alcoholics, will also be described. These approaches were chosen because they are representative of the research and clinical work currently being conducted with alcoholics and their families. In addition each has a particular theory/philosophy with which it is identified, and research designed to assess its efficacy. The current chapter will serve as an evaluative review of the literature on behavioral and systems approaches to treating alcohol abuse. Thus, the scope of the current chapter does not include an exhaustive review of all studies relevant to these two approaches to family therapy of alcohol problems. For example, the role of the family in the development of drinking problems will not be discussed, except where specifically relevant to treatment.

The move to include family members in treatment is an acknowledgment of the reciprocal relationship between an alcoholic's behavior and the consequences experienced by members of his/her family. The effects of the dysfunctions experienced by the alcoholic are often shared by individuals with whom she or he interacts. Thus, the family unit is usually the primary group to directly experience maladaptive drinking behavior and its consequences. Coping with these consequences may produce a variety of psychological and social reactions in individual family members as well as in the family unit as a whole (Moos, Finney & Gamble, 1982). Further, issues within the family can maintain or increase problem drinking behavior (Jacob, Dunn, & Leonard, 1983; Wiseman, 1981). Since cause–effect relationships are difficult to disentangle and specify, researchers and clinicians have begun to focus on working with the alcoholic and his/her family.

Other reasons for the shift to family therapy include: (1) reports of a better response to treatment on the part of the alcoholic when other family members (particularly spouses) are included; (2) minimization of the isolation experienced by alcoholics in treatment by themselves; (3) exposure of other problem areas that may also require treatment (e.g., communication, parenting issues, sexual problems); and (4) a shared common goal for members of the family unit (Janzen, 1977). The broader focus and goals of family-oriented treatment might also allow the family to experience successes in nondrinking areas. Thus, even if the alcoholic is not totally abstinent, gains may be made in areas such as quality of communication, employment, and better parenting.

ROLE OF THE FAMILY ENVIRONMENT IN TREATMENT OUTCOME

There are a number of factors that can enhance the response to family treatment. For example, alcoholics from a positive family environment involving cohesion and active recreational activities had better treatment outcomes than those from environments in which there was more emphasis on conflict and control (Moos, Bromet, Tsu, & Moos, 1979). Similarly, alcoholics who reported more problems related to the nuclear family (e.g., strained or conflictual family relations) or problems related to interaction with the father tended to have poorer treatment outcomes (Vannicelli, Gingerich, & Ryback, 1983). In the latter study, improvements in nondrinking areas (e.g., job status) occurred for families presenting with an emphasis on communication problems.

Comparisons of alcoholic, recovered alcoholic, and nonalcoholic families also illustrate the reciprocal relationships among drinking behavior, spouse and family functioning, and treatment outcome. Moos and his colleagues have assessed aspects of these complex relationships in their program of research on family functioning of alcoholics (e.g., Finney Moos, Cronkite, & Gamble, 1983; Moos et al., 1979; Moos, Finney & Chan, 1981; Moos et al., 1982; Moos & Moos, 1984). For example, Moos et al. (1982) compared the predominantly female spouses of relapsed and recovered alcoholics with nonalcoholic community controls. Although they found no significant differences in social competence and the use of coping strategies among the three groups of spouses, the spouses of relapsed alcoholics reported the most stress. Stress was related to increased experience of negative life events, decreased participation in social activities, and less family cohesion. The spouses of both relapsed and recovered alcoholics were emotionally (anxiety, depression) and physically (number of minor symptoms) affected by their partner's drinking, whereas the control spouses' functioning was not related to partner variables. A 2-year follow-up of this sample focused on role functioning and family environment (Moos & Moos, 1984). Results indicated similar levels of cohesion, expressiveness, organization, and conflict in the family environments of recovered alcoholics and nonalcoholic controls. However, there was more conflict and poorer functioning in the families of relapsed alcoholics, particularly those currently drinking. Finney et al. (1983) have proposed and tested a conceptual model in which stress, exemplified by impairment of the alcoholic (e.g., drinking, anxiety and depression, occupational functioning) was an important determinant of the functioning of the nonalcoholic spouse. The alcoholic's nondrinking impairment (e.g., occupational functioning) also had a significant impact on spouse's impairment (e.g., physical symptoms, depression).

The duration of the alcoholic's sobriety can also have an impact on family functioning (Roberts, Floyd, O'Farrell, & Cutter, 1985). Roberts et al. found that the marital interactions of "high sobriety" (sober for $\geq$ 2 years) couples were less conflictual (fewer disagreements and aggressive behaviors, more talkative) than were "low sobriety" (sober for $\leq$ 4 months) couples. These results were interpreted as indicating that "longer durations of sobriety for alcoholic husbands would be associated with fewer struggles for control and less conflict in the marital interactions of alcoholics and their wives" (p. 310).

Steinglass, Tislenko, and Reiss (1985) studied family interaction and drinking patterns of alcoholics over a longer (2-year) period. They reported no significant differences in the home interaction patterns of families of alcoholics with either of three patterns of drinking (stable wet—families where drinking continued for the 2 years; stable dry—families where sobriety was maintained for the 2 years; alternators—families where drinking fluctuated between wet and dry periods). However, there was a trend for less family cohesion and greater marital instability in stable wet families. Jacob and Leonard (1988) found that "steady" alcoholics and their spouses exhibited better problem solving skills and less negativistic patterns of interactions than "episodic" alcoholics and their spouses. The seemingly inconsistent findings of these two studies are related to their differential designation of types of alcoholics. For the purposes of this review, these studies are of interest because they indicate that different patterns of abusive drinking have a differential impact on family functioning. A more extensive discussion of the research on the interaction patterns of alcoholic families is presented in Leonard's chapter in this volume.

Preli and Protinsky (1988) reported differences in the structure of families with an actively alcoholic member, a recovered alcoholic member, or nonalcoholic members. Families with an active or recovered alcoholic member showed pathological relationship structures involving reversals in the family hierarchy, and alcoholic families had the greatest proportion of cross-generational (mother–child) coalitions.

Clearly, these results illustrate that a drinking spouse can adversely affect the functioning of his/her nonalcoholic partner and other family members, as well as general family interaction. The nonalcoholic partner's functioning in turn has been cited as a factor in the alcoholic's recovery (Orford et al., 1975; Wright & Scott, 1978). Thus, a cycle of reciprocal negative influences between the alcoholic and the nonalcoholic partner can be set into motion.

Taken together these studies suggest that important reciprocal relationships exist between the family environment and the alcoholic's drinking status. Some of these effects are evident in the structure of family interactions (Moos & Moos, 1984; Preli & Protinsky, 1988; Roberts et al., 1985), while others are evident in the functioning of particular family members (Moos et al., 1982). An actively drinking alcoholic can have a deleterious effect on his/her spouse, including reports of increased levels of stress (Moos et al., 1982; Moos & Moos, 1984) as well as physical symptoms and depression (Finney et al., 1983). More positive family environments are related to more positive treatment outcomes (Finney et al., 1983; Moos et al., 1979; Vannicelli et al., 1983). However, the cause–effect nature of this relationship is not easily disentangled.

THE BEHAVIORAL APPROACH

Behavioral theory subscribes to the basic tenet that behavior is learned and maintained via principles of reinforcement and therefore is amenable to being unlearned. Within the behavioral approach, social learning theory incorporates aspects of the stimulus–response models of operant and classical conditioning, but expands beyond these models to include cognitive processes (George & Marlatt, 1983). Over the years a number of researchers in the alcohol treatment field have applied behavioral principles to working with couples as well as with a wider range of family members. Generally families are seen as providing three types of consequences: "(a) reinforcement for drinking behavior in the form of attention or care taking, (b) shielding the alcoholic from experiencing the negative consequences of drinking, and (c) punishing drinking behavior" (McGrady, 1986, p. 310). The guiding principles of the application of behavioral techniques in family treatment of alcohol abuse is to increase and reinforce positive behaviors/interactions among family members and to decrease negative behaviors/interactions related to drinking.

Behavioral treatment encompasses a variety of techniques, many of which have been incorporated into family treatment of alcohol abuse. Assessment usually begins with a functional analysis of problem areas (Vuchinich,

Tucker, & Harllee, 1988). Specific targets for intervention are then identified. The selection of treatment techniques is based on the results of the functional analysis thereby allowing for the tailoring of interventions to specific areas of need. Treatment often includes "homework" assignments (e.g., monitoring of behavior, engaging in pleasurable activities that serve as alternatives to drinking) to be performed between sessions.

Research on behavioral family-oriented treatment of alcohol abuse can be placed in three categories: (1) demonstrations of the use of behavioral techniques as core elements or adjuncts to treatment; (2) comparisons of treatment techniques within a behavioral framework; and (3) comparisons between behavioral techniques and other approaches. Each will be described in turn below.

Demonstrations of the Use of Behavioral Techniques

A study by Hunt and Azrin (1973) is an early example of the application of a comprehensive behavioral program to family treatment of alcohol abuse. Employing a "community reinforcement approach" based on operant reinforcement, the program was designed to improve the client's functioning in areas other than drinking (e.g., family interactions, vocational and recreational activities, social contacts). Sixteen male alcoholics were randomly assigned to either the experimental group or a matched (e.g., age, education, previous hospitalizations) control group. Alcoholics in the control condition received standard hospital treatment including alcohol education and Alcoholics Anonymous (AA). Subjects in the experimental group received standard treatment plus assistance in a variety of areas (e.g., finding a job, improving social relationships) including marital and family counseling. At the 6-month follow-up, the experimental group functioned significantly better than the control group in all areas including marital satisfaction and drinking behavior.

Azrin (1976) extended the design of this study to include more subjects (10 per condition). In addition to the community reinforcement approach previously described, subjects in the experimental group also received the drug disulfiram (Antabuse) and participated in a buddy system in which former alcoholics served as "peer-advisors." The matched control group received standard treatment including Antabuse. This second study also included a more extensive follow-up of 2 years. Results indicated that during the first 6 months alcoholics in the experimental group drank on a smaller percentage of days, were less often absent from home, spent less time in institutions (e.g., hospital, prison), and were employed for more time than the control group. These benefits were maintained through the 2-year follow-up.

These two studies are methodologically noteworthy for a number of reasons. They employed a paraprofessional staff, including ex-alcoholics, to serve as advisors and focused on practical constraints to satisfactory life adjustment (jobs, legal problems), beyond those directly linked to family interaction. Although the small sample sizes are a limitation of these studies, they achieved excellent results, especially given the fact that the alcoholics in the study possessed characteristics previously linked to a poor prognosis for treatment (e.g., low SES, unemployed). In terms of research methodology, each study included a matched control group, objective assessment of outcome, and an adequate follow-up period. Although the results are promising, these studies have not yet been replicated and/or extended to larger samples, a possible constraint being the time and resource intensiveness of the experimental intervention. Nevertheless, these studies are comprehensive and effective models of behavioral family treatment of alcohol problems.

Behavioral approaches have also been used to train spouses to motivate alcoholics to begin treatment (Sisson & Azrin, 1986) and to comply with an Antabuse regimen (Keane, Foy, Nunn, & Rychtarik, 1984). Sisson and Azrin (1986) found behavioral strategies useful in teaching nonalcoholic women to encourage their alcoholic partners to seek treatment and achieve sobriety. The reinforcement program consisted of a variety of strategies including providing positive consequences for not drinking and negative consequences for intoxication, organizing alternative nonalcoholic activities, and providing joint counseling if the alcoholic responded to persuasion and entered treatment. The reinforcement program was compared to a "traditional" program based on alcohol education, supportive counseling, and referral to Al-Anon. Compared to the alcoholic partners of women in the traditional program, the alcoholic partners of women in the reinforcement program were more successful in decreasing drinking behavior (number of drinking days, days intoxicated, volume consumed/drinking episode) and increasing use of Antabuse. While interesting, this study too is best viewed as a demonstration project in which a small number of subjects (seven in reinforcement and five in traditional) were provided with intensive interventions.

Keane et al. (1984) compared two behavioral approaches to a control condition for increasing compliance with use of Antabuse. Twenty-five men who had completed an inpatient treatment program were randomly assigned to three conditions. The two behavioral conditions were contracting/recording (subjects signed a contract to take Antabuse in the spouse's presence and recorded drug ingestion) and contracting/recording plus positive reinforcement (contacting as well as encouragement to experience weekly treats). The control condition involved explanation of the use of Antabuse, but did not include contracting/recording. The subjects and their nonalcoholic partners participated in an extended discharge session in which the behavioral intervention was presented. Results indicated a high rate of compliance with the Antabuse regimen (88%) and less abusive drinking in the two behavioral conditions than in the control condition. Clinical application of contracting for compliance with taking Antabuse also has been included in other behavioral marital treatment programs (cf. O'Farrell & Cutter, 1984).

Comparisons Among Behavioral Family-Oriented Treatment and Other Approaches

In comparison with other family oriented approaches, behavioral marital therapy is generally effective for a variety of clinical problems (Hahlweg & Markman, 1988). Behavioral marital therapy for alcoholics is one of the most extensively studied aspects of family treatment for alcohol abuse. Behavioral interventions for couples have typically been conducted on an outpatient basis (Keane et al., 1984; McCrady et al., 1986; O'Farrell, Cutter, & Floyd, 1985). The goals of treatment have focused on changes in drinking behavior (McCrady et al., 1986) as well as family functioning (e.g., marital satisfaction, changes in patterns of interaction; O'Farrell et al., 1985). The treatment techniques have included communication training to enhance the clarity and quality of verbal interactions, training in problem solving, and sex therapy (O'Farrell & Cutter, 1984).

O'Farrell and Cutter (1984) described a comprehensive set of clinical procedures that can be employed in a behavioral marital therapy program for alcoholics. The focus of their treatment program is improvement in the couple's marital functioning as a route to improving the drinking behavior of the alcoholic. Assessment is conducted during the first two to three sessions during which couples complete measures on drinking behavior and their marital and sexual relationship, and provide a videotaped sample of communication related to discussion of a marital problem. Subsequent interventions are designed to change conditions that maintain drinking and enhance conditions that promote sobriety. In this 10-week program, alcoholics commit to a goal of abstinence, contract to use Antabuse, and discuss how to prevent or cope with a relapse. Spouses monitor positive behaviors (such as expressions of caring), plan and engage in shared recreational activities, learn and practice communication skills, and practice skills related to negotiating and maintaining agreements. Homework assignments related to these areas of change are assigned and progress is monitored on a weekly basis. Therapists are trained and supervised in their implementation of the treatment techniques.

The results of the application of these strategies have been quite positive. O'Farrell et al. (1985) compared behavioral marital therapy, interaction therapy (mutual support, problem solving), and a no-marital-therapy control condition for male alcoholics who had just completed a 28-day standard inpatient treatment program. Relative to couples who did not receive marital therapy, couples receiving behavioral marital therapy reported greater marital satisfaction and stability while showing improvements in specific areas targeted for intervention (communication, emotional distress, use of Antabuse). Couples receiving interaction therapy showed improvement in some areas of marital functioning, but alcoholics who received behavior therapy also showed better drinking outcomes.

Comparisons of Treatment Techniques Within a Behavioral Framework

Along with the outcome studies just described, research within the behavioral approach has included evaluation of the relative efficacy of specific strategies for family treatment. Hedberg and Campbell (1974) compared behavioral family therapy (reinforcement, assertiveness training, behavioral contracting) to three standard behavioral treatments provided to the alcoholic (systematic desensitization, covert sensitization, or electric shock). They found family therapy to be the most efficacious in changing drinking behavior up to a 6-month follow-up (74% of clients achieved their goal of abstinence or controlled drinking).

McCrady et al. (1986) compared different approaches to couples treatment within a behavioral framework. Couples were randomly assigned to outpatient treatment consisting of either a minimal spouse involvement (MSI; spouse present to provide understanding and support), alcohol-focused spouse involvement (AFSI; couples learn skills related to modifying drinking behavior), or alcohol behavioral marital therapy (ABMT; interventions from MSI and AFSI as well as marital therapy). Results through a 6-month follow-up indicated that although treatment was effective in achieving abstinence and decreasing heavy drinking, there were no differences among the three groups in frequency of drinking. During treatment the MSI and AFSI groups reported significantly greater marital satisfaction than the ABMT group. At the 6-month follow-up there were no differences in marital satisfaction among the three groups and all groups reported improvements in their relationships. McCrady et al.'s comparison of treatment strategies within the behavioral framework suggests that behaviorally based couples treatment is generally effective in reducing drinking and increasing marital satisfaction, but that no single technique produces a superior outcome.

Conclusion

While several studies indicate that behavioral marital therapy can be effective in changing both the interaction patterns and drinking behavior of alcoholics, the pattern of results across studies does not yet conclusively indicate the efficacy of this approach. The early demonstration studies often produced excellent outcome, but these occurred only with intensive intervention applied to small samples of subjects. These studies were innovative in their use of nonprofessionals and extended family members (Azrin, 1976; Hunt & Azrin, 1973) and suggested that behavioral approaches are effective in motivating alcoholics to seek treatment (Sisson & Azrin, 1986) and use Antabuse (Keane et al., 1984). However, no attempts have been made to replicate or extend the demonstration studies.

Couples who received behavioral marital therapy have shown somewhat better outcomes in drinking behavior and marital functioning than subjects receiving interactional therapy or no treatment (O'Farrell et al. 1985). Comparisons of techniques within a behavioral framework have generally indicated that family therapy is better than nonfamily approaches (Hedberg & Campbell, 1974), but variations in the nature of family treatment did not produce different outcomes (McCrady et al., 1986).

FAMILY SYSTEMS APPROACH

Family systems theory encompasses a set of general tenets from which a wide variety of treatment techniques has been derived. As outlined by Steinglass (1982), adherents to the family systems approach subscribe to the following core ideas:

1. The family is viewed as an organizational unit in which members relate and interact in a reciprocally deterministic fashion. When applied to alcohol abuse, this tenet suggests that just as the alcoholic's drinking has an impact on the family, so too does the family play a role in the maintenance of the drinking problem.

2. Families seek to establish and maintain a sense of equilibrium. While this equilibrium is not necessarily indicative of healthy interactions within the unit, the familiarity/comfort of the state of equilibrium leads to resistance to changes in behavior. Alcohol may serve to stabilize certain families; thus even adaptive changes in drinking behavior may be resisted because such changes are seen as destabilizing the family's interaction patterns.

3. The member of the family who manifests clinical symptoms (e.g., alcoholism) is the "identified patient." This individual is "selected by the family system to express for the entire family the particular piece of disturbance represented by the symptom selected" (p. 131). The identified patient protects or stabilizes the functioning of all members of the family unit through the expression of his/her pathological symptoms.

4. Communication within the family can serve to establish/reinforce patterns of interaction indicative of the family system.

5. Family interaction occurs within boundaries that may be either rigid and impermeable or highly permeable with respect to the outside world.

Rigid boundaries create a sense of isolation while highly permeable boundaries interfere with family cohesion. Families of alcoholics are said to maintain rigid boundaries, thus functioning within a sphere of isolation.

Family systems therapy has been applied to the treatment of a variety of addictive behaviors (e.g., Stanton et al., 1982, in the area of drug abuse treatment), and application of family systems techniques has included a variety of "schools" of therapy. As a major exponent of the family systems approach to alcohol abuse, Steinglass (cf., Steinglass, Bennett, Wolin, & Reiss, 1987) has focused on studying patterns of interaction in alcoholic families. Some of these ideas have been tested in an experimental program designed to demonstrate the value of the interactionist approach as a mode of intervention. Steinglass (1979) described a 6-week intensive treatment program administered to a sample of 10 couples. The program was divided into three phases. The first phase consisted of 2 weeks during which couples met in groups for 3 sessions/week. The second phase included a 10-day conjoint hospitalization during which couples were provided with access to alcohol and the focus of treatment was on changing patterns of interaction. In the third phase, which lasted 3 weeks, patients participated in twice weekly outpatient group therapy. Group meetings were also conducted every 6 weeks during the 6-month follow-up. Assessments occurred in the four general areas of individual drinking behavior, psychiatric symptoms, social functioning, and marital interaction.

Results for the eight alcoholics who remained in treatment showed a moderate decrease in drinking behavior, the only variable on which alcoholics and their nonalcoholic spouses could be distinguished. This latter finding was said to provide support for the hypothesis that pathology related to alcohol abuse is manifested in family members other than the identified alcoholic. Interestingly, a reduction in drinking by the alcoholic was associated with a reduction in the psychiatric symptomatology of the nonalcoholic partner. The program was most effective in changing marital interaction. However, Steinglass concluded that the program may need a longer time frame so that changes in interaction can become solidified.

Steinglass (1979) demonstrated that an interactionist-based treatment for alcoholism can produce positive outcomes. A variety of objective measures was employed to assess functioning in diverse areas and the program had a strong theoretical base. However, the small sample of selected alcoholics and the lack of a control group limits interpretation and generalization of the results of this study.

McCrady and colleagues (McCrady, Paolino, Longabaugh, & Rossi, 1979) compared an interactionist-based marital therapy approach to individualized treatment. Results indicated that inclusion of the spouse in treatment enhanced its efficacy, but all groups (joint admission, couples therapy, individual therapy) showed improvements in drinking behavior and marital satisfaction. These results were maintained at a 4-year follow-up (McCrady, Moreau, Paolino, & Longabaugh, 1982).

While the results of early research were promising, little systematic treatment outcome research employing a systems framework has been undertaken. Most recently, Zweben, Pearlman, and Li (1988) compared a brief (single session) advice intervention with a more comprehensive 8-week systems-oriented conjoint treatment for a relatively nondistressed sample of 218 couples in which one member reported a moderately severe drinking problem. Both the Advice Counseling and the Conjoint Therapy conditions focused on interpersonal aspects of drinking behavior and the marital relationship. In the Advice Counseling condition couples were assisted with the identification of specific areas for change, goals of treatment, and strategies for achieving the goals. The Conjoint Treatment emphasized clarification of communication, problem solving, and practice of skills targeted to achieving treatment goals. Results were reported for 116 couples of the total sample (a 47% attrition rate), who were followed for 18 months after initial intake. The results indicated very few significant differences between the conditions. Both groups showed similar levels of improvement in drinking behavior (59% of the combined sample were classified as "greatly improved" in drinking) and marital satisfaction.

The results of Zweben et al.'s study suggest that even a relatively brief systems-oriented intervention can be moderately effective. This study is noteworthy for its large sample of subject, the use of psychometrically rigorous measures, systematic presentation of treatment techniques by trained therapist's, and an adequate follow-up period. However, there is neither an adequate control condition nor was a comparison made to non-systems-oriented treatment, and the attrition rate of 47% was quite high. If replicated, these results suggest that resources dedicated to intensive treatment might be better employed in brief interventions focused on achieving and maintaining specific goals.

Although not within an interactionist perspective, previous research on "advice" versus comprehensive alcoholism treatment for couples has also indicated no significant differences in outcome. Edwards et al. (1977) reported that at the 1-year follow-up, a single session of "advice" to an alcoholic and his spouse was just as effective as a broad-spectrum program that included the spouse. A 2-year follow-up of this sample indicated a significant interaction between the nature of the intervention and treatment outcome. Alcoholics receiving intensive treatment were more likely to be abstainers and alcoholics receiving brief advice were more likely to be controlled drinkers (Orford, Oppenheimer, & Edwards, 1976).

Conclusion

In direct comparisons, interactional marital treatment for alcoholics has proven as effective as individualized treatment (McCrady et al., 1979; Mc-

Crady et al., 1982) and less effective than a behavioral approach (O'Farrell et al., 1985). Current research within the interactionist approach suggests that a brief intervention is just as effective as intensive treatment (Zweben et al., 1988). While suggestive of techniques that might prove effective, the paucity of research on systems-oriented family treatment for alcoholics is indicative of the fact that while descriptions of systems approaches to treating alcoholic families abound, the body of methodologically sound empirical research on systems approaches is relatively limited. Thus one must concur with Jacobson, Holtzworth-Munroe, and Schmaling's (1989) conclusion that "the discrepancy between the predominance of systemic notions leading us to believe in the promise of marital treatments and the dearth of research on the efficacy of systemic approaches is striking" (p. 9). Further research to identify active ingredients in systems-oriented family therapy as well as tests of its efficacy seems necessary.

AL-ANON

One of the most readily available approaches to including family members in alcohol abuse treatment is Al-Anon. Al-Anon focuses on self-help rather than the involvement of treatment professionals. Its appeal seems to reside with its focus on self-help, the fact that groups are widely available, and that Al-Anon is affiliated with Alcoholics Anonymous (AA), even to the extent of subscribing to AA's 12 Steps. As with AA, Al-Anon subscribes to a disease model of alcoholism in which the tenets of being powerless over alcohol, but having the power to change alcohol-related behavior, are central. All of this occurs within a context in which the individual is encouraged to subscribe to a higher spiritual power of his/her own choosing. Although the alcoholic is held responsible for his/her own drinking behavior, the partner's role is said to be that of unintentional facilitator of the illness of alcoholism by responding to the alcoholic's drinking with anxiety and anger. Adherence to the disease model is said to remove hostility and guilt related to having an alcoholic spouse. In Al-Anon, the nonalcoholic partner is confronted with the fact that change in drinking is the responsibility of the alcoholic. She or he is encouraged to focus on developing her/ his own areas of fulfillment while becoming detached from involvement with the alcoholic's maladaptive drinking. By focusing on developing independent areas of interest and satisfaction, the nonalcoholic partner has the potential to experience some areas of happiness even within the context of an alcoholic marriage/family. This type of change in the partner can facilitate changes in the alcoholic when or if she or he decides to abstain from drinking.

Al-Anon is designed to provide support to the nonalcoholic partner (usually wife) or relative within a group framework where discussion of issues is emphasized. Ablon's (1974) participant observation studies of Al-Anon indicated that the majority of participants were white, middle-class women between the ages of 30 and 50. Although Al-Anon groups vary in their characteristics, meetings typically involve a sharing of experiences and strategies for coping with having an alcoholic spouse and adhering to the tenets of Al-Anon. An essential component of Al-Anon is the provision of social support among group members. This occurs both in the context of interaction within the group and telephone and social contacts outside of group meetings. In many cases Al-Anon serves as a source of friendship and camaraderie for women who have become socially isolated as a result of their preoccupation with their husband's alcohol abuse.

Research on Al-Anon is limited but some assessments of its efficacy do exist. Gorman and Rooney (1979) achieved a 73% response rate to a questionnaire mailed to 168 wives involved in Al-Anon. Results were consistent with the tenets of Al-Anon, in that the duration of membership in Al-Anon was associated with a decrease in negative coping behaviors (e.g., covering up for the alcoholic, nagging, and coaxing). It was concluded that "wives of alcoholics are capable of modifying their behavior regardless of their spouses' drinking" (p. 1037), a conclusion which contrasts with the interactionist approach which describes the functioning of families of alcoholics as being linked to the alcoholics' drinking. Even if this limited support of Al-Anon's principles did not suffer from the obvious biases of self-selection of participants and lack of a comparison group it is not clear that Al-Anon can be universally applied to all partners of alcoholics. The narrow range of demographic characteristics encompassed by Al-Anon members (Ablon, 1974) as well as the "spiritual" nature of its philosophy may place some limits on its appeal.

While not directly focusing on participation in Al-Anon, a number of researchers have assessed the coping skills of the wives of alcoholics. Rychtarik's chapter in this volume suggests that a major methodological limitation of this research is the poor measurement of coping skills. Even given this limitation, this area of research provides insight into an important component of Al-Anon: learning practical strategies for dealing with an alcoholic spouse. The results of these studies suggest that membership in Al-Anon could be an important adjunct to treatment. For example, Orford et al. (1975) reported that wives' coping behaviors that actively discouraged drinking (e.g., hiding alcoholic beverages) were related to a good prognosis for their alcoholic husbands. Coping behaviors that indicated avoidance and withdrawal from the marriage were related to a poorer drinking outcome for the alcoholic husbands. Wright and Scott (1978) reported a significant difference in the abstinence rate of alcoholics whose wives were involved in outpatient counseling as well as Al-Anon, concluding that "as an alcoholic's illness is a family illness, treating a spouse is a way of treating an alcoholic" (p. 1581). Most recently, Rychtarik,

Carstensen, Alford, Schlundt, & Scott (1988) reported that Al-Anon experienced wives performed significantly better on an inventory of alcohol-related coping skills than did wives who were not Al-Anon experienced.

Conclusion

Given the fact that Al-Anon contains ingredients shown to be effective in other approaches to treatment (e.g., social support, problem solving, use of adaptive coping strategies) it could serve as an effective intervention for the spouses of alcoholics. However, since no methodologically rigorous empirical validation of its efficacy exists, knowledge concerning the role of participation in Al-Anon must remain at the level of testimonials and isolated descriptions of outcome.

EVALUATION OF EXISTENT RESEARCH

In their assessment of the scientific foundations of family therapies Bednar, Burlingame, and Masters (1988) examined extant research on systems and behavioral approaches with regard to basic scientific considerations of: (1) semantic and measurement precision, (2) research methodology, and (3) potential for results having an influence on the development of knowledge. They concluded that systems and behavioral approaches are at different points in their development with regard to establishing a base of scientific knowledge. Systems approaches were found to be wanting in all three areas. Criticisms included the failure to clearly delineate theoretical constructs, the failure to operationalize distinct treatment techniques, and an overly ambitious attempt to evaluate efficacy empirically even before fulfilling the need for more fundamental descriptive information that would help to address the limitations cited.

Behavioral approaches were viewed as being at a more advanced level of knowledge gathering in that definitions of constructs are precise and measurable, methodology is more rigorous, and there is reciprocity between developments in theory and in research. Given the pluses of behavioral approaches, "one can place greater confidence in their conclusions than in those of the systems oriented approaches" (p. 427). Bednar et al.'s conclusion represents a relative judgment concerning the research on family treatment for a variety of problems, and is consistent with previous reviews of empirical research on the efficacy of behavioral (Hahlweg & Markman, 1988) and nonbehavioral family therapy methods (Wells & Dezen, 1978).

Bednar et al.'s conclusion can also be applied to the literature on family treatment of alcohol abuse. Janzen's (1977) review of the literature on family treatment of alcoholism concluded that for the most part such treatment can be successful. However, he cited limitations in the data that made it difficult to "show that family treatment is as good or better than other forms of treatment for alcoholism" (p. 128). Some 12 years later a similar conclusion can be drawn, particularly for nonbehavioral approaches.

The methodological limitations of research on family treatment of alcohol abuse have been outlined in previous reviews (Janzen, 1977; Jacobson et al., 1989). Generally, these reviews conclude that the research on family treatment does not meet the criteria appropriate for determining comparative efficacy. These criteria include random assignment to conditions, the need for adequate control conditions, and the specification of interventions (Kazdin, 1980). Nor does the conceptualization of treatment necessarily match current theory on family processes. Instead the research can often best be described as a creative and rather eclectic mix of clinical lore and available resources. Some of these limitations are clearly linked to the complexities of assessing and treating the variety of areas that are affected by alcohol abuse as well as general problems inherent in doing clinical research.

Given the developmental differences between systems and behavioral approaches, evaluation of comparative efficacy of family treatment of alcohol abuse seems premature. In order to improve the current state of research, attention must be given to the quality of the efforts to assess the efficacy of both behavioral and family systems approaches.

IMPROVING THE METHODOLOGY OF RESEARCH ON FAMILY TREATMENT FOR ALCOHOL ABUSE

Until more rigorous definition of constructs, specification of testable hypotheses, and methodologically sound research is forthcoming, it is difficult to have confidence in the findings concerning family systems approaches to alcohol abuse. The results of behavioral studies show promise, although the active ingredients of change and issues related to maintenance of treatment gains require more specification and investigation.

Given the methodological limitations cited, adherence to some rudimentary guidelines for conducting research would improve the quality of research on family treatment of alcohol abuse. The attempt to improve the quality of research should include a focus on the development of scientific knowledge within treatment approaches as well as evaluation of the comparative efficacy of different approaches. While not exhaustive, the following are some basic guidelines for improved methodology for research on family treatment of alcohol abuse.

1. Development of theoretical constructs: At the most fundamental level there is a lack of specification of theoretical constructs in much of family treatment. Often the defining characteristic of family treatment is that two or more members of a family meet to discuss family problems, suggesting that "families may profit from therapy, not because of any new treatment considerations, but simply because all family members are present in a discussion about family problems" (Bednar et al., 1988, p. 417). Without a conceptual framework in which the active ingredients and boundary conditions of family treatment of alcohol abuse can be specified, statements such as the above cannot be refuted.

2. *Expand the definition of the family:* A related issue is the definition of what constitutes "a family." Much of the research to date has focused on the marital dyad. Clearly, reciprocal relationships between the alcoholic and other family members can also impact on treatment outcome. The work of Azrin and colleagues (Azrin, 1976; Hunt & Azrin, 1973; Sisson & Azrin, 1986) has encompassed broader definitions of "family" including parents or other relatives and close friends of the alcoholic. However, none of the research to date has included the children of alcoholics in family treatment. As research with members of marital dyad progresses, there is also a need for systematically testing the effect of including a variety of other family members in alcohol treatment.

3. *Descriptive research is integral to theory development:* Conducting research at the descriptive level can be important to the systematic development of theory (Bednar et al., 1988). However, even at this level some systematic assessment of specific needs and use of quantifiable methods of observation is necessary. The work of researchers such as Steinglass and colleagues (Steinglass et al., 1987) and Jacob and colleagues (Jacob & Krahn, 1988; Jacob & Leonard, 1988) is exemplary in that it includes careful observation, description, and quantification of family interaction. This attention to detail can provide a basis for developing and refining family treatment techniques. Once these techniques are established, then comparisons with techniques of proven efficacy can be made.

4. *Include control and comparison groups:* Given the relative infancy of this area of research, there is a need to employ research designs that include control groups. Traditional control conditions (e.g., waiting list or no treatment) may be practically and ethically disadvantageous since some subjects may continue to experience the negative effects of alcohol abuse while participating in research. In some cases, placebo control groups (treatment condition minus the essential therapeutic ingredient being tested) may be feasible. In addition, Basham (1986) has suggested the use of comparative designs in which "one compares two or more treatments without conceptualizing either as a formal control group" (p. 90). These designs are particularly useful in situations in which the essential ingredients of a treatment package cannot easily be specified. In such designs the differences between two or more treatments are compared in relative terms. Comparative designs have been employed in research on family treatment

of alcoholism (e.g., McCrady et al., 1986; O'Farrell et al., 1985, Zweben et al., 1988) and expansion of their use is recommended. When comparison/control groups are included in a research design, random assignment to conditions and independent assessment of outcome are important to minimize bias in outcome (Kazdin, 1980).

5. *Include objective outcome data:* A related issue is the need for objective assessment of outcome and functioning. While convenient, easy to collect, and reliable under certain circumstances (Sobell et al., 1988), reliance on self-report data limits the validity of research findings. This is especially true if such findings are based on measures lacking rigorous psychometric evaluation. Objective sources of information (institutional records, ratings of independent judges, use of validated behavioral criteria) is a necessary part of methodologically rigorous designs for studying family treatment of alcohol abuse.

6. *Broaden outcome measures:* Improvements in drinking behavior are not necessarily related to improvements in other areas of the alcoholic's functioning (Pattison, 1976). Thus, one obvious need in family treatment is a broader range of outcome variables. Even if drinking behavior is the focus of treatment, assessment of individual and family functioning in a variety of areas (e.g., ability to effectively maintain roles, social interactions, employment, finances, marital satisfaction) provides rich sources of information about outcome.

7. *Specify the goals of treatment:* Specification of the goal of family treatment is paramount. Research to date has had one of two foci: use family treatment to directly influence drinking behavior and thereby indirectly improve family interaction (e.g., Hedberg & Campbell, 1974; McCrady et al., 1986), or use family treatment to directly improve family interaction and thereby indirectly influence drinking behavior (e.g., Cadogan, 1973; Hunt & Azrin, 1973; O'Farrell et al., 1985; Steinglass, 1979). Both the nature of treatment and its expected outcome vary based on the choice of a focus, but this is often not clearly articulated. By specifying the primary goal of treatment researchers can more clearly understand the nature of the change process and the boundary conditions for the use of particular interventions. Direct comparisons of interventions representative of these two foci also might be very informative.

8. *Include long-term follow-up:* The duration of the response to treatment is an important indicator of treatment efficacy. Long-term follow-up of responses to family treatment is essential. While longer follow-ups of 18 months or more have been reported (Azrin, 1976; McCrady, et al., 1982; Zweben et al., 1988) the more common case is a limited follow-up of 6 months or less (McCardy et al., 1986; O'Farrell et al., 1985; Steinglass, 1979). Again the more comprehensive the follow-up assessment (including a variety of objective measures), the better.

NEW DIRECTIONS FOR RESEARCH

Nature of Social Support Provided by the Family

The family treatment approach is built in part on the notion that families serve as a positive source of social support, and that is typically the case (Colletti & Brownell, 1982; McCrady, 1986). There is also much to suggest that the family can serve as a source of stress with regard to recovery and/or sabotage treatment (Collins, Emont, & Zywiak, 1988; Coyne, Wortman, & Lehman, 1985). The family systems approach implicitly assumes that the family can play a negative role in treatment (Steinglass, 1982). It acknowledges family member's resistance to behavior change on the part of the identified patient as one of the reasons for working with the entire family unit rather than the individual. The role of negative social influence is likely to be more of a problem for behavioral approaches, where this issue is not explicitly acknowledged, than it is for the family systems approach. However both approaches should further study the role of the family as a source of negative and positive social influence, with respect to drinking behavior. In particular, knowledge of negative processes will help to elucidate potential barriers to effective treatment.

Gender of the Alcohol Abuser

The lack of distinction based on the gender of the client has been cited as a limitation of family-oriented behavioral treatment (Gurman & Klein, 1984) and of family systems theories (Hare-Mustin, 1987). Therefore, it is no surprise that one of the issues that must be addressed in future research is the differential effect of alcohol abuse based on gender of the alcoholic. Currently much of the family treatment of alcoholism literature focuses on the male drinker (as spouse and/or father) (e.g., Hunt & Azrin, 1973; O'Farrell et al., 1985) or combines treatment for male and female alcoholics making no distinction in family dynamics related to gender, family role, etc., of the alcoholic (McCrady et al., 1979; Vanicelli et al., 1983; Zweben et al., 1988). Employing either of these strategies means that the familial impact of the impaired female drinker (as spouse and/or mother) is often overlooked. Yet, for example, familial pressure to return home has been cited as a factor in women dropping out of an inpatient treatment program (Berger, 1981).

Williams and Klerman (1984) reviewed research on the familial effects of female drinking across the life stages, highlighting the different purposes served by alcohol as developmental changes occur over time. While calling attention to the relative paucity of research on women's abuse of alcohol, their review also indicated the complex of sociocultural issues that may become expressed in excessive drinking. These issues also affect the nature of family interaction and other dynamics related to having a female problem drinker as a family member.

Adolescence is the time when drinking typically begins. During this stage, risk factors for alcohol abuse include exposure to alcohol use as a maladaptive coping strategy in the family of origin and inadequate parenting or unstable families if parents are alcoholic. Young adulthood is the time when many women report experiencing the most alcohol problems (Wilsnack, Wilsnack, & Klassen, 1984). As women move to choosing partners, alcoholic women may be more likely to choose heavy drinking partners/husbands who facilitate maintenance of their own drinking. In addition, child bearing and rearing may introduce conflicts and stress with regard to multiple roles related to meeting work and family demands as well as fulfilling personal needs. As adulthood proceeds, issues related to the loss of social status and support related to marital disruption, and the "empty nest" when children leave home, can contribute to further drinking. The elderly female faces issues of loneliness related to changes in role and/or death of a spouse. Continuing changes in women's social roles in the 1990s are likely to include more exposure to alcohol. Thus, the need to focus on women's alcohol use and abuse, as well as the "family" constellation in which their drinking occurs, may be even greater in the future.

The foregoing discussion raises concerns that go beyond the issue of the gender of the alcoholic to include a call for the expansion of treatment research to examination of the role of alcohol abuse by different family members. At another level, expansion of the narrow range of demographic characteristics represented in the typical samples employed in research on family treatment for alcohol abuse would be welcome. Much of the current research is on white, middle-class, male alcoholics. Sociocultural differences among ethnic/racial groups are likely to include different norms and expectations related to family roles and interaction that impact on the response to family treatment (Finney et al., 1983; Patterson, Charles, Woodward, Roberts, & Perk, 1981). Inclusion of a variety of sociocultural groups and consideration of features unique to and/or common among these groups would enhance our understanding of the complex interaction of sociocultural factors in the response to family treatment.

Similarities Among Dysfunctional Families

Alcohol abuse represents but one of a number of areas of dysfunction that impacts on families. There is a need for more information on the functioning of alcoholic families, particularly as they compare to dysfunctional non-alcoholic families of similar background and socioeconomic status. As described by Cronkite et al. in this volume, Moos and colleagues have studied families in which either alcoholism or depression contributed to family dysfunction. Their results suggest that although there are some aspects of family interaction that are unique to alcoholism, maladaptive interaction patterns are found in other types of families containing a dysfunctional member. Jacob and his colleagues (e.g., Jacob & Krahn, 1988) have also studied interaction patterns in families with a depressed member as a control for alcoholic member. The results of both programs of research suggest that the specific nature of the individual's impairment may be a less potent contributor to family dysfunction than is the fact that the family contains an impaired member. Clearly then, the information gleaned from studies on different types of dysfunctional families can provide a basis for generating ideas related to conceptualizing the specific role of alcohol (as compared to other forms of impairment) in family functioning, developing family-oriented treatment for alcohol abusers, and specifying appropriate criteria for treatment outcome.

Can Family Interventions Serve as a Prevention Strategy?

Typically, family treatment is implemented once an individual has been identified as having an alcohol problem and/or the family is experiencing the negative consequences of such a problem. Family-oriented interventions could play a role in prevention or early intervention with problem drinking. For example, Yates (1988) has outlined an experimental program designed to help family members identify and bring into treatment individuals in the early stages of their drinking problem. In his sample of 30 cases, approximately one-half of the drinkers had never received any former intervention for their drinking problem. For many of these cases the family-oriented program was successful in preventing a drinking problem from developing beyond its initial stages.

As identification of individuals at high risk for alcohol abuse becomes increasingly common, even earlier points of intervention may become evident. For example, both research and clinical experience suggest that growing up in a family environment in which alcohol abuse is present may place an individual at risk for learning maladaptive drinking behavior. It is possible that work with families containing an identified alcoholic can not only serve as treatment for the alcoholics, but might also serve as a means of preventing problem drinking in their offspring. Assessment of drinking outcomes with individuals other than the identified alcoholic (e.g., spouse, offspring) would be an excellent start to answering the question of whether family treatment can serve prophylactic purposes (Orford, 1984).

GENERAL CONCLUSION

The inclusion of family members in treatment for alcohol abuse coincides with both theoretical and clinical notions concerning the reciprocal relationships between the alcoholic and other family members. Irrespective of their appeal, the promise of these notions has not been borne out in the results of the research to date. The outcome of both behavioral and systems-oriented research on family treatment does not clearly indicate that the inclusion of family members enhances treatment efficacy. This is particularly true when long-term follow-ups are conducted (e.g., McCrady et al., 1982). Although disappointing, this should not be seen as cause for alarm. Research on family-oriented treatment of alcohol abuse is in its infancy and the results of the research to date should not be seen as conclusive. Instead, these results are indicative of areas for future growth and refinement. Creative and methodologically sound extensions of many of the studies reviewed here would do much to enhance knowledge about the effective implementation of family-oriented treatment programs for alcohol abuse. As representative of initial forays into a complex area of research, the studies reviewed provide excellent starting points for future research. The important concern at this juncture is that future research employ the appropriate methodology and include consideration of the array of issues that impact on the efficacy of family treatment.

Acknowledgments. The author wishes to thank Gerard J. Connors, William M. Lapp, and John S. Searles for their comments on an earlier draft of this chapter.

REFERENCES

Ablon, J. (1974). Al-Anon family groups. *American Journal of Psychotherapy, 28,* 30–45.

Azrin, N. H. (1976). Improvements in the community reinforcement approach to alcoholism. *Behaviour Research and Therapy, 14,* 339–348.

Basham, R. B. (1986). Scientific and practical advantages of comparative design in psychotherapy research. *Journal of Consulting and Clinical Psychology, 54,* 88–94.

Bednar, R. L., Burlingame, G. M., & Masters, K. S. (1988). Systems of family treatment: Substance or semantics. *Annual Review of Psychology, 39,* 401–434.

Berger, A. (1981). Family involvement and alcoholics' completion of a multiphase treatment program. *Journal of Studies on Alcohol, 42,* 517–521.

Cadogan, D. A. (1973). Marital group therapy in the treatment of alcoholism. *Quarterly Journal of Studies on Alcohol, 34,* 1187–1194.

Colletti, G., & Brownell, K. D. (1982). The physical and emotional benefits of social support: Application to obesity, smoking, and alcoholism. In M. Hersen, R. M. Eisler, & P. M. Miller (Eds.), *Progress in behavior modification,* vol. 13 (pp. 109–178). New York: Academic Press.

Collins, R. L., Emont, S. L., & Zywiak, W. H. (1988, November). *The role of social support in smoking cessation.* Paper presented at the annual meeting of the Association for Advancement of Behavior Therapy, New York, NY.

Coyne, J. C., Wortman, C. B., & Lehman, D. (1985, August). *The other side of support: Emotional overinvolvement and miscarried helping.* Paper presented at the annual convention of the American Psychological Association, Los Angeles, CA.

Edwards, G., Orford, J., Egert, S., Guthrie, S., Hawker, A., Hensman, C., Mitcheson, M., Oppenheimer, E., & Taylor, C. (1977). Alcoholism: A controlled trial of "treatment" and "advice". *Journal of Studies on Alcohol, 38,* 1004–1031.

Finney, J. W., Moos, R. H., Cronkite, R. C., & Gamble, W. (1983). A conceptual model of the functioning of married persons with impaired partners: Spouses of alcoholic patients. *Journal of Marriage and the Family, 45,* 23–34.

George, W. H., & Marlatt, G. A. (1983). Alcoholism: The evolution of a behavioral perspective. In M. Galanter et al. (Eds.), *Recent advances in alcoholism,* vol. 1, (pp. 105–138). New York: Plenum.

Gorman, J. M., & Rooney, J. F. (1979). The influence of Al-Anon on the coping behavior of wives of alcoholics. *Journal of Studies on Alcohol, 40,* 1030–1038.

Gurman, A. S., & Klein, M. H. (1984). Marriage and the family: An unconscious male bias in behavioral treatment? In E. A. Blechman (Ed.), *Behavior modification with women* (pp. 170–189). New York: Plenum.

Hahlweg, K., & Markman, H. J. (1988). Effectiveness of behavioral marital therapy: Empirical status of behavioral techniques in preventing and alleviating marital distress. *Journal of Consulting and Clinical Psychology, 56,* 440–447.

Hare-Mustin, R. T. (1987). The problem of gender in family therapy theory. *Family Process, 26,* 15–27.

Hedberg, A. G., & Campbell, L. (1974). A comparison of four behavioral treatments of alcoholism. *Journal of Behavior Therapy and Experimental Psychiatry, 5,* 251–256.

Hunt, G. M., & Azrin, N. H. (1973). A community-reinforcement approach to alcoholism. *Behaviour Research and Therapy, 11,* 91–104.

Jacob, T., Dunn, N., & Leonard, K. (1983). Patterns of alcohol abuse and family stability. *Alcoholism: Clinical and Experimental Research, 7,* 382–385.

Jacob, T., & Krahn, G. (1988). Marital interaction of alcoholic couples: Comparison with depressed and nondistressed couples. *Journal of Consulting and Clinical Psychology, 56,* 73–79.

Jacob, T., & Leonard, K. E. (1988). Alcoholic–spouse interaction as a function of alcoholism subtype and alcohol consumption interaction. *Journal of Abnormal Psychology, 97,* 231–237.

Jacobson, N. S., Holtzworth-Munroe, A., & Schmaling, K. B. (1989). Marital therapy and spouse involvement in the treatment of depression, agoraphobia, and alcoholism. *Journal of Consulting and Clinical Psychology, 57,* 5–10.

Janzen, C. (1977). Families in the treatment of alcoholism. *Journal of Studies on Alcohol, 38,* 114–130.

Kazdin, A. E. (1980). *Research design in clinical psychology.* New York: Harper & Row.

Keane, T. M., Foy, D. W., Nunn, B., & Rychtarik, R. G. (1984). Spouse contracting to increase Antabuse compliance in alcoholic veterans. *Journal of Clinical Psychology, 40,* 340–344.

McCrady, B. S. (1986). The family in the change process. In W. E. Miller & N.

Heather (Eds.), *Treating addictive behaviors: Processes of change* (pp. 305–318). New York: Plenum.

McCrady, B. S., Moreau, J., Paolino, T. J., & Longabaugh, R. (1982). Joint hospitalization and couples therapy for alcoholism: A four year follow-up. *Journal of Studies on Alcohol, 43,* 1244–1250.

McCrady, B. S., Noel, N. E., Abrams, D. B., Stout, R. L., Nelson, H. F., & Hay, W. M. (1986). Comparative effectiveness of three types of spouse involvement in outpatient behavioral alcoholism treatment. *Journal of Studies on Alcohol, 47,* 459–467.

McCrady, B. S., Paolino, T. J., Longabaugh, R., & Rossi, J. (1979). Effects of joint hospital admission and couples' treatment for hospitalized alcoholics: A pilot study. *Addictive Behaviors, 4,* 155–165.

Moos, R. H., Bromet, E., Tsu, V., & Moos, B. (1979). Family characteristics and the outcome of treatment for alcoholism. *Journal of Studies on Alcohol, 40,* 78–88.

Moos, R. H., Finney, J. W., Chan, D. A. (1981). The process of recovery from alcoholism: I. Comparing alcoholic patients and matched community controls. *Journal of Studies on Alcohol, 42,* 383–402.

Moos, R. H., Finney, J. W., & Gamble, W. (1982). The process of recovery from alcoholism: II. Comparing spouses of alcoholic patients and spouses of matched community controls. *Journal of Studies on Alcohol, 43,* 888–909.

Moos, R. H., & Moos, B. S. (1984). The process of recovery from alcoholism: III. Comparing families of alcoholics and matched control families. *Journal of Studies on Alcohol, 45,* 111–118.

O'Farrell, T. J., & Cutter, H. S. G. (1984). Behavioral marital therapy couples groups for male alcoholics and their wives. *Journal of Substance Abuse Treatment, 1,* 191–204.

O'Farrell, T. J., Cutter, H. S. G., & Floyd, F. J. (1985). Evaluating behavioral marital therapy for male alcoholics: Effects of marital adjustment and communication from before to after treatment. *Behavior Therapy, 16,* 147–167.

Orford, J. (1984). The prevention and management of alcohol problems in the family setting: A review of work carried out in English-speaking countries. *Alcohol and Alcoholism, 19,* 109–122.

Orford, J., Guthrie, S., Nicholls, P., Oppenheimer, E., Egert, S., & Hensman, C. (1975). Self-reported coping behavior of wives of alcoholics and its association with drinking outcome. *Journal of Studies on Alcohol, 36,* 1254–1267.

Orford, J., Oppenheimer, E., & Edwards, G. (1976). Abstinence or control: The outcome for excessive drinkers two years after consultation. *Behaviour Research and Therapy, 14,* 409–418.

Patterson, E. T., Charles, H. L., Woodward, W. A., Roberts, W. R., & Perk, W. E. (1981). Differences in measures of personality and family environment among black and white alcoholics. *Journal of Consulting and Clinical Psychology, 49,* 1–9.

Pattison, E. M. (1976). A conceptual approach to alcoholism treatment goals. *Addictive Behaviors, 1,* 177–192.

Preli, R., & Protinsky, H. (1988). Aspects of family structures in alcoholic, recovered, and nonalcoholic families. *Journal of Marital and Family Therapy, 14,* 311–314.

Roberts, M., Floyd, F. J., O'Farrell, T. J., & Cutter, H. (1985). Marital interactions and the duration of alcoholic husbands' sobriety. *American Journal of Drug and Alcohol Abuse, 11,* 303–313.

Rychtarik, R. G., Carstensen, L. L., Alford, G. S., Schlundt, D. G., & Scott, W. O. (1988). Situational assessment of alcohol-related coping skills in wives of alcoholics. *Psychology of Addictive Behavior, 2,* 66–73.

Sisson, R. W., & Azrin, N. H. (1986). Family-member involvement to initiate and promote treatment of problem drinkers. *Journal of Behavior Therapy and Experimental Psychiatry, 17,* 15–21.

Sobell, L. S., Sobell, M. B., Riley, D. M., Schuller, R., Pavan, D. S., Cancilla, A., Klajner, F., & Leo, G. I. (1988). The reliability of alcohol abusers' self-reports of drinking and life events that occurred in the distant past. *Journal of Studies on Alcohol, 49,* 225–232.

Stanton, M. D., Todd, T. C., & Associates (1982). *The family therapy of drug abuse and addiction.* New York: Guilford.

Steinglass, P. (1979). An experimental treatment program for alcoholic couples. *Journal of Studies on Alcohol, 40,* 159–182.

Steinglass, P. (1982). The roles of alcohol in family systems. In J. Orford & J. Harwin (Eds.), *Alcohol and the family* (pp. 127–150). London: Croom Helm.

Steinglass, P., Bennett, L., Wolin, S. J., & Reiss, D. (1987). *The alcoholic family.* New York: Basic Books.

Steinglass, P., Tislenko, L., & Reiss, D. (1985). Stability/instability in the alcoholic marriage: The interrelationships between course of alcoholism, family process and marital outcome. *Family Process, 24,* 365–376.

Vannicelli, M., Gingerich, S., & Ryback, R. (1983). Family problems related to the treatment and outcome of alcoholic patients. *British Journal of Addiction, 78,* 193–204.

Vuchinich, R. E., Tucker, J. A., & Harllee, L. M. (1988). Behavioral assessment. In D. M. Donovan & G. A. Marlatt (Eds.), *Assessment of addictive behaviors* (pp. 51–83). New York: Guilford.

Wells, R. A., & Dezen, A. E. (1978). The results of family therapy revisited: The nonbehavioral methods. *Family Process, 17,* 251–274.

Williams, C. N., & Klerman, L. V. (1984). Female alcohol abuse: Its effects on the family. In S. C. Wilsnack & L. J. Beckman (Eds.), *Alcohol problems in women* (pp. 280–312). New York: Guilford.

Wilsnack, R. W., Wilsnack, S. C., & Klassen, A. D. (1974). Women's drinking and drinking problems: Patterns from a 1981 National Survey. *American Journal of Public Health, 74,* 1231–1238.

Wiseman, J. (1981). Sober comportment: Patterns and perspectives on alcohol addiction. *Journal of Studies on Alcohol, 42,* 106–126.

Wright, K. D., & Scott, T. B. (1978). The relationship of wives' treatment to the drinking status of alcoholics. *Journal of Studies on Alcohol, 39,* 1577–1581.

Yates, F. E. (1988). The evaluation of a "Co-operative Counselling" alcohol service which uses family and affected others to reach and influence problem drinkers. *British Journal of Addiction, 83,* 1309–1319.

Zweben, A., Pearlman, S., & Li, S. (1988). A comparison of brief advice and conjoint therapy in the treatment of alcohol abuse: The results of the Marital Systems study. *British Journal of Addiction, 83,* 899–916.

12

Remission Among Alcoholic Patients and Family Adaptation to Alcoholism: A Stress and Coping Perspective

RUTH C. CRONKITE, JOHN W. FINNEY, JAMIE NEKICH, and RUDOLF H. MOOS

Stress and coping theory provides a useful framework for understanding the challenges faced by families with an alcoholic member. This theoretical perspective, which focuses on stressful life circumstances, social resources, and individual coping responses, can shed light on both the processes of remission and relapse for alcoholics in family settings and the processes by which family members adapt to an alcoholic partner or parent. These processes are two sides of the same coin: Patients may benefit from certain types of positive posttreatment family situations; family members may benefit from the remission of patients' symptoms. We have been conducting research that addresses both processes. We summarize that research here; more details are recorded in Moos, Finney, and Cronkite (1990) and in earlier research reports that are cited at appropriate points.

A STRESS AND COPING PERSPECTIVE

Our approach to patient remission and to family adaptation is broad. In order to adequately understand family influences on patient remission and

This chapter is adapted from R. H. Moos, J. W. Finney, and R. C. Cronkite, *Alcoholism treatment: Process and outcome*. New York: Oxford University Press. Copyright 1990 Oxford University Press. Adapted by permission.

relapse, we believe it is necessary to embed patient functioning in a more comprehensive model that includes the effects of a broad range of stressors and resources and of patients' coping responses. An alcoholic's life context can provide a supportive milieu for continued improvement, cushion the impact of stressors, or trigger a relapse (Brown, 1985; Marlatt & Gordon, 1985; Vannicelli, Gingerich, & Ryback, 1983). Although stressors are risk factors, they do not necessarily precipitate a relapse or lead to a decline in functioning. That is, individuals typically face some situations that are stressful; it is how they appraise these situations—as challenging or threatening—as well as their personal and social resources that determine whether stressors lead to a relapse (Samsonowitz & Sjoberg, 1981). For example, a cohesive family may contribute to good treatment outcome by fostering reliance on effective coping responses, such as taking direct action to deal with modifiable stressors. Further, treatment can help patients learn coping skills that can improve the quality of their life contexts and help minimize the negative impact of life stressors (O'Farrell & Cutter, 1984).

Similarly, in order to understand how spouses and children adapt to an alcoholic partner or parent, we believe that the effects of factors other than the functioning of the alcoholic person must be considered. Although an actively alcoholic family member typically represents a significant stressor, the impact on a spouse may depend on the spouse's prior functioning, the quality of the family environment, and the spouse's coping responses. Similarly, children's functioning in families with an alcoholic parent can be better understood if research also considers the functioning of the nonalcoholic parent and the overall quality of the family environment.

The model in Figure 12.1 shows the connections among seven sets of factors associated with the adaptation of a member of an alcohol-impaired family. When the focal family member is the alcoholic patient, the model reflects the factors that influence the processes of remission and relapse: the patient's demographic characteristics, personal resources, and functioning at intake; treatment program and treatment experiences; life context factors (the functioning of other family members, life stressors, social resources); and the patient's coping responses. This model can also be used to examine how demographic characteristics, prior functioning, and life context factors affect the adaptation of a spouse or child in a family with an alcohol-impaired member (although treatment experiences shown in Panel III are not as directly involved in spouse and child adaptation).

In this chapter, we first summarize our research on factors associated with the posttreatment functioning of a sample of alcoholic patients in family settings. We emphasize the role of family influences—in particular, aspects of the family environment that may be considered stressors and re-

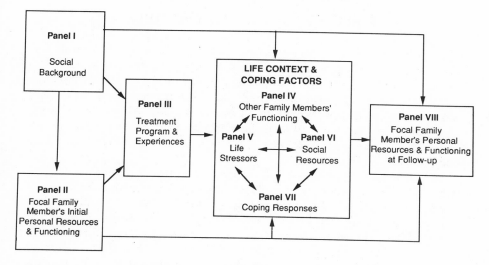

FIGURE 12.1. A stress and coping model of the determinants of functioning of members of an alcohol-impaired family.

sources and may impede or facilitate remission. We compare the families of remitted and relapsed patients on these factors with those of matched, non-problem-drinking community controls. We then examine the influence of patient, treatment, family, stressor, and personal coping factors on patient functioning.

Next, we turn to the issue of how well spouses and children adapt to an alcoholic partner or parent. Although intuitively one might expect that a spouse and/or children would benefit from their alcoholic partner's/parent's remission, Steinglass (1981) has argued that sobriety may bring non-drinking-related aspects of family dysfunction to the foreground. To address this issue, we first compare the functioning of spouses of remitted and relapsed patients with spouses of non-problem-drinking community controls. Then we examine the adaptation of spouses within a broader conceptual framework that includes not only the functioning of the alcoholic partner, but also the spouse's initial functioning, exposure to life stressors, and the spouse's coping responses.

Similarly, we compare the functioning of children of remitted and relapsed patients with that of children in families without drinking problems, and then try to understand children's functioning more completely by embedding it in a broad conceptual model. Finally, we discuss the implications of research for the treatment of alcoholic persons and their spouses as well as future research.

PATIENT AND FAMILY SAMPLES

We studied patients who sought treatment for alcoholism in one of five residential treatment facilities. Both nonprofit and for-profit programs were included. Of an initial sample composed of approximately 500 patients, 157 returned to family settings. We asked these patients if they and their families would participate in an extended study. Altogether, 124 patients and their families (79% of those eligible) agreed to participate. Of these, 113 patients (98% of the 118 persons still living) were followed 18 months later.[1]

At intake to treatment, the 113 patients were mostly middle-aged (74% were 40 years or older), white (88%), and educated beyond high school (68%), although only 19% were college graduates. There were 88 men and 25 women. During the month before entry into the program, most patients (75%) reported drinking daily, with a mean alcohol consumption of more than 13 ounces of ethanol from all beverages on a typical drinking day. Almost half (43%) of these patients had been hospitalized for alcoholism in the previous 3 years.

We selected matched community control families from the same census tract as each treated family. We excluded families that had a member who had been treated for alcoholism or who was a heavy drinker. The 113 community controls matched the patient sample on sex, age, ethnicity, religion, education, and family size.

REMISSION AND RELAPSE AMONG PATIENTS IN FAMILY SETTINGS

Families with an actively alcoholic family member are often characterized by heightened conflict, marital disruption, disturbed communication, and role dysfunction (Jacob & Seilhamer, 1987; Steinglass & Robertson, 1983; Zweben, 1986). Some research shows that abstinence rarely brings quick relief and can be painful for the alcoholic and his or her immediate family—at least over the short run (Vaillant, 1983; Wiseman, 1981). Recovering alcoholics often experience difficulty as they try to renegotiate occupational and family responsibilities. Such findings have led some investigators to speculate that the identified patient's alcohol abuse may not be the family's major problem and that family functioning may continue to be marginal even when the alcoholic member recovers (Steinglass, 1981; Steinglass, Bennet, Wolin, & Reiss, 1987). Thus, a relatively stressor-free, supportive milieu and effective coping skills may be necessary to maintain remission during the initial recovery phase, particularly if treatment has not addressed nondrinking-related deficiencies in the alcoholic and his or her family system (Rosenberg, 1983).

We examined these issues by comparing relapsed and remitted patients and their families with matched community controls and their families on two broad domains of variables: (1) family and social functioning (household role performance, family social activities, and informal social contacts), and (2) life stressors and coping responses. (See Moos et al., 1990, for more details on the measurement of these variables.) First, we compared the community controls with remitted and relapsed alcoholic patients; subsequently, we compared the patients' spouses and children with the controls' spouses and children.

On the basis of their drinking behavior during the 2 years after treatment, we divided the patients contacted at the 2-year follow-up into remitted and relapsed groups (Moos, Finney, & Chan, 1981). These are the two global categories most often used in describing alcoholism treatment outcome and provide a way to compare patients who are doing well or poorly in terms of their drinking behavior with community residents who do not have alcohol-related problems. Information about the adaptation and life contexts of matched community controls provides a realistic baseline to judge the extent to which remitted patients are functioning adequately and have achieved relatively benign life situations.

Patients in the remitted group met each of five criteria at both the 6-month and 2-year follow-ups: (1) no rehospitalization for alcoholism; (2) no inability to work because of alcoholism; (3) abstaining or consuming fewer than 5 ounces of 100% ethanol on a typical drinking day in the month prior to the follow-up[2]; (4) an average consumption of fewer than 3 ounces of 100% ethanol per day; and (5) no problems from drinking, with the exception of family arguments. There were 55 individuals in the remitted group; the remaining 58 individuals were classified as relapsed.

Mood, Health-Related, and Occupational Functioning

Although the remitted patients were as self-confident and had similar levels of depression and physical symptoms as the community controls, they were functioning less well in some areas than the controls. That is, remitted patients reported more anxiety, consumed more medications (primarily vitamins and tranquilizers), visited doctors more frequently, and were more likely to have been hospitalized. Some remitted alcoholics may have had residual medical disorders that required continuing treatment. Alcoholic patients are more likely than nonalcoholic individuals to report medical problems, incur accidents, and use health care services (Roghmann, Roberts, Smith, Wells, & Wersinger, 1981). The remitted patients were comparable to the controls in their occupational functioning.

In contrast, the relapsed patients consistently functioned more poorly in mood- and health-related areas than either the remitted patients or community controls at the 2-year follow-up. Relapsed alcoholics reported more depression, anxiety, physical symptoms, and medication use; they also showed less self-confidence, lower income, and poorer occupational functioning. Only 38% of the relapsed patients were employed full-time compared to about 60% of the remitted patients and controls (see Moos et al., 1981, and Moos et al., 1990).

Family and Social Functioning

How did the family situations of remitted and relapsed patients compare with those of community controls? In general, families of remitted patients were comparable to those of community controls. The family environments of remitted alcoholics were as cohesive, expressive, well-organized, and free of conflict as the families of community controls. Together with the fact that remitted alcoholics reported fewer family arguments, these findings are consistent with the idea that families of remitted alcoholics avoid conflict and tension for fear of triggering renewed drinking. The remitted alcoholics and their spouses had similar levels of household role performance and as much agreement about family functioning and the family climate as the community controls and their spouses. Although the remitted patients and their families were not quite as active socially nor as recreationally oriented as the community controls, the differences were relatively small. About 75% of these patients had been abstinent in the month prior to the 2-year follow-up, and they may have reduced their social contacts to avoid being tempted to drink.

Relapsed alcoholics' family functioning was considerably poorer than that of community controls. At the 2-year follow-up, the families of relapsed alcoholics showed less cohesion, expressiveness, recreational orientation, and organization, and more disagreement about their family climate. In addition, the families of the heavier-drinking relapsed patients experienced even more conflict and less expressiveness and organization, and participated in fewer social activities. Moreover, the alcoholic member in the relapsed families participated in fewer household tasks, while the spouse performed a larger share of them.

Overall, our findings are consistent with those of Roberts, Floyd, Farrell, and Cutter (1985), who found that more conflicted marital interactions and more struggles for control were associated with a shorter period of sobriety for alcoholic husbands. Our findings also corroborate prior research (Jacob & Seilhamer, 1987; Wiseman, 1981) indicating that families with an alcoholic member experience considerable strain, which diminishes when the alcohol abuser controls his or her drinking.

Life Stressors and Coping Responses

At the 2-year follow-up, remitted patients were more likely than community controls to experience positive life events. In contrast, relapsed patients experienced significantly more negative and fewer positive events than did members of the other two groups.

The remitted alcoholics and the community controls did not differ on their coping responses. In contrast, the relapsed alcoholics were more likely to rely on avoidance coping responses and less likely to use active cognitive coping responses than either the remitted patients or the controls. In general, cognitive coping seems to increase the likelihood of stable remission, while avoidance coping is related to continuing dysfunction and relapse after treatment.

Overall, these findings show that some stably remitted alcoholics and their partners can attain normal personal and family functioning. Our results do not support the assertion that families of remitted patients attain only marginal levels of adaptation or that family functioning deteriorates because previously suppressed problems emerge after the patient achieves abstinence or nonproblem drinking. Instead, our results suggest that remitted patients try to obtain help from physicians and others in the community, who are likely to respond supportively to an alcoholic who is making a concerted effort at recovery. These successfully treated alcoholic patients and their families have managed to create relatively benign circumstances that may contribute to long-term recovery (for more information on the long-term recovery of these patients, see Moos et al., 1990).

The process of remission may not necessarily go smoothly. In an incisive paper, Wiseman (1980) pointed out that alcoholic men typically feel tense, irritable, and depressed and are more sensitive to physical aches and pains during moderate-term sobriety. Many recovering alcoholics describe this as a difficult period. Their wives may ventilate pent-up anger over their husband's past irresponsible and aggressive behavior. With longer-term sobriety, some men become model husbands and fathers, but a minority are lethargic and withdrawn and tend to create a somber home atmosphere. In either case, wives are tense and fearful of stimulating outbursts and renewed drinking episodes. None of the alcoholics or wives of alcoholics Wiseman studied felt that their lives fully returned to normal.

THE PROCESSES OF REMISSION AND RELAPSE IN A FAMILY CONTEXT

To better understand the effects of family and other life context and coping factors on patient posttreatment functioning, we examined their interrelationships within the overall model described earlier (see Figure 12.1). Patient intake characteristics were expected to affect treatment experiences, life context factors, and posttreatment functioning. In general, patients who were more socially advantaged and less seriously impaired prior to treatment were expected to have more benign circumstances and to function better following treatment. We wanted to examine to what extent these pretreatment factors impacted on patients' posttreatment life context factors (stressors, resources, and coping responses). We felt these latter factors might mediate the effects of treatment, as well as exert independent effects on posttreatment functioning. We discuss findings based primarily on analyses at the 2-year follow-up. Moos et al. (1990) discuss results of analyses predicting patient functioning at the 10-year follow-up.

Relationships Among Patient, Treatment, and Life Context Factors

We found only a few significant relationships among the patient, treatment, and extratreatment factors. More advantaged and less impaired patients were more likely to receive treatment in one of the private programs. Patient and treatment variables did not predict life stressors or family resources.

Only stressful life conditions influenced the family environment; more stressors were related to fewer family resources. More intensive treatment did not lead to an improved family environment. This finding is not surprising in that the treatment programs we studied offered little family-oriented treatment. In examining coping responses, we found that coping was not related to patients' social background, intake functioning, or amount of treatment. However, patients who had more family resources used a broader range of active coping responses. We next wanted to identify how each of these sets of factors influences treatment outcome (Cronkite & Moos, 1980).

Life Stressors and Posttreatment Functioning

Stressful life events, spouse dysfunction, and children's health problems were associated with poorer 2-year treatment outcome. Patients who experienced more negative events reported more physical symptoms and depression, and were less likely to be abstinent. Patients whose spouses drank more and reported more physical symptoms drank more themselves and experienced more physical symptoms and depression. In addition, patients whose spouses were more depressed did less well in all areas except social functioning; patients whose children had more health problems consumed more alcohol and were more depressed.

Our findings suggest that a spouse's drinking behavior can significantly influence how an alcoholic mate functions following treatment. In addition, a spouse's poor mood and physical complaints can be a chronic source of stress and lead to more family conflict, thus exacerbating the detrimental influence of the spouse. Moreover, poorer functioning spouses tend to use more avoidance coping styles, such as withdrawal and acting out, which also predict poorer outcome for the patient (Gorman & Roony, 1979; Orford et al., 1975). Conversely, a well-functioning spouse who abstains from alcohol can be a vital source of social support, thus increasing the patient's chance of successful recovery (see Moos et al., 1990).

Family Resources and Posttreatment Functioning

Several aspects of family climate were related to 2-year treatment outcome. In general, we found that patients in cohesive, expressive, well-organized, and recreationally active families functioned better in both the drinking and nondrinking areas. In contrast, family conflict was associated with poorer outcome, particularly with more physical symptoms and more depression.

Our findings are consistent with those of Orford and his colleagues (1975). In a predictive study of men patients and their wives, they reported that high marital cohesion at the beginning of treatment is related to better treatment outcome 1 year later. A good prognosis was based on emotional closeness between the spouses, the husband's involvement in family tasks, and the wife's positive view of the future of the marriage and of her husband when he was sober. Similarly, Ward (1981) noted that patients' pretreatment satisfaction with their family roles and their spouses was predictive of better drinking behavior and interpersonal attitudes at a 5-month follow-up. Conversely, Vannicelli et al. (1983) found that lack of family involvement and high family strain and conflict at treatment intake predicted poor treatment outcome.

Coping Responses and Posttreatment Functioning

As expected, patients who relied on active cognitive and active behavioral coping had better outcomes, whereas the use of avoidance coping was linked to worse outcomes. Thus, even though coping responses are somewhat situation-specific, they seem to capture an aspect of stable personal tendencies that are associated with long-term functioning. Only a few other studies have examined the connections between coping responses and the recovery process. Litman, Eiser, Rawson, and Oppenheim (1979) found that successful (remitted) patients were more likely than relapsed patients to use cognitive control (stopping to examine motives, remembering past difficulties due to drinking) as a coping strategy and to show more flexible coping in high-risk situations. In addition, Jones and Lanyon (1981) found that alcoholic patients' ability to use active problem-solving strategies and resist being compliant or passive in a stressful situation also was associated with better adjustment after treatment. Finally, Sjoberg and Samsonowitz (1985) reported that alcohol abusers who used more coping techniques to help them give up drinking were more successful (see also Chaney & Roszell, 1985).

Together, these findings support the idea that stressful life conditions can contribute to relapse, whereas good family relationships and active coping responses tend to facilitate the recovery process. They imply that some effects that have been attributed to patient demographic factors in earlier studies may actually reflect patients' return to a less stressful and more supportive family context, as well as acquiring the skills to manage difficult life conditions more effectively. In fact, these extratreatment factors accounted for more of the variation in alcohol consumption, abstinence, physical symptoms, and depression than did patient background, intake functioning, and treatment combined, thus confirming their importance in the recovery process. More specifically, family resources and use of active coping skills promote remission, whereas stressful life conditions and avoidance coping responses increase the likelihood of relapse. These context and coping factors affect mood- and health-related functioning as well as drinking outcomes (Brown, 1985; Cronkite & Moos, 1980; Marlatt & Gordon, 1985).

Summary of Research on Remission and Relapse

Our findings support the idea that family, other life context, and personal coping factors are intimately involved in the processes of remission and relapse, and that substantial benefits may accrue when individuals curtail their alcohol abuse. At the 2-year follow-up, remitted alcoholics reported they had more family cohesion and organization, less family conflict, and more extensive social support networks than the relapsed patients. Moreover, they experienced no more life stressors than the community controls and were somewhat more likely to experience positive events.

In contrast, most of the relapsed alcoholics apparently were trapped in a vicious cycle in which stressful life conditions, which may have been exacerbated by their alcohol abuse, contributed to its continuation. A pattern may have been established in which the stressors were amplified and more heavy drinking ensued. This process was no doubt fostered by the high conflict and lack of cohesion and structure in the relapsed patients' families, and by their recurrent lack of employment and frequent job changes. The combination of more life stressors, inadequate social resources, and reliance on less effective coping responses seems to have made it especially hard for the relapsed patients to break their destructive drinking patterns.

Our findings are consistent with those of other studies. Rosenberg (1983) noted that remitted alcoholic patients experienced fewer negative and more positive life events, were less compliant in high-risk situations, and enjoyed more social support from family and friends. Large and dense social networks composed of close friends who do not drink heavily tend to discourage excessive drinking and encourage alcoholics to enter and continue treatment (Strug & Hyman, 1981). In fact, a 20-year follow-up of treated men alcoholics by Nordstrom and Berglund (1986) found that more than 70% of recovered patients attributed their recovery to changes in social circumstances, social pressure to stop drinking, and negative social consequences of alcohol abuse. More generally, positive changes in a person's family and work settings are associated with the process of natural recovery and the maintenance of remission after treatment (Ogborne, Sobell, & Sobell, 1985).

SPOUSES OF ALCOHOLIC PATIENTS

How spouses adapt to an alcoholic mate is of interest in its own right. Recently, some researchers have addressed the issues of whether spouses of impaired individuals differ from spouses of controls, and how spouses adapt to and cope with an alcohol-impaired partner. The growing interest in these issues cuts across a number of disorders, including drug abuse, depression, schizophrenia, and varied medical conditions (Beardslee, Bemporad, Keller, & Klerman, 1983; Emery, Weintraub, & Neale, 1982; Leff & Vaughn, 1985; Orford & Harwin, 1982).

Three theoretical orientations have dominated research on spouses of alcoholic patients: the personality perspective, the stress perspective, and the coping perspective. Research on the spouses of alcoholics began with the assumption that these spouses suffer from long-standing personal deficits; it culminated in attempts to delineate personality traits that predispose individuals to select a mate who is alcoholic. A second line of research focused on the stressors associated with being married to an alcoholic partner and how they contribute to spouses' dysfunction. This approach assumes that spouses are essentially normal individuals who experience severe intermittent strain. Finally, a new line of research involves identifying the ways spouses cope with an alcoholic partner and maintain a satisfactory life-style despite being enmeshed in a disturbed marriage. This approach acknowledges that some spouses cope more effectively with the stressors that confront them and thus are able to lead essentially normal lives (for reviews, see Jacob, 1986; Kaufman & Pattison, 1982; Orford & Harwin, 1982; Paolino & McCrady, 1977).

Research based on the personality perspective implied that a spouse's dysfunction preceded the partner's abusive drinking. A deficient personality in the spouse was thought to create the need for an alcoholic partner and deterioration or "decomposition" of the spouse's functioning if this need was no longer met because the partner stopped drinking. However, there is no empirical support for either the disturbed personality or the decompensation hypothesis (for reviews see Nace, 1982; Paolino & McCrady, 1977).

The stress hypothesis has been examined by comparing spouses whose alcoholic mates were currently abstinent with spouses of currently heavy-drinking alcoholics. However, an alcoholic patient's return to sobriety does not necessarily alleviate stress-related disturbances in other family members. Residual dysfunction of the alcoholic partner, such as depression or social withdrawal, can create ongoing strain for the spouse. Accordingly, finding that spouses of remitted alcoholics do not function as well as spouses of nonalcoholics may be consistent with the stress perspective and does not necessarily imply that spouses of alcoholics are emotionally dependent on the continued dysfunction of their partner.

The coping perspective emphasizes spouses' personal resources and coping skills. Orford and his colleagues (1975) identified ten styles of wives' coping behavior, some of which were associated with a good prognosis for the alcoholic partner. Active behavioral coping responses that imply some bond exists between the partners, such as the wife's pleading, were related to improvement in the husband's drinking behavior (Gorman & Rooney, 1979). In contrast, some wives create an independent existence for themselves while remaining married. Thus, wives of alcoholics modify their coping strategies in response to changes in their husband's drinking behavior. In turn, the coping patterns adopted by spouses may affect their own adaptation (see also Gorman & Rooney, 1979; Wiseman, 1980).

Spouses of Stably Remitted and Relapsed Alcoholics

In our study, we compared the spouses of stably remitted and relapsed patients with the matched spouses of community controls. We first examined whether spouses of remitted patients can attain normal lives and normal levels of functioning. We then compared adaptation among spouses of relapsed alcoholics with that among matched spouses of controls and of remitted alcoholics (Moos et al., 1981).

We identified few differences between the spouses of remitted alcoholics and those of community controls. The spouses of remitted patients were less likely to have consumed alcohol during the past month, and they reported fewer social contacts and recreational pursuits. Otherwise, these spouses achieved comparable levels of occupational functioning, stressors, and social resources, and coped with ongoing stressors just as well. Thus, spouses of remitted alcoholics function as well as demographically matched spouses of nonalcoholic community controls.

The disadvantages associated with having a relapsed partner, however, were evident in the spouse's functioning, family environment, and stressors. Spouses of relapsed patients reported more alcohol consumption and depression, experienced more life stressors, and saw their family environments as less cohesive and recreationally oriented compared to spouses of control and/or remitted patients.

Our findings are most consistent with the stress and coping perspectives. We found no support for the idea that spouses of alcoholics are likely to suffer from underlying personality or coping resource deficits, nor was there support for the idea that they are harmed by their partner's successful control of alcohol abuse. Spouses whose alcoholic partners were drinking heavily experienced much more dysfunction than spouses of controls or remitted patients. We conclude that spouses of alcoholics are basically normal individuals trying to cope with disturbed marriages and dysfunctional partners. These spouses experience cyclical crisis situations and severe strain created by their life with an alcoholic partner, but these consequences abate when the partner makes a concerted effort to control his or her abusive drinking (Moos et al., 1981).

An Integrated Perspective on Spouses of Impaired Partners

We tried to integrate and extend prior research on spouses of alcoholic patients by drawing again on the conceptual model in Figure 12.1. The model can be applied to current spouse adaptation just as it was applied to patient adaptation. In this case, the focal family member is the spouse of the alcoholic patient (Panels II and VIII), and the alcoholic patient's functioning corresponds to Panel IV. Spouse functioning can be affected by the alcoholic partner's level of functioning in both drinking and nondrinking areas (e.g., anxiety, depression, and occupational functioning). In addition, the model reflects the mutual influence marital partners have on each other. Moreover, family social resources and a spouse's coping responses can mediate the effects of stressors on spouse functioning (Finney, Moos, Cronkite, & Gamble, 1983).

Looking first at the relationships among the predictors of spouse functioning in the conceptual model, we found that spouses who functioned better initially experienced fewer life stressors and functioned better at the 2-year follow-up, but spouse social background and initial functioning were not associated with the alcoholic partner's impairment. More important, a high level of impairment of the alcoholic partner was associated with spouses' reports of more life stressors and fewer social resources. There was little relationship between spouses' social background or initial functioning and their family resources. Finally, spouses who had better social backgrounds and reported more positive family environments tended to use more active cognitive or active behavioral coping.

Consistent with our predictions and with stress and coping theory, the alcoholic partner's impairment was strongly related to poorer spouse functioning. Because patients who reduce or eliminate their alcohol consumption may not function better psychosocially, we examined the influence of both the alcoholic partner's drinking and other areas of partner dysfunction (Steinglass, 1981; Steinglass et al., 1987); specifically, we separated drinking from other aspects of impairment. While the alcoholic partner's drinking did not have an independent influence on spouse functioning, the alcoholic's social and psychological impairment did have a significant independent effect on spouse depression and physical symptoms.

We found that the influence of the alcoholic partner's drinking problems on spouse functioning is mediated by the alcoholic partner's impairment in other areas. Thus, information about the alcoholic partner's drinking behavior provides only a partial account of the impact an alcoholic partner has on his or her spouse. The symptoms of the nonalcoholic spouse may be linked more closely to the social and behavioral consequences of drinking than to the level of alcohol consumption itself (Steinglass, 1981; but see Jacob, Dunn, Leonard, & Davis, 1985). At least in the short run, spouses of sober alcoholics may experience some strain caused by their alcoholic partner's continuing psychosocial dysfunction (Wiseman, 1981).

Negative life events were also associated with increased alcohol consumption among spouses. Contrary to expectation, life stressors had relatively little impact on other aspects of spouse functioning. The influence of negative events on spouses' alcohol consumption suggests that the spouses were quite labile in their drinking habits.

Spouses in families that lacked cohesion reported more physical symptoms, while those in highly conflicted families experienced more depression and physical symptoms. As might be expected, spouses in less expressive families were more depressed. A moral-religious emphasis was related to more physical symptoms, probably because health problems often stimulate a search for deeper understanding (Moos, 1984).

Spouses' coping responses were related to their level of adaptation. Prior research has shown that a spouse's reliance on avoidance coping is related to poorer treatment outcome for the alcoholic partner (Gorman & Rooney, 1979; Orford et al., 1975); our findings indicate that the use of avoidance coping to manage stressors is also associated with poorer spouse functioning. Specifically, spouses who rely more on avoidance coping report poorer mood and health and use more medications than spouses who rely less on them, even after the partner's level of alcohol consumption is considered. Spouses who use mainly active coping strategies when their partner is drinking heavily function better than those who use avoidance responses (see also Gorman & Rooney, 1979). Thus, some spouses of alcoholics may amplify the effects of stressful life conditions by employing ineffective methods to deal with them.

Our conceptualization of the determinants of spouse functioning is one of many that can be formulated. There may be better indicators of personal resources, and there may be alternative connections among the predictors we have examined. Additionally, some predictors are likely to have a mutual influence on each other—especially the functioning of individuals married to each other. More generally, to provide a comprehensive account of functioning of members of an alcohol-impaired family, we need to look beyond the alcoholic member's drinking to other factors that affect family members.

CHILDREN OF ALCOHOLIC PARENTS

Alcoholism has a pervasive influence not only on spouses, but also on children. The prevalence of alcohol-related problems is more than twice as high among children of alcoholic parents than among children of normal-drinking parents (Goodwin, 1985). Both genetic and environmental factors are involved in these familial associations (Cloninger, Bohman, & Sigvardsson, 1981; Gabrielli & Plomin, 1985).

Some of the health and behavior problems experienced by children of heavy drinkers may foreshadow subsequent development of alcoholism (Knop, Teasdale, Schulsinger, & Goodwin, 1985). Such problems include impulsivity, rebellious behavior, hyperactivity, a disturbed school career, lack of verbal proficiency, and poor academic achievement. Compared to children of moderate-drinking or abstaining parents, children of heavy-drinking parents are also more likely to experience such physical and emotional problems as insomnia, nightmares, depression, and low self-esteem, and to visit physicians more frequently (for overviews, see Adler & Raphael, 1983; Deutsch, 1982; Knop et al., 1985). The insidious impact of parental alcohol abuse is clear, but little is known about how it is mediated or how it can be overcome.

Although the literature mainly addresses dysfunction among children of alcoholics, the majority of these children adapt normally without developing serious drinking problems (West & Prinz, 1987). Constitutional factors and the early family environment can buffer the risks of parental alcoholism. For example, Werner's 18-year longitudinal study (1986) identified personal characteristics and qualities of the caregiving environment as factors that differentiated children of alcoholic parents into those who did and those who did not develop serious problems. Almost 60% of the children in Werner's study were functioning quite well at age 18, indicating a high degree of resiliency in this age group. Resilient children tended to receive more attention from their caretaker in the early years, experience fewer stressful events during their first two years of life, and develop better communication skills and more positive self-regard overall.

The adverse impact of excessive parental drinking on children has clearly been established (for reviews, see Adler & Raphael, 1983; Deutsche, 1982; Knop et al., 1985). Factors such as disrupted communication and parenting abilities, parent–child conflict and rejection, and lack of family cohesion may mediate the impact of the parental disorder, as well as have important independent effects of their own (Adler & Raphael, 1983; West

& Prinze, 1987). Stressful life events, marital conflict, and family disorganization comprise a set of additional risk factors, whereas family cohesion, expressiveness, and recreational activities are resources that may offset the adverse effect of abusive drinking on children. In a study of "superkids"—children who appear to be invulnerable to parental psychiatric disorders—Kauffman, Grunebaum, Cohler, & Gamer (1979) found that cohesive yet independent relationships with the mother and positive social contacts with adults outside the family mitigated the influence of serious parental psychopathology.

These ideas led us to apply our conceptual model (Figure 12.1) in a way that depicts the influence of family and other life context factors on children's adaptation. Family demographic factors, such as size and socioeconomic status, and a child's personal resources, such as self-esteem, can influence the child's adaptation. More specifically, we expected that the severity of the impaired parent's dysfunction would have a major impact on the child's well-being. Thus, a child is likely to be more affected when the alcoholic parent is a heavier drinker. We thought that the alcoholic parent's impairment in areas other than drinking also would have a detrimental influence on the child, just as it had on the spouse. Because a child's observation and modeling of a parent's ineffective problem-solving behavior may make the child more vulnerable, we posited that the parent's tendency to use avoidance coping also would create problems for the child. In this respect, the child is affected by both the parent's general mood and health and the parent's daily behavior. Because each parent's health and functioning affect the child, the model reflects the influence of the nonalcoholic as well as the alcoholic parent.

Children in Alcoholic-Parent and Matched Control Families

We first compared children in the families of remitted ($N = 28$) and relapsed ($N = 23$) alcoholic patients with children in families of the matched community controls ($N = 59$). Emotional disturbance in children was reported more than twice as often among relapsed (52%) as among control (22%) families. Compared to children in control families, children in families of relapsed alcoholics suffered from more depression and anxiety, experienced more indigestion and nightmares, and were more likely to have serious physical and mental problems. In contrast, physical health and emotional functioning among children in families of remitted alcoholics were comparable to that among children in control families (Moos & Billings, 1982).

Compared with families of controls, families of relapsed alcoholics with children living at home were less cohesive and expressive, and less likely to foster independence, achievement, intellectual and recreational pursuits, and a moral-religious orientation. In addition, the relapsed families were less well organized and the parents disagreed more about the family climate.

These aspects of the family environment are closely linked to adaptation among young children and adolescents. The family climate of the remitted alcoholics was similar to that of the controls. Baer, Garmezy, McLaughlin, Pokorny, and Wernick (1987) found that lack of family cohesion and expressiveness and more family conflict were related to more alcohol use among students in junior high school. In contrast, a family emphasis on personal growth within the context of supportive parent–child relationships, clear rules, and well-defined limits (Moos & Moos, 1986) seems to benefit children.

Because it helps to shape a child's temperament, the family environment may increase susceptibility to alcoholism in adulthood. Tarter, Alterman, and Edwards (1985) have suggested that the risk for alcoholism is increased by high emotionality, short attention span, and sustained arousal after stimulation. These characteristics of temperament are more likely to develop among infants in families that are highly conflicted and that lack cohesion, expressiveness, and an emphasis on independence and intellectual and recreational pursuits (Plomin & DeFries, 1985). As we have noted, these are the qualities that characterize families of alcoholic parents, especially those with ongoing serious drinking problems. By fostering a family climate that promotes certain temperament characteristics, parental alcoholism may increase a child's risk for alcohol abuse and other behavioral dysfunctions.

The stress-related influence of parental alcoholism on children seems to diminish or disappear when the parent succeeds in controlling his or her alcohol abuse. This finding is consistent with our observation of normal mood and health among the spouses of remitted alcoholics. It strengthens the conclusion that an alcoholic family system need not continue to place undue strain on its members when the identified patient's alcohol abuse has been remitted for an extended period (see also Callan & Jackson, 1986).

Although the children of remitted alcoholics were found to be functioning normally, they may be at increased risk over the long term. Some children of alcoholics may remain symptom-free until they reach adulthood and encounter stressors that touch on areas of latent vulnerability. In any case, our findings imply that the alcoholic parent's remission and other compensatory family factors may offset these long-term risks.

Determinants of Functioning of Children of Alcoholic Parents

We next examined children's functioning within the broader conceptual framework outlined in Figure 12.1. Specifically, we used parent functioning, family stressors, and family resources to predict the emotional and physical functioning of the child after controlling group membership (alcoholic and control) and family size. Parent functioning was assessed by alcohol consumption, drinking problems, anxiety, depression, physical symptoms, occupational functioning, and use of avoidance coping. The stressors were negative life events, family arguments, and parental disagreement about the family environment; the resources were family cohesion and organization.

In general, the indices of parental and family dysfunction were related to children's depression and emotional problems, but not to their physical problems. Aside from the expected influence of the alcoholic parent's drinking problems, the emotional dysfunction (especially depressed mood) of *both* parents and their use of avoidance coping were associated with more emotional problems among their children. The alcoholic parent's physical symptoms and occupational functioning were predictably related to children's adaptation. Stressful life events and family conflict, spouses' disagreement, and lack of family cohesion and organization also predicted children's emotional symptoms.

Risk and Resistance Factors

We considered the extent to which a parent's drinking problems and depression, the nonalcoholic parent's reliance on avoidance coping, and lack of family support were independent risk factors associated with children's multiple health problems. We defined multiple health problems as present when children in a family had three or more problems out of a total of twelve emotional or physical problems. We compared the prevalence of multiple health problems among children exposed to as many as four risk factors: parental drinking problems, parental depression, an unsupportive family environment, and the nonalcoholic or control-match parent's reliance on avoidance coping.

The proportion of families with multiproblem children increased with the number of risk factors. There were no multiproblem children in any of the families that had no risk factors. The prevalence of multiple problems in children was 28% in families with one risk factor and 46% in families with two or more risk factors.

Whereas parental dysfunction and an unsupportive family place children's health at risk, low stress and high support appear to function as protective factors. The presence of these resistance factors was associated with lower rates of multiple problems among children of an alcoholic parent. Fifty percent of the alcoholic-parent families with no resistance factors had children with three or more problems. This rate dropped to 15% among families in which neither parent was depressed, and to 8% among those who also enjoyed high cohesion. There were no families with multiple problems among children when the nonalcoholic parent also did not rely on avoidance coping. Thus, we were able to identify a group of alcoholic-parent families that had relatively healthy children, as evidenced by a comparatively low rate of multiple health problems.

We have highlighted how a family-oriented conceptual paradigm can help to understand some of the determinants of child functioning. Clair and Genest (1987) found that a similar paradigm helped to understand adjustment among young adult children of alcoholic fathers. Compared to children of nonalcoholic parents, children of alcoholic fathers reported more conflict and less cohesion, organization, and intellectual orientation in their family of origin. In addition, they were more prone to depression and more likely to endorse emotion-focused coping strategies such as wishful thinking and avoidance coping. High family conflict and a lack of family cohesion, expressiveness, and independence were related to depression proneness and low self-esteem. Benson and Heller (1987) emphasized how family cohesion and support contribute to good adjustment among young adult daughters of alcoholic and problem-drinking fathers.

FUTURE DIRECTIONS

We have described a research program that focused on life context and coping factors in families with a treated alcoholic member. Our perspective points to the risk and resistance factors involved in the processes of patients' remission and relapse; moreover, it applies to spouses and children as they try to adapt to an alcoholic partner or parent. The findings that emerge from our research imply that life context factors—including spouse functioning and overall family climate—play an important role in the posttreatment process of recovery for patients and their families. They also suggest that if an alcoholic patient achieves remission for two years, the functioning levels of his or her spouse and children generally return to normal.

Implications for Assessment, Diagnosis, and Treatment

As we have shown, patients' life contexts and coping skills play a continuing role in the posttreatment course of alcohol abuse. Although clinicians usually focus on an individual's demographic factors and initial levels of functioning, it is the life context and coping factors that are more pervasive and intense, and that still have a strong impact long after treatment (Orford, 1985).

Our findings indicate that treatment should be oriented toward strengthening the natural recovery process and improving the life contexts of patients and their ability to manage these contexts (see also Edwards, 1984;

Mulford, 1984; Vaillant et al., 1983). The idea of shaping formal interventions to enhance natural recovery is supported by research on other substance abuse disorders, as well as by studies of the psychosocial outcomes of a variety of psychiatric and medical conditions (Moos, 1985).

Comprehensive Assessment and Diagnosis

We recommend that more emphasis be placed on identifying potentially alterable characteristics of patients and their life contexts and on using this information in the treatment process. Because patients and their spouses and children influence each other, it is important to evaluate the status and functioning of the alcoholic's family and other social environments. Information about current and expected stressors can identify situations that may increase the risk of relapse; information about patients' coping styles may help clinicians teach patients how to minimize stressors and adapt more effectively. Routine evaluations of patients' life contexts, especially their family and work settings, can be used to monitor the outcome of patients' efforts to improve their everyday environments.

In sum, more comprehensive and conceptually focused measures of life stressors, social resources, and coping responses will foster more accurate predictions of treatment outcome and facilitate more effective clinical interventions. Accordingly, we have developed a Life Stressors and Social Resources Inventory, which assesses ongoing life circumstances and new life events in eight important domains, including spouse/partner, children, extended family, physical health, financial, and work (Moos, Fenn, Billings, & Moos, 1989; Moos & Moos, 1988). We have also constructed a Coping Responses Inventory that taps appraisal-focused, problem-focused, and emotion-focused coping responses (Moos, 1988). (These Inventories can be used to develop profiles that depict patients' life contexts and coping responses; they may also have some value in planning and evaluating alcoholism treatment.)

Family-Oriented Treatment

Our findings point to the pivotal influence of family functioning on treatment outcome. We believe that family-oriented therapy should be considered as a component in the treatment of alcoholic patients who live in a family setting; we think it is clinically appropriate for a large proportion of such patients. Clinicians are developing effective interpersonal or systems approaches and behavioral approaches to family treatment (Hazelrigg, Cooper, & Borduin, 1987); some are being used with alcoholic patients (O'Farrell, Cutter, & Floyd, 1985). In structuring the initial stages of family treatment, clinicians will need to consider the quality of preexisting family relationships (Ford, Bashford, & De Witt, 1984; Vannicelli, Gingerich,

& Ryback, 1983). As the specific aspects of family functioning associated with relapse are identified, clinicians can develop targeted treatment programs to change them. This process has proven fruitful in the development of family treatment for schizophrenia and depression (Goldstein, Hand, & Hahlweg, 1986).

Coping Skills Training

Clinicians and researchers are beginning to recognize the central role that inadequate coping skills play in perpetuating alcohol abuse, and are developing cognitive and behavioral skills training programs that show positive short-term results (Marlatt & Gordon, 1985). Most coping skills programs emphasize behavioral strategies, but our findings show that cognitive strategies are at least as effective in preventing relapse. In fact, cognitive coping can be used in all kinds of circumstances, including those in which behavioral options are not available. Cognitive coping strategies are also less under situational control and thus not as likely to be disrupted by increased life stressors or reduced social support as are behavioral responses (Oei & Jackson, 1982). These ideas are consistent with the secondary prevention program formulated by Sanchez-Craig, Wilkinson, and Walker (1987), who noted that problem drinkers trying to reduce their alcohol consumption relied on cognitive coping at least as much as on behavioral coping. Accordingly, Sanchez-Craig and her colleagues (1987) developed an outpatient skills training program for early-stage problem drinkers; they have also applied the program to other client groups such as drug abusers.

Spouses and Children

A stress and coping perspective can be applied to spouses and children as well as to the alcoholic patient. Our research has shown that to understand spouse and child functioning, one must look beyond the alcoholic patient's functioning and examine other life stressors and coping resources that affect the alcoholic patient's spouse and children.

Spouses

Researchers might consider several issues in planning future studies of spouses of alcohol abusers. First, integration of personality theories and stress and coping theory will allow for a more comprehensive perspective on the many facets of spouse functioning. Even though most prior research supports the idea that a spouse's dysfunction is linked primarily to current stressors, personal factors are likely to be important as well. For example, our findings imply that some spouses of alcoholics tend to rely more heavily on avoidance coping responses to manage current stressors. Similarly, in their study of alcoholic men, O'Farrell, Harrison, and Cutter (1981) found that the wives who were shy as children were more likely than their more outgoing counterparts to endure their husband's verbal abuse of them and their children. Thus, personal and contextual factors may be mutual determinants of spouse functioning.

A second issue is how alcoholics and their spouses may be alike in some personal and behavioral characteristics. deBlois and Steward (1983) identified assortative mating among alcoholics and their spouses, that is, rebellious and unconventional young women were more likely to marry men with these same traits who later became alcoholic. However, spouse similarity also may be attributed to environmental factors such as common life conditions and the postmarital influence of the spouses on each other (Hall, Hesselbrock, & Stabenau, 1983; Merikangas, 1982). Again, a comprehensive perspective on spouse functioning should consider personal as well as contextual factors.

A third issue concerns the potential adaptive consequences of heavy drinking in some families. Most families function better when the alcoholic member regains sobriety, especially if that person is a violence-prone binge drinker. Among steady in-home drinkers, however, high alcohol consumption may be associated with more marital satisfaction and fewer symptoms among some spouses (Dunn, Jacob, Hummon, & Seilhamer, 1987; Jacob, Dunn, & Leonard, 1983). As Wiseman (1981) noted, some sober alcoholics are tense, irritable, and depressed and create a dreary home life. From a different perspective, a newly abstinent partner may upset a carefully crafted pattern of spouse and family adaptation to a "missing" husband or wife (Steinglass, 1981). From this perspective, treatment providers should consider how sobriety may impact family functioning and consider treatment of dysfunction in nondrinking areas when drinking has been used to cope with or mask these areas.

Spouse Interventions

Our findings have implications for and support certain interventions for spouses of alcoholics. Such interventions can be directed toward enabling a spouse to better deal with the distress of being married to an alcoholic partner and/or enabling the spouse to assist the alcoholic partner in overcoming alcohol abuse.

Our findings indicate that being married to an alcoholic partner is a significant source of spouse dysfunction. The analyses also suggest, however, that certain family climate factors and approaches to dealing with this stressor can help to mitigate some of its deleterious effects. Family-oriented interventions that teach communication skills that help to establish and maintain a less conflicted, more cohesive family climate can reduce the negative impact on the spouse. Because avoidance coping strategies appear to be detrimental, interventions that lead to more effective active coping responses, both cognitive and behavioral, also may be beneficial.

With respect to spouse influences on an alcoholic partner, McCrady (1986) distinguishes between alcohol-specific family influences and general family factors related to drinking behavior. In the former category, she includes reinforcing the alcoholic's drinking behavior through attention and caretaking, protecting the alcoholic from the consequences of problem drinking, and punishing the alcoholic for his or her drinking behavior. All three types of responses are hypothesized to increase the likelihood of the alcoholic's drinking. McCrady suggests that a spouse can be taught to reinforce the alcoholic partner for appropriate behaviors (e.g., reducing alcohol consumption) and to withhold positive reinforcement when relapse occurs. Sisson and Azrin (1986) provide evidence of the effectiveness of such approaches. Although our findings do not address how these spouse behaviors are related to a partner's drinking behavior, they are relevant to another category of spouse response suggested by McCrady: modeling appropriate drinking behavior. The relationship we found between a spouse's alcohol consumption and that of the alcoholic partner suggests that interventions to help spouses reduce their alcohol intake may positively affect the alcoholic partner's drinking.

In considering general family influences on an alcoholic's drinking behavior, McCrady (1986) includes poor communication and problem-solving skills that lead to unclear and inconsistent communications and hostile interactions in alcoholic couples. McCrady suggests that interventions be directed toward improving communication skills and increasing the frequency of positive exchanges between the spouse and the alcoholic partner. McCrady also advocates that the family spend time together in activities that are positive experiences but not compatible with alcohol use (see Sisson & Azrin, 1986). Our findings regarding the impact of family cohesion and recreational orientation on patient functioning support such approaches.

Children

We have found that parental disorder, stressful conditions, and the quality of family life influence children's health. The stress and coping perspective can be used to integrate findings from studies of children with other risk factors such as parental divorce, depression, or chronic physical illness (Peters & Esses, 1985). We need conceptually comparable studies of children who have been exposed to different types of parental disorders so that we can identify both general and disorder-specific factors that affect children. Such studies should examine the family stressors and resources that serve to accentuate or ameliorate the impact of a family member's dysfunction.

To fully understand the determinants of family functioning and how they join with parental dysfunction to affect children, we need to consider the broader social context. A setting can affect a person even though he or she is not directly involved in it. For example, a parent's work setting can affect how that parent interacts with his or her children. Future research on the impact and moderators of parental dysfunction should be guided by a conceptual framework that encompasses the interconnections among family, work, school, and peer influences (Moos, 1987). Such research may identify general processes by which impaired parents influence their children and how these processes can be modified by beneficial factors in family and extrafamily contexts.

CONCLUSION

Our data point to complex reciprocal relationships between an alcoholic patient's functioning and the functioning of the patient's spouse and children. A patient who returns to more benign family circumstances generally does better; in addition, the functioning of the patient's spouse and children, and therefore the posttreatment environment, influences the patient's functioning. Conversely, the spouse and children of an alcoholic patient are affected by the patient's adjustment. In this regard, our findings indicate that two years after a patient's remission has begun, nonalcoholic family members do not appear to suffer from this change in the family system. Thus, although family homeostasis may be disrupted at earlier stages in the remission process, any negative effects of a recovering patient's sobriety on other family members seem to be resolved within two years. Spouses and children benefit considerably from their partner's/parent's remission. In fact, a child often is a dual beneficiary of an alcoholic patient's remission— the child experiences direct positive effects from the alcoholic parent's remission as well as the indirect effects of having a more adequately functioning, nonalcoholic parent.

Overall, our data support the value of a stress and coping framework for studying alcoholism in a family context. The framework can guide future research to achieve a better understanding of the processes of patient remission and relapse, and the processes by which nonalcoholic family members adapt to remitted and relapsed alcoholic parents or partners.

Acknowledgment. The research was supported by NIAAA Grants AA02863 and AA06699 and by Department of Veterans Affairs Medical and Health Services Research and Development Service research funds. Adrienne Juliano, Saori Kamano, and Bernice Moos helped with manuscript preparation.

Notes

1. Seven other individuals whose families declined to participate at the 6-month follow-up did participate, along with their families, at the 2-year follow-up. These patients were the heads of their households (husband or wife). Seven persons in the longitudinal sample who participated in the follow-ups at both 6 months and 2 years were not heads of household. The analyses comparing patients and their families with community controls and their families focused on the 113 patients who were heads of their households. The analyses focusing on the processes of remission and relapse among the family-based patients focused on the 113 patients who had complete data at the 6-month and 2-year follow-ups.

2. Our measure of ounces of ethanol consumed on drinking days is "liberal" in that it is the sum of the usual ethanol intake from beer, wine, and spirits when each beverage is consumed. Thus, it reflects the unrealistic assumption that the individual consumes all three beverages on a drinking day. Our second drinking behavior measure of the ounces of ethanol consumed per day, on average, takes into account how often each of the three beverages is consumed, but it does not capture the heavy consumption on intermittent drinking days of a binge drinker.

REFERENCES

Adler, R., & Raphael, B. (1983). Children of alcoholics. *Australian and New Zealand Journal of Psychiatry, 17,* 3–8.

Baer, P. E., Garmezy, L. B., McLaughlin, R. J., Pokorny, A. D., & Wernick, M. J. (1987). Stress, coping, family conflict, and adolescent alcohol use. *Journal of Behavioral Medicine, 10,* 449–466.

Beardslee, W. R., Bemporad, J., Keller, M. B., & Klerman, G. L. (1983). Children of parents with major affective disorder: A review. *American Journal of Psychiatry, 140,* 825–832.

Benson, C. S., & Heller, K. (1987). Factors in the current adjustment of young, adult daughters of alcoholic and problem-drinking fathers. *Journal of Abnormal Psychology, 96,* 305–312.

Brown, S. (1985). Reinforcement expectancies and alcoholism treatment outcome after a one-year follow-up. *Journal of Studies on Alcohol, 46,* 304–308.

Callan, V. J., & Jackson, D. (1986). Children of alcoholic fathers and recovered alcoholic fathers: Personal and family functioning. *Journal of Studies on Alcohol, 47,* 180–182.

Chaney, E. F., & Roszell, D. K. (1985). Coping in opiate addicts maintained on methadone. In S. Shiffman & T. A. Wills (Eds.), *Coping and substance use* (pp. 267–293). New York: Academic Press.

Clair, D., & Genest, M. (1987). Variables associated with the adjustment of offspring of alcoholic fathers. *Journal of Studies on Alcohol, 48,* 345–355.

Cloninger, C. R., Bohman, M., & Sigvardsson, S. (1981). Inheritance of alcohol abuse. *Archives of General Psychiatry, 38,* 861–868.

Cronkite, R. C., & Moos, R. H. (1980). The determinants of posttreatment functioning of alcoholic patients: A conceptual framework. *Journal of Consulting and Clinical Psychology, 48,* 305–316.

deBlois, C. S., & Stewart, M. A. (1983). Marital histories of women whose first husbands were alcoholic or antisocial. *British Journal of Addiction, 78,* 205–213.

Deutsch, C. (1982). *Broken bottles, broken dreams: Understanding and helping the children of alcoholics.* New York: Columbia University Press.

Dunn, N. J., Jacob, T., Hummon, N., & Seilhamer, R. A. (1987). Marital stability in alcoholic-spouse relationships as a function of drinking pattern and location. *Journal of Abnormal Psychology, 96,* 99–107.

Edwards, G. (1984). Drinking in longitudinal perspective: Career and natural history. *British Journal of Addiction, 79,* 175–183.

Emery, R. E., Weintraub, S., & Neale, J. M. (1982). Effects of marital discord on the school behavior of children of schizophrenic, affectively disordered, and normal parents. *Journal of Abnormal Child Psychology, 10,* 215–228.

Finney, J., Moos, R., Cronkite, R., & Gamble, W. (1983). A conceptual model of the functioning of married persons with impaired partners: Spouses of alcoholic patients. *Journal of Marriage and the Family, 45,* 23–34.

Ford, J. D., Bashford, M. B., & DeWitt, K. N. (1984). Three approaches to marital enrichment: Toward optimal matching of participants and interventions. *Journal of Sex and Marital Therapy, 10,* 41–48.

Gabrielli, W. F., & Plomin, R. (1985). Drinking behavior in the Colorado adoptee and twin sample. *Journal of Studies on Alcohol, 46,* 24–31.

Goldstein, M. J., Hand, I., & Hahlweg, K. (1986). *Treatment of schizophrenia: Family assessment and intervention.* Berlin: Springer Verlag.

Goodwin, D. W. (1985). Alcoholism and genetics. *Archives of General Psychiatry, 42,* 171–174.

Gorman, J., & Rooney, J. (1979). The influence of Al-Anon on the coping behavior of wives of alcoholics. *Journal of Studies on Alcohol, 40,* 1030–1038.

Hall, R. L., Hesselbrock, V. M., & Stabenau, J. R. (1983). Familial distribution of alcohol use: II. Assortative mating of alcoholic probands. *Behavior Genetics, 13,* 373–382.

Hazelrigg, M. D., Cooper, H. M., & Borduin, C. M. (1987). Evaluating the effectiveness of family therapies: An integrative review and analysis. *Psychological Bulletin, 101,* 428–442.

Jacob, T. (1986). Alcoholism: A family interaction perspective. In C. Rivers (Ed.), *Nebraska Symposium on Motivation, 34.* Lincoln, NE: University of Nebraska Press.

Jacob, T., Dunn, N. J., & Leonard, K. (1983). Patterns of alcohol abuse and family stability. *Alcoholism: Clinical and Experimental Research, 7,* 382–385.

Jacob, T., Dunn, N. J., Leonard, K., & Davis, P. (1985). Alcohol-related impairments in male alcoholics and the psychiatric symptoms of their spouses: An attempt to replicate. *American Journal of Drug and Alcohol Abuse, 11,* 55–67.

Jacob, T., & Seilhamer, R. A. (1987). Alcoholism and family interaction. In T. Jacob (Ed.), *Family interaction and psychopathology: Theories, methods, and findings* (pp. 535–580). New York: Plenum.

Jones, S., & Lanyon, R. (1981). Relationship between adaptive skills and outcome of alcoholism treatment. *Journal of Studies on Alcohol, 42,* 521–525.

Kauffman, C., Grunebaum, H., Cohler, B., & Gamer, E. (1979). Superkids: Competent children of psychotic mothers. *American Journal of Psychiatry, 136,* 1398–1402.

Kaufman, E., & Pattison, E. M. (1982). The family and alcoholism. In E. M. Pattison & E. Kaufman (Eds.), *Encyclopedic handbook of alcoholism* (pp. 663–672). New York: Gardner.

Knop, J., Teasdale, T. W., Schulsinger, F., & Goodwin, D. W. (1985). A prospective study of young men at high risk for alcoholism: School behavior and achievement. *Journal of Studies on Alcohol, 46,* 273–278.

Leff, J., & Vaughn, C. (1985). *Expressed emotion in families: Its significance for mental illness.* New York: Guilford.

Litman, G., Eiser, J., Rawson, N., & Oppenheim, A. (1979). Towards a typology of relapse: Differences in relapse precipitants and coping behaviours between alcoholic relapsers and survivors. *Behaviour, Research and Therapy, 17,* 89–94.

Marlatt, G. A., & Gordon, J. R. (Eds.) (1985). *Relapse prevention: Maintenance strategies in addictive behavior change.* New York: Guilford.

McCrady, B. S. (1986). The family in the change process. In W. R. Miller & N. Heather (Eds.), *Treating addictive behaviors* (pp. 305–319). New York: Plenum.

Merikangas, K. R. (1982). Assortative mating for psychiatric disorders and psychological traits. *Archives of General Psychiatry, 39,* 1173–1180.

Moos, R. H. (Ed.) (1984). *Coping with physical illness: New directions.* New York: Plenum.

Moos, R. (1985). Evaluating social resources in community and health care contexts. In P. Karoly (Ed.), *Measurement strategies in health psychology* (pp. 433–459). New York: Wiley.

Moos, R. (1987). Person-environment congruence in work, school, and health care settings. *Journal of Vocational Behavior, 31,* 231–247.

Moos, R. (1988). *Coping Responses Inventory manual.* Palo Alto, CA: Social Ecology Laboratory, Stanford University and Department of Veterans Affairs Medical Center.

Moos, R., & Billings, A. (1982). Children of alcoholics during the recovery process: Alcoholic and matched control families. *Addictive Behaviors, 7,* 155–163.

Moos, R., Fenn, C., Billings, A., & Moos, B. (1989). Assessing life stressors and social resources: Applications to alcoholic patients. *Journal of Substance Abuse, 1,* 135–152.

Moos, R., Finney, J., & Chan, D. (1981). The process of recovery from alcoholism: I. Comparing alcoholic patients and matched community controls. *Journal of Studies on Alcohol, 42,* 383–402.

Moos, R., Finney, J., & Cronkite, R. (1990). *Alcoholism treatment: Context, process, and outcome.* New York: Oxford University Press.

Moos, R., & Moos, B. (1986). *Family Environment Scale manual,* 2nd ed. Palo Alto, CA: Consulting Psychologists Press.

Moos, R., & Moos, B. (1988). *Life Stressors and Social Resources Inventory preliminary manual.* Palo Alto, CA: Social Ecology Laboratory, Stanford University and Department of Veterans Affairs Medical Center.

Mulford, H. A. (1984). Rethinking the alcohol problem: A natural processes model. *Journal of Drug Issues, 14,* 31–43.

Nace, E. P. (1982). Therapeutic approaches to the alcoholic marriage. *Psychiatric Clinics of North America, 5,* 543–564.

Nordstrom, G., & Berglund, M. (1986). Successful adjustment in alcoholism: Relationships between causes of improvement, personality, and social factors. *Journal of Nervous and Mental Disease, 174,* 664–668.

Oei, T. P. S., & Jackson, P. (1982). Social skills and cognitive behavioral approaches to the treatment of problem drinking. *Journal of Studies on Alcohol, 43,* 532–547.

O'Farrell, T. J., & Cutter, H. S. G. (1984). Behavioral marital therapy for male alcoholics: Clinical procedures from a treatment outcome study in progress. *American Journal of Family Therapy, 12,* 33–46.

O'Farrell, T. J., Cutter, H. S. G., & Floyd, F. J. (1985). Evaluating behavioral marital therapy for male alcoholics: Effects on marital adjustment and communication from before to after treatment. *Behavior Therapy, 16,* 147–167.

O'Farrell, T. J., Harrison, R. H., & Cutter, H. S. G. (1981). Marital stability among wives of alcoholics: An evaluation of three explanations. *British Journal of Addiction, 76,* 175–189.

Orford, J. (1985). *Excessive appetites: A psychological view of addictions.* New York: Wiley.

Orford, J., Guthrie, S., Nicholls, P., Oppenheimer, E., Egert, S., & Hensman, C. (1975). Self-reported coping behavior of wives of alcoholics and its association with drinking outcome. *Journal of Studies on Alcohol, 36,* 1255–1267.

Orford, J., & Harwin, J. (Eds.) (1982). *Alcohol and the family.* London: Croom Helm.

Paolino, T., & McCrady, B. (1977). *The alcoholic marriage: Alternative perspectives.* New York: Grune & Stratton.

Peters, L. C., & Esses, L. M. (1985). Family environment as perceived by children with a chronically ill parent. *Journal of Chronic Disease, 38,* 301–308.

Plomin, R., & DeFries, J. (1985). *Origins of individual differences in infancy: The Colorado Adoption Project.* New York: Academic Press.

Roberts, M., Floyd, F., O'Farrell, T., & Cutter, H. (1985). Marital interactions and the duration of alcoholic husbands' sobriety. *American Journal of Drug and Alcohol Abuse, 11,* 303–313.

Roghmann, K., Roberts, J., Smith, T., Wells, S., & Wersinger, R. (1981). Alcoholics' versus nonalcoholics' use of services of a health maintenance organization. *Journal of Studies on Alcohol, 42,* 312–322.

Rosenberg, H. (1983). Relapsed versus non-relapsed alcohol abusers: Coping skills, life events, and social support. *Addictive Behaviors, 8,* 183–186.

Samsonowitz, V., & Sjoberg, L. (1981). Volitional problems of socially adjusted alcoholics. *Addictive Behaviors, 6,* 385–398.

Sanchez-Craig, M., Wilkinson, D. A., & Walker, K. (1987). Theory and methods for secondary prevention of alcohol problems: A cognitively based approach. In W. M. Cox (Ed.), *Treatment and prevention of alcohol problems: A resource manual* (pp. 287–331). New York: Academic Press.

Sisson, R. W., & Azrin, N. H. (1986). Family member involvement to initiate and promote treatment of problem drinkers. *Journal of Behavior Therapy and Experimental Psychiatry, 17,* 15–21.

Sjoberg, L., & Samsonowitz, V. (1985). Coping strategies and relapse in alcohol abuse. *Drug and Alcohol Dependence, 15,* 283–301.

Steinglass, P. (1981). The alcoholic family at home: Patterns of interaction in dry, wet, and transitional stages of alcoholism: *Archives of General Psychiatry, 38,* 578–584.

Steinglass, P., Bennet, L. A., Wolin, S. J., & Reiss, D. (1987). *The alcoholic family.* New York: Basic Books.

Steinglass, P., & Robertson, A. (1983). The alcoholic family. In B. Kissin & H. Begleiter (Eds.), *The pathogenesis of alcoholism: Vol. VI. Psychosocial factors* (pp. 243–307). New York: Plenum.

Strug, D. L., & Hyman, M. M. (1981). Social networks of alcoholics. *Journal of Studies on Alcohol, 42,* 855–884.

Tarter, R., Alterman, A., & Edwards, K. (1985). Vulnerability to alcoholism in men: A behavior/genetic perspective. *Journal of Studies on Alcohol, 46,* 329–356.

Vaillant, G. E. (1983). *The natural history of alcoholism: Causes, patterns, and paths to recovery.* Cambridge, MA: Harvard University Press.

Vaillant, G. E., Clark, W., Cyrus, C., Milofsky, E. S., Kopp, J., Wulsin, V. W., & Mogielnicki, N. P. (1983). Prospective study of alcoholism treatment: Eight-year follow-up. *American Journal of Medicine, 75,* 455–463.

Vannicelli, M., Gingerich, S., & Ryback, R. (1983). Family problems related to the treatment and outcome of alcoholic patients. *British Journal of Addiction, 78,* 193–204.

Ward, D. (1981). The influence of family relationships on social and psychological functioning: A follow-up study. *Journal of Marriage and the Family, 43,* 807–815.

Werner, E. E. (1986). Resilient offspring of alcoholics: A longitudinal study from birth to age 18. *Journal of Studies on Alcohol, 47,* 34–40.

West, M. O., & Prinz, R. J. (1987). Parental alcoholism and childhood psychopathology. *Psychological Bulletin, 102,* 204–218.

Wiseman, J. (1980). The "home treatment": The first steps in trying to cope with an alcoholic husband. *Family Relations, 29,* 541–549.

Wiseman, J. (1981). Sober comportment: Patterns and perspectives on alcohol addiction. *Journal of Studies on Alcohol, 42,* 106–126.

Zweben, A. (1986). Problem drinking and marital adjustment. *Journal of Studies on Alcohol, 47,* 167–172.

13

The Marital Relationship and Alcoholism Treatment

BARBARA S. McCRADY

This chapter will provide an overview of major research advances related to the understanding of alcoholism in the context of the marital relationship. It will highlight work done by the author, in the context of contemporary research with alcoholics and their spouses. This work spans a decade and a half in which major changes have occurred in the degree of interest and emphasis on the role of the family in both the etiology and treatment of alcoholism. When this work began, terms such as "co-dependency" (Cermak, 1986) were unknown, there was little concern for the impact of parental alcoholism on children, and few alcoholism treatment programs had developed family aspects of their treatment. In the last 15 years, however, significant changes have occurred in several research and clinical domains related to the alcoholic family, three of which will be covered here: the functioning of the nonalcoholic spouse of the alcoholic: the nature of the relationship between the alcoholic and his or her partner; and the effectiveness of approaches to treatment for these couples.

THE NONALCOHOLIC SPOUSE

Clinical and research interest in the role of the family in the etiology and treatment of alcoholism dates back to the 1930s when clinical social workers first began to report their observations of women married to alcoholic men (Lewis, 1937). In those early reports, the problems of alcoholic couples were conceptualized in psychodynamic terms, with a focus on the individual psychopathology of each partner. The "disturbed personality hypothesis" described women married to alcoholics as having neurotic conflicts with control, dependency, or anger, who resolved these conflicts through marriage to an alcoholic man. If the alcoholic were to successfully resolve his drinking problem, it was believed that the woman would decompensate to more severe psychopathology, because the defense of being married to an alcoholic had been removed (reviewed in Paolino & McCrady, 1977).

By the 1950s, these early models began to be scrutinized, and alternative conceptualizations were offered (Jackson, 1954). The behavior of women married to alcoholic men, while still seen as dysfunctional, was conceptualized not as "disturbed," but rather as an understandable reaction to a chronically stressful environment. Our own early research in this area (Paolino, McCrady, Diamond, & Longabaugh, 1976) assessed the functioning of spouses of hospitalized alcoholics, and found that these spouses scored within the normal range on general measures of psychiatric severity (the Alienation scale from the Psychological Screening Inventory (PSI), Lanyon, 1973) and generalized anxiety and stress (the Discomfort scale from the PSI). However, these spouses also scored significantly higher than normal controls on a measure of defensiveness (the Defensiveness scale from the PSI). These findings provided little support for the early "disturbed personality hypothesis" in that the spouses showed no marked psychopathology early in their partners' hospitalization. The increase in defensiveness may well derive from the guilt and self-blaming often seen among families of alcoholics.

In the 1960s, Kogan and Jackson (1965) tested Jackson's model by assessing the functioning of women married to currently drinking or abstinent alcoholics, comparing them to control women who were married to nonalcoholic men. By controlling for the current drinking status of the alcoholic, they were able to assess whether or not the woman's distress was higher or lower when her husband was abstinent. Their research strongly supported the stress hypothesis in finding that the women whose husbands were abstinent were most similar in functioning to the controls.

Kogan and Jackson's work was limited by its retrospective nature. The differences among the women could have been a result of preabstinence differences in the wives, rather than differences as a consequence of abstinence. To examine spouse functioning prospectively rather than retrospectively, we followed the spouses in our previous study, assessing their functioning immediately (6 weeks) and 6 months after treatment began (Paolino, McCrady & Kogan, 1978). Alcoholic partners in the study significantly decreased their drinking over time, to a mean daily intake of 0.10 ounces of ethanol. Spouses showed significant decreases in anxiety and depression, as measured by the Multiple Affect Adjective Checklist (Zuckerman & Lubin, 1965). No changes were observed in measures of general psychopathology, which had been in the normal range at baseline.

Subsequent to our longitudinal study, Moos, Finney and Gamble (1982) used a more sophisticated longitudinal design with a larger sample of treated alcoholics, who were carefully matched to community controls. Two years after treatment, they compared the functioning of spouses of community controls with spouses of those alcoholics who had recovered and those who had relapsed. Their results showed that the spouses of recovered alcoholics were indistinguishable from spouses of community controls, while the spouses whose husbands continued to drink problematically continued to show significant levels of subjective distress.

In summary, research on the functioning of the nonalcoholic partner consistently supports a stress/adaptation model, which suggests that these spouses are responding to a chronic stressor by experiencing a variety of types of discomfort or disturbance, and that these symptoms are closely tied to the drinking status of the partner. There is no evidence from the research of an underlying personality disturbance among partners of alcoholics that exists independent of the active drinking status of the alcoholic. These research findings seriously raise questions about the current emphasis on "codependency" as a personality disorder (Cermak, 1986).

THE NATURE OF THE ALCOHOLIC MARITAL RELATIONSHIP

Models of Interactional Behavior

As family systems and behavioral interactional models of family functioning were articulated in the 1970s, researchers and clinicians began to conceptualize the behavior of couples in alcoholic relationships from an interactional rather than an individual psychopathology perspective. This perspective suggested a reciprocal relationship between alcoholism and marital functioning, in which drinking and relationship behaviors were integrally intertwined. Early research deriving from an interactional perspective examined the nature of actual interactions between alcoholics and their partners or other family members, and included observations of the impact of alcohol on these interactions. Using an inpatient research unit as their experimental setting, Steinglass and his colleagues (Steinglass, Weiner & Mendelson, 1971; Weiner, Tamerin, Steinglass & Mendelson, 1971) studied interactions between an alcoholic father and son, and a pair of alcoholic brothers. They observed certain predictable changes in interactional behavior associated with drinking, which led them to perceive drinking as reinforcing, or having "adaptive consequences" for, the relationship (Davis, Berenson, Steinglass, & Davis, 1974).

Other researchers also began to examine sources of reinforcement for drinking within the alcoholic marriage. Peter Miller and his colleagues (Becker & Miller, 1976; Hersen, Miller & Eisler, 1973) studied spouse behavior when couples discussed alcohol or another, neutral topic. They reported that wives of alcoholic men looked at their husbands more when discussing alcohol than another topic, and that the husbands talked more during alcohol than non-alcohol-related interactions. Their data suggested that spouses might actually be reinforcing drinking by paying more attention to alcohol-related conversation. We continued this line of research by examining differences in interactional behavior when discussing alcohol, another problem area, or a neutral topic, positing that the increased attention might be related to the greater salience of the alcohol topic when compared to a neutral topic. Our results indicated that wives paid the most attention to the alcohol topic, and that couples emitted the highest frequency of problem solving statements when discussing alcohol (McCrady & Wiener, 1978), thus supporting the hypothesis that couples' interactions may be particularly reinforcing when discussing drinking itself, not just a problem area in the relationship.

Subsequent to these early studies, a number of interactional studies have reported increases in positive interactional behaviors associated with drinking (e.g., Billings, Kessler, Gomberg & Weiner, 1979; Frankenstein, 1982). These studies are important in recognizing that, despite the negative aspects of alcoholism for a marriage, there are positive changes in the marital relationship associated with drinking. Clinically, these findings suggest that treatment might be more effective if a couple is assisted in obtaining these same positive interactions without the presence of alcohol. This hypothesis was tested in some of our treatment outcome research (discussed below).

Gender Differences in Alcoholic Marriages

One area of marital interaction that has been poorly researched, and which is important to the development of conjoint treatments for alcoholism, has been the study of the marital relationships of couples where the husband or the wife is alcoholic. Higher separation and divorce rates characterize alcoholic women's marriages, and alcoholic women's mates are more likely to be alcohol or drug abusers themselves (reviewed in McCrady, 1988). Despite these known differences in alcoholic women's marriages, little empirical information is available about them. In the context of a treatment outcome study, we examined the nature of the relationships for alcoholic men ($n = 33$) and women ($n = 12$) in intact marriages (Noel & McCrady, 1982). We found that the women were more likely to have begun to drink and to have developed their drinking problems subsequent to the marriage, rather than prior to or early in the marriage. In addition, we found generally higher marital satisfaction among the alcoholic women and their husbands than among the alcoholic men and their wives. The alcoholic women also exhibited more positive verbal communication behavior than the alcoholic men, whereas the alcoholic men were more likely to engage in nonverbal negative behavior. Despite this overall picture of less distressed relationships for the alcoholic women, in the area of sexual functioning these couples showed significant distress. For the women, the more severe their drinking problems, the less frequently they had sexual intercourse. There also was a significant, negative relationship between the alcoholic woman's and her husband's sexual satisfaction, while the alcoholic men and their wives' reports of sexual satisfaction were positively correlated.

Thus, this single study suggests different patterns in alcoholic women's and alcoholic men's relationships. If the women are able to maintain a marital relationship, it appears that the relationship has significant strengths not seen in the alcoholic men's marriages—more marital satisfaction, more positive communication, and a longer period of marriage before the alcoholism enters the picture. These observations suggest that alcoholism may play a less central role in these relationships than in the relationships of alcoholic men. However, these couples seem to play out their marital conflicts in the sexual area, suggesting the special importance of attention to sexual functioning during treatment of alcoholic women.

These studies of the marital relationships of alcoholics suggest the importance of conjoint therapy as an approach to alcoholism treatment. Attention to changing communication patterns to achieve more positive interactions when sober, and to attending to specific relationship problems, such as sexual functioning, would appear to be important components of therapy. The next section reviews some of our research on the treatment of alcoholics and their spouses.

EFFECTIVENESS OF CONJOINT TREATMENT FOR ALCOHOLISM

Research on the treatment of alcoholic couples has derived from three different theoretical perspectives—the family disease model (e.g., Laundergan & Williams, 1979), family systems models (Steinglass, Wolin, Bennett & Reiss, 1987), and social learning model (McCrady & Hay, 1987). Although a description of each model is beyond the scope of this chapter, it is important to note that each model assumes the importance of involving the spouse in the treatment process, and each assumes that changes must occur in multiple areas of functioning, not just in the consumption of alcohol. Our research has derived from family systems and behavioral perspectives.

Family Systems Perspectives and Treatment Studies

Family systems perspectives on alcoholism have incorporated many of the core concepts of family systems theory, such as homeostasis, boundaries, circular causality, and feedback, into models of the alcoholic family system. Family systems models focus on the interaction of the family as a whole, rather than on the behavior of individual family members, as in the disease model, or behavior of spouses, as in behavioral models. Steinglass and his colleagues (Steinglass et al., 1987) posit a family developmental model of alcoholism, in which alcohol plays unique and distinct roles at different stages in the development and evolution of the family. Alcoholism is seen as an organizing principle for some alcoholic families, with the presence or absence of alcohol being the most important variable defining interactional behavior in the family.

Family-systems-oriented treatment of alcoholic families utilizes a variety of techniques to affect interactions. Therapy focuses on the interactional, rather than the individual level, and discussion of the presenting problem (drinking) is directed to a collaborative, interactional level, rather than an individual level. Attempts are made to redefine roles, realign alliances, and change patterns of communication within the family. Understanding changes in family interactional behavior when the alcoholic is drinking is crucial to the therapy. Family therapists also stress the importance of attention to the individual clinical needs of the alcoholic, such as detoxification, medical treatment, and an individual treatment component to support changes in drinking (Kaufman, 1985).

In 1977, Steinglass reviewed research on couples' treatments for alcoholism. He noted a number of clinical reports of the application of family therapy techniques to alcoholism treatment, but noted that there was a "remarkable paucity of studies dealing with family therapy for alcoholism" (p. 116) and states that there was "very little hard evidence . . . demonstrating the efficacy of family therapy" (p. 116).

Our own early research represents one of the few controlled studies of systems-oriented alcoholism treatment. In this early work (McCrady, Paolino, Longabaugh, & Rossi, 1979), we hypothesized that if alcoholism was so integral to family functioning, an intensive intervention would be necessary to effect significant changes in the marital relationship. We developed an approach to treatment, the joint hospitalization, which derived from similar work with neurotic mothers and their infants (Main, 1958), and schizophrenic patients and their families (Bowen, 1961). In the joint hospitalization, alcoholics and their spouses were jointly admitted to a psychiatric hospital, and participated in all aspects of the treatment together. In addition to structured therapeutic activities such as couples and individual group therapy for each partner, the couples participated in the therapeutic milieu, and met with unit staff members on a regular basis to receive feedback on interactions which the staff had observed, and to receive help to change maladaptive interactions. In addition, couples sought out staff when conflicts arose in order to gain an understanding of these and to generate more constructive ways of resolving them.

Couples were randomly assigned, on a two-to-one basis, to either the joint hospitalization condition, or one of two comparison conditions, a couples-involved condition without joint hospitalization, or a condition that involved only the alcoholic partner in treatment. All subjects for the study were selected from among alcoholic inpatients at a psychiatric facility. Subjects in the couples condition participated in couples group therapy and in separate groups for each partner, while subjects in the alcoholics-only condition participated in a different therapy group.

Couples were evaluated at 6–8 weeks and 6–8 months after hospital discharge, using multiple measures of drinking, drinking-related problems, marital happiness, and general life functioning. All groups showed significant decreases in the number of reported marital problems, depression, anxiety, other psychological symptoms, and decreased impairment from use of alcohol, with no differences among the three groups on any of these measures. The distribution of results on the alcohol consumption measure necessitated the use of nonparametric statistics which did not allow direct comparisons among the three treatment conditions on actual drinking. The nonparametric analyses found that only the joint admission and couples group conditions showed significant decreases in quantity of alcohol consumed, although the consumption level in the alcoholics-only group was similar to that of the other two groups at the 6-month follow-up point.

Couples were then reevaluated 4 years after the initiation of treatment (McCrady, Moreau, Paolino & Longabaugh, 1982). Through multiple tracking procedures, at least one member of each couple was located, although complete data could not be obtained for five subjects. Overall, there were no differences in long-term outcome among the three groups, in terms of marital, residential, or employment status, subjective or objective drinking status, or negative consequences of drinking. We also attempted to identify differences between subjects who were abstinent or markedly improved and those who were not. Improved/abstinent subjects were significantly older, had been married longer, and had more hospitalizations for drinking problems.

Overall, the results of the joint admission study guided our later research in several respects. First, it was apparent that it was possible to intensively involve couples in treatment, and that many spouses were willing to go to extraordinary lengths to attempt to facilitate their partner's recovery. However, while the joint hospitalization was feasible, there were no data that supported the superior effectiveness of a hospital level of care for family members over outpatient models of spouse involvement. Results from Steinglass's work (Steinglass, 1979) with a joint hospitalization study for alcoholic couples also suggested no dramatic benefits from the intensive, residential level of care. The results also indicated improvements in drinking habits only for the couples-involved group, lending some support to previous findings of the superior effectiveness of spouse-involved over individual-only treatment (e.g., Cadogan, 1973; Corder, Corder & Laidlaw, 1972; Gliedman, Rosenthal, Frank & Nash, 1956). These three major findings from the study led us to decide to continue to research couples models of alcoholism treatment, but to focus attention on outpatient, rather than the more intensive and costly inpatient, models.

Behavioral Models and Treatment Studies

At the same time that we were completing the joint admission study, several researchers were applying behavioral models to alcoholism treatment, with some very positive results (e.g., Azrin, 1976; Hunt & Azrin, 1973; Sobell & Sobell, 1973). These results, combined with the emergence of behavioral marital therapy models (e.g., O'Leary & Turkewitz, 1978; Weiss, 1978), suggested that treatment based on behavioral models might yield more positive results than the more broadly interactional approach taken in the joint admission study. Three major models began to characterize conjoint behavioral treatments: treatments to train spouses to change alcohol-related behaviors; use of spouses as reinforcers of positive treatment behaviors; and use of behavioral marital therapy techniques to change marital interactions.

Spouse Behavior Change

Like family disease model clinicians, behavioral clinicians have observed that spouses of alcoholics engage in a variety of dysfunctional behaviors related to their partners' drinking. These behaviors include such actions as nagging about drinking, attempting to control drinking, providing alcohol or drinking in the presence of the alcoholic, and reinforcing the drinking through attention or other positive behaviors. In contrast to family disease models, behavioral clinicians do not posit an underlying condition (codependency) which leads to these behaviors. Rather, they view the behaviors as ineffective attempts to cope with a highly stressful problem. The ways that spouses attempt to cope are seen as influenced by multiple factors, including the severity of the partner's alcoholism, the type and range of social supports available, the types of attributions that the spouse makes about the drinking, the general repertoire of coping skills that the spouse has available, and the types of coping that the spouse learned from his or her family of origin (Finney, Moos, Cronkite, & Gamble, 1983).

An early behavioral program (Cheek, Franks, Laucius, & Burtle, 1971) attempted to teach wives of alcoholics to modify the consequences of the alcoholic's drinking, and to become less distressed by situations with their partner that produced tension or anxiety. The study was limited by the low participation rate (17%) and the lack of a control group. For those wives that participated, posttests revealed modest changes in communication and coping, as measured by the spouses' self-reports. A more comprehensive program (Thomas & Santa, 1982), Unilateral Family Therapy, described a three-component approach to spouse treatment: teaching spouses to cope with drinking and other life problems; changing the family's functioning through therapy with the individual; and teaching the spouse techniques to facilitate sobriety. These two studies formed the basis for the spouse interventions developed in our next couples study (described below). After we had completed this study, Sisson and Azrin (1986) reported a study which lent added support to the effectiveness of the spouse component of the treatment. They compared the effectiveness of two approaches to spouse treatment: behavioral reinforcement training, and a traditional program emphasizing education and supportive counseling. The reinforcement counseling resulted in a larger proportion of alcoholic partners seeking treatment, and was associated with greater reductions in drinking. The study is limited by very small samples (12 subjects total), and a short follow-up of only 5 months.

Use of Spouses as Reinforcers of Treatment

An alternative approach to spouse involvement which is unique to behavioral approaches is the enlistment of the spouse as a monitor of treatment. Two recent studies have reported on the effectiveness of spouse contracting in increasing compliance with taking disulfiram. Azrin, Sisson, Meyers, and Godley (1982) reported a 6-month follow-up study of 43 subjects treated at a rural, outpatient alcoholism treatment clinic. Subjects all agreed to take disulfiram, and then were randomly assigned to experimental conditions, which varied in the amount of spouse involvement and the amount of treatment provided beyond a minimum of five counseling sessions. Where spouses (or other partners) were involved, the client agreed to take disulfiram in the presence of the partner each day, and the couple role-played situations in which either partner might be noncompliant with the agreement. Six months after treatment, significant differences among the groups were found. Subjects who received minimal treatment and no spouse involvement reported drinking on an average of 16.4 days of the previous month, compared to 7.9 days for those with the partner involved, and 0.9 for those who received broad spectrum behavior therapy as well as partner involvement.

A similar study (Keane, Foy, Nunn, & Rychtarik, 1984) evaluated the effectiveness of spouse contracting for observing use of disulfiram. A 3-month follow-up found somewhat better disulfiram compliance when the spouse was involved in monitoring, but no statistical analyses were reported. Although the use of a spouse as a specific monitor of disulfiram compliance has not been a component of our treatment protocol, the use of the spouse to reinforce change has been an integral component of the treatment.

Behavioral Marital Therapy

A third behavioral approach has viewed the marital relationship as integral to the maintenance of changes in drinking behavior, and has evaluated treatment interventions that include behavioral marital therapy as one component of the treatment.

Our recent research has evaluated the effectiveness of behavioral approaches to involving the spouse in outpatient treatment. The PACT (Project for Alcoholic Couples Treatment) study evaluated different types of spouse-involved outpatient alcoholism treatment (McCrady et al., 1986; McCrady, Stout, Noel, Abrams, & Nelson, 1987). Subjects were 45 alcoholics and their partners. Subjects were included in the study if they were between 21 and 65 years of age, legally married, not abusing other drugs, had no concomitant major psychiatric disorder, and agreed not to participate in other forms of treatment during the active treatment phase of the study.

Couples were randomly assigned to one of three treatment conditions, which varied in the degree of spouse involvement and the degree of focus on marital relationship issues. In all three treatment conditions, which included 15 treatment sessions, each 1½ hours long, the alcoholic partner learned a variety of behavioral self-control skills to achieve and maintain abstinence from alcohol. In the Minimal Spouse Involvement (MSI) condition, the spouse attended all treatment sessions, but participated only by hearing what the alcoholic partner was learning during treatment, and by providing information relevant to the treatment. In the Alcohol-Focused Spouse Involvement (AFSI) condition, the spouse was also present for all treatment sessions, and learned a variety of techniques for responding to drinking behavior, handling drinking situations and feelings related to past drinking, and providing reinforcement to his/her alcoholic partner for positive behavior change. The spouse-focused techniques in this condition drew heavily from the work of Sisson & Azrin (1986), Thomas and Santa (1982), and Cheek et al. (1971). In the Alcohol Behavioral Marital Therapy (ABMT) condition, each partner learned the individual skills taught in the AFSI condition, and the couple also received behavioral marital therapy, which included reciprocity enhancement techniques, as well as communication and problem-solving training (Jacobson & Margolin, 1979). By systematically varying the degree and type of spouse involvement, the study could separate out the effects of spouse involvement, the spouse learning new skills, and directly modifying the marital relationship.

During treatment, couples in the three treatment conditions showed a differential pattern of involvement in treatment, and a differential pattern of change in drinking (McCrady, Noel, et al., 1986). The Minimal Spouse Involvement condition had a substantial dropout rate (53%), compared to less than 20% in the other two treatment conditions. There were also significant differences in compliance with homework assigned for couples to complete together—couples in the ABMT condition were much more likely to complete conjoint assignments than AFSI couples (there were no conjoint assignments for the MSI couples, since the spouse was not asked to make any behavioral changes during the treatment). By the end of treatment, those alcoholics who received behavioral marital therapy as part of the treatment showed significant decreases in the frequency of drinking, not shown in those subjects who received treatment that focused solely on alcohol-related coping.

Over the 18 months after treatment, couples who received marital therapy showed a substantially different pattern of outcomes than those who did not (McCrady et al., 1987). Couples in the ABMT condition showed a significant, positive linear increase in the proportion of abstinent days over time. In contrast, couples in the MSI condition showed a significant, negative linear decrease in the proportion of abstinent days over time. The two linear regressions were significantly different. Couples in the marital therapy condition were more likely to experience relapses early after treatment, but showed gradual improvement, with increasingly longer periods of abstinence, and shorter relapses, if relapses occurred. Couples whose spouses were minimally involved in the treatment showed the opposite pattern of results—better abstinence right after treatment, but a gradual increase in drinking over time. The pattern of change in the AFSI condition was unclear. Couples in the marital therapy condition also were less likely to report marital separations, and reported significantly higher marital satisfaction than other couples. The alcoholic partners in the ABMT condition also reported significantly more positive subjective well-being than subjects in the other two conditions. There were no differences among the three conditions on rehospitalizations, use of other treatment supports, or occupational or legal status.

A similar pattern of gradual improvement after treatment with behaviorally oriented marital therapy was reported from the BETA (Butler Environmental Treatment of Alcoholism) project (Stout, McCrady, Longabaugh, Noel & Beattie, 1987). In this study, linear time trend analyses were used to compare the percentage of abstinent days for 3-month blocks of time after entry into the study. Follow-ups for 1 year revealed that those alcoholics who received individually oriented treatment had better outcomes initially, but showed a substantial and continuing decline in abstinent days throughout the follow-up. In contrast, subjects whose partners were involved in treatment showed some decrease in abstinent days over the first 6 months, then a gradual improvement thereafter.

The specific findings from the PACT and BETA studies are complemented by the work of O'Farrell and his colleagues. Project CALM (Classes on Alcoholic Marriages) (O'Farrell, Cutter & Floyd, 1985) was a couples aftercare program associated with an inpatient Veterans Administration alcoholism treatment program. Subjects were 36 male alcoholics and their wives, randomly assigned to interactional couples group therapy, behavioral couples group therapy, or a no-spouse-involved control group. Although 18 months of follow-up have been completed, only the data from an immediate posttreatment evaluation have been published. Results suggested that couples in the behavioral condition showed significant improvements on marital satisfaction and marital communication, which were significantly greater than that of the controls. Alcoholics in the behavioral condition reported fewer drinking days than subjects in the other two conditions.

Overall, behavioral approaches to couples treatment appear to show promise. Several different types of spouse-involved treatment have been studied. These studies seem to suggest that techniques for spouse involvement deriving from behavioral principles are more effective than alternatives in increasing compliance with treatment, in terms of the decision to enter treatment, remain in treatment, comply with treatment requirements, and in maintaining positive changes in drinking behavior. Those treatments that focus on unilateral spouse involvement have provided the least data, although the Sisson and Azrin (1986) study suggests such an approach may increase the alcoholic's willingness to become involved with treatment. Treatment that uses the spouse as a monitor and support for taking disulfiram has shown promise in maintaining compliance with disulfiram, but the follow-ups are relatively short (3–6 months), and few studies have been reported. Behavioral approaches to marital therapy with alcoholics also appear to increase compliance with treatment. These studies also suggest that attention to the marital relationship may yield better long-term outcomes than more alcohol- or individually-focused treatment, but that short-term results are less positive. The reasons for the pattern of outcomes observed across these two studies are unclear. It is possible that the marital therapy initially creates increased stress on the couple, as they become aware of a variety of marital problems in addition to the drinking problem. As they are attempting to use many new skills, they may have more difficulty in the first months after treatment, accounting for more frequent relapses. However, as they consolidate their new learning, relapses decrease. Family systems models would suggest that the marital therapy disrupts the family system, which would show more signs of strain until a new homeostasis is achieved.

RELATIONSHIPS BETWEEN MARITAL FUNCTIONING AND TREATMENT OUTCOME

Treatment studies raise theoretical questions about the relationships between drinking and the marital relationship. Among these are (1) the degree to which marital functioning predicts change in drinking, (2) the degree to which changes in drinking predict changes in marital functioning, and (3) the degree and manner in which the relationship recovers as the alcoholism resolves.

In the PACT study, we examined the first of these questions by studying the interrelationships between drinking and marital functioning (McCrady, Stout, & Noel, 1986). We found significant, positive relationships between pretreatment marital satisfaction and positive drinking outcomes (significant correlations ranged from .30 to .58, depending on the variables examined). Correlations were higher for spouse than subject marital satisfaction, and were higher for heavy drinking than abstinence. We also found a significant, positive relationship between improved marital satisfaction during treatment and both increases in abstinence and decreases in heavy drinking.

A study by Steinglass, Tislenko, and Reiss (1985) is most relevant to the second question, the degree to which changes in drinking predict marital functioning. They reported that abstinence was an important predictor of marital stability—2-year follow-ups found 50% separation rates among couples where one partner was actively drinking. In addition, they found that families with a higher degree of involvement and interaction were more likely to remain together than those with lower levels of engagement. These data suggest that successful resolution of drinking problems contributes strongly to marital stability, but that the quality of the relationship also has an important role.

Other studies have examined the course of change in the marriages of alcoholics after treatment. Moos and Moos (1984) found, two years after treatment, that the marriages of recovered alcoholics were significantly different from those of relapsed alcoholics, with more joint sharing of household responsibilities, fewer arguments, and more agreement between the partners. Our data suggest that the course of change in the relationship may not be a simple, linear, positive relationship. In the PACT data (McCrady, Stout & Noel, 1986), a significant, *negative* relationship between positive communication by the alcoholic after treatment and abstinence was found, which lasted up to the 1-year follow-up point. There were also significant, positive relationships between *increased* negative behavior from the alcoholic and the spouse, and increased abstinence immediately after treatment. One year after treatment, the relationship between negative behavior and abstinence reversed.

These findings seem to suggest that there may be phases of change in couples' relationships during recovery. First, it appears that couples go through a period of being more direct and honest with each other. This directness is reflected in more negative interpersonal behavior, and less positive behavior by the alcoholic. Why this occurs is a matter of speculation, but may in part be accounted for by both partners feeling the need to discuss problems directly and openly, something which they were unable to do when the alcoholic was actively drinking. As the couple is relatively unpracticed in having direct conversations, there may be a negative quality to the interactions. As recovery progresses, the alcoholic also may feel less need to try to be "nice" as a way to make up for guilt and remorse about drinking, and be more willing to express a range of feelings more directly. The spouse, who may have learned to be quiet and compliant, or to avoid the drinking partner while actively drinking, may feel more comfortable in being direct about negative feelings. By a year after treatment, the marriages of couples with the best drinking outcomes begin to look like the best functioning marriages, with couples being able to be more positive with each other, and more able to use effective problem-solving skills. The couples apparently have learned how to deal with problems, have resolved some major issues, and are happier in the marriages.

CONCLUSIONS

This chapter has focused on the author's own work, in the context of the larger body of contemporary research on alcoholism and marriage. Several lines of research have been reviewed, focusing on the functioning of the nonalcoholic spouse, the marital relationship, and the use methods to change that relationship.

The picture that emerges from this body of literature suggests two major themes. First, coping models provide a framework for understanding many recent findings. Spouses of alcoholics appear to be coping with highly stressful, complex environments, and show the strain of those experiences. If the stress is removed through the successful resolution of the partner's drinking problem, the spouses are more able to function, and appear no more (or less) anxious, depressed, or unhappy than partners who have not had to cope with alcoholism. Coping models also provide a framework for understanding the recovery of the marital relationships of alcoholics. In the early months after treatment, couples have to cope with a broad array of new problems, related both to the relationship and the recovery. They may have difficulty facing and successfully resolving their problems. Their new communication skills may be incompletely learned, and they face a variety of problems that they had not addressed while the alcoholic partner was drinking problematically. As a result, the alcoholic may experience relapses, and the couple may experience negative feelings that they had previously avoided. As they develop skills to cope with these major problems, drinking decreases or stops, and the marital relationship improves.

The second theme that emerges is that the nature of treatment appears to have some impact on the course of change in alcoholics. Couples-involved treatment yields a more positive treatment outcome than individual-only treatment. Behavioral interventions appear to result in increased compliance with treatment. Treatments that focus specifically on the marital relationship result in improved communication, and, over time, in better drinking outcomes as well.

Many questions about the nature and mechanisms of change in alcoholic marriages remain unanswered. Among these are: What are the most effective means to help couples avoid or manage relapse episodes? What are effective ways to combine couples' interventions with self-help approaches? What are the commonalities and dissimilarities between alcoholics and their partners in terms of expectancies about alcohol and change in drinking, and to what degree do these shared or dissimilar beliefs differentially predict treatment success? These questions are being addressed in current research.

REFERENCES

Azrin, N. (1976). Improvements in the community-reinforcement approach to alcoholism. *Behavior Research and Therapy, 14*, 339–348.

Azrin, N. H., Sisson, R. W., Meyers, R., & Godley, M. (1982). Alcoholism treatment by disulfiram and community reinforcement therapy. *Journal of Behavior Therapy and Experimental Psychiatry, 13*, 105–112.

Becker, J. V., & Miller, P. M. (1976). Verbal and nonverbal marital interaction patterns of alcoholics and nonalcoholics. *Journal of Studies on Alcohol, 37*, 1616–1624.

Billings, A. G., Kessler, M., Gomberg, C. A., & Weiner, S. (1979). Marital conflict resolution of alcoholic and nonalcoholic couples during drinking and non-drinking sessions. *Journal of Studies on Alcohol, 40*, 183–195.

Bowen, M. (1961). The family as the unit of study and treatment. *American Journal of Orthopsychiatry, 31*, 40–60.

Cadogan, D. A. (1973). Marital group therapy in the treatment of alcoholism. *Quarterly Journal of Studies on Alcohol, 34*, 1187–1194.

Cermak, T. (1986). *Diagnosing and treating co-dependence*. Minneapolis, MN: Johnson Institute Books.

Cheek, R. E., Franks, C. M., Laucius, J., & Burtle, V. (1971). Behavior-modification training for wives of alcoholics. *Quarterly Journal of Studies on Alcohol, 32*, 456–461.

Corder, B. F., Corder, R. F., & Laidlaw, N. D. (1972). An intensive treatment program for alcoholics and their wives. *Quarterly Journal of Studies on Alcohol, 33*, 1144–1146.

Davis, D. I., Berenson, D., Steinglass, P., & Davis, S. (1974). The adaptive consequences of drinking. *Psychiatry, 37*, 209–215.

Finney, J., Moos, R., Cronkite, R., & Gamble, W. A. (1983). A conceptual model of the functioning of married persons with impaired partners: Spouses of alcoholic patients. *Journal of Marriage and the Family, 45*, 23–34.

Frankenstein, W. (1982). Alcohol intoxication effects on alcoholics' marital interactions for three levels of conflict intensity. (Unpublished Masters thesis, Rutgers University.)

Gliedman, L. H., Rosenthal, D., Frank, J. D., & Nash, H. T. (1956). Group therapy of alcoholics with concurrent group meetings of their wives. *Quarterly Journal of Studies on Alcohol, 17,* 655–670.

Hersen, M., Miller, P. M., & Eisler, R. M. (1973). Interactions between alcoholics and their wives: A descriptive analysis of verbal and nonverbal behavior. *Quarterly Journal of Studies on Alcohol, 34,* 516–520.

Hunt, G., & Azrin, N. (1973). The community reinforcement approach to alcoholism. *Behaviour Research and Therapy, 11,* 91–104.

Jackson, J. K. (1954). The adjustment of the family to the crisis of alcoholism. *Quarterly Journal of Studies on Alcohol, 15,* 562–586.

Jacobson, N. S., & Margolin, G. (1979). *Marital therapy.* New York: Brunner/ Mazel.

Kaufman, E. (1985). *Substance abuse and family therapy.* Orlando, FL: Grune & Stratton.

Keane, T. M., Foy, D. W., Nunn, B., & Rychtarik, R. G. (1984). Spouse contracting to increase Antabuse compliance in alcoholic veterans. *Journal of Clinical Psychology, 40,* 340–344.

Kogan, K., & Jackson, J. K. (1965). Alcoholism: The fable of the noxious wife. *Mental Hygiene, 49,* 428–437.

Lanyon, R. I. (1973). *Psychological Screening Inventory Manual.* Goshen, NY: Research Psychologists Press.

Laundergan, J. C., & Williams, T. (1979). Hazelden: Evaluation of a residential family program. *Alcohol, Health and Research World, 3,* 13–16.

Lewis, M. L. (1937). Alcoholism and family casework. *Social Casework, 35,* 8–14.

Main, T. F. (1958). Mothers with children in a psychiatric hospital. *Lancet, 2,* 845–847.

McCrady, B. S. (1988). Behavioral medicine and the woman alcoholic. In E. Blechman & K. Brownell, (Eds.), *Behavioral medicine and the woman patient* (pp. 356–368). NY: Plenum.

McCrady, B. S., & Hay, W. (1987). Coping with problem drinking in the family. In: J. Orford (Ed.), *Coping with disorder in the family* (pp. 86–116). London: Croom Helm.

McCrady, B. S., Moreau, J., Paolino, T. J., Jr., & Longabaugh, R. L. (1982). Joint hospitalization and couples therapy for alcoholism; a four-year follow-up. *Journal of Studies on Alcohol, 43,* 1244–1250.

McCrady, B. S., Noel, N. E., Abrams, D. B., Stout, R. L., Nelson, H. F., & Hay, W. M. (1986). Comparative effectiveness of three types of spouse involvement in outpatient behavioral alcoholism treatment. *Journal of Studies on Alcohol, 47,* 459–467.

McCrady, B. S., Paolino, T. J., Jr., Longabaugh, R. L. & Rossi, J. (1979). Effects of joint hospital admission and couples treatment for hospitalized alcoholics; a pilot study. *Addictive Behaviors, 4,* 155–165.

McCrady, B. S., Stout, R. L., & Noel, N. E. (1986, August). Interrelationships between drinking and marital functioning in alcoholic couples. Paper presented at the Annual Meeting of the American Psychological Association, Washington, DC.

McCrady, B. S., Stout, R. L., Noel, N. E. Abrams, D. B. & Nelson, H. F. (1987)

(unpublished). Comparative effectiveness of three types of spouse involved behavioral alcoholism treatment: Outcomes 18 months after treatment.

McCrady, B. S., & Wiener, J. (1978, November). Verbal and nonverbal marital interactions in male and female alcoholics. Paper presented at the Annual Meeting of the Association for Advancement of Behavior Therapy, Chicago, IL.

Moos, R. H., Finney, J. W., & Gamble, W. (1982). The process of recovery from alcoholism. II. Comparing spouses of alcoholic patients and matched community controls. *Journal of Studies on Alcohol, 43,* 888–909.

Moos, R. H., & Moos, B. S. (1984). The process of recovery from alcoholism. III. Comparing functioning of families of alcoholics and matched control families. *Journal of Studies on Alcohol, 45,* 111–118.

Noel, N. S., & McCrady, B. S. (1982, August). Differences in marital functioning of male and female problem drinkers. Paper presented at the Annual Meeting of the American Psychological Association, Washington, DC.

O'Farrell, T. J., Cutter, H. S. G., & Floyd, F. J. (1985). Evaluating behavioral marital therapy for male alcoholics: Effects on marital adjustment and communication from before to after treatment. *Behavior Therapy, 16,* 147–167.

O'Leary, K. D., & Turkewitz, H. (1978). Marital therapy from a behavioral perspective. In T. J. Paolino, Jr., & B. S. McCrady (Eds.), *Marriage and marital therapy* (pp. 240–297). NY: Brunner/Mazel.

Paolino, T. J., Jr. & McCrady, B. S. (1977). *The alcoholic marriage: Alternative perspectives.* NY: Grune & Stratton.

Paolino, T. J., Jr., McCrady, B., Diamond, S., & Longabaugh, R. (1976). Psychological disturbances in spouses of alcoholics. An empirical assessment. *Journal of Studies on Alcohol, 37,* 1600–1607.

Paolino, T. J., Jr., McCrady, B. S., & Kogan, K. B. (1978). Alcoholic marriages: A longitudinal empirical assessment of alternative theories. *British Journal of Addiction, 73,* 129–138.

Sisson, R. W., & Azrin, N. (1986). Family-members involvement to initiate and promote treatment of problem drinkers. *Journal of Behavior Therapy and Experimental Psychiatry, 17,* 15–21.

Sobell, M. B., & Sobell, L. C. (1973). Alcoholics treated by individualized behavior therapy: One year treatment outcome. *Behavior Research and Therapy, 11,* 599–618.

Steinglass, P. (1977). Experimenting with family treatment approaches to alcoholism, 1950–1975: A review. *Family Process, 15,* 97–123.

Steinglass, P. (1979). An experimental treatment program for alcoholic couples. *Journal of Studies on Alcohol, 40,* 159–182.

Steinglass, P., Tislenko, L., & Reiss, D. (1985). Stability/instability in the alcoholic marriage: The interrelationships between course of alcoholism, family process, and marital outcome. *Family Process, 24,* 365–376.

Steinglass, P., Weiner, S., & Mendelson, J. H. (1971). Interactional issues as determinants of alcoholism. *American Journal of Psychiatry, 128,* 275–279.

Steinglass, P., Wolin, S., Bennett, L., & Reiss, D. (1987). *The alcoholic family.* New York: Basic Books.

Stout, R. L., McCrady, B. S., Longabaugh, R., Noel, N. E., & Beattie, M. C. (1987). Marital therapy helps to maintain the effectiveness of alcohol treatment: Replication of an outcome crossover effect. *Alcoholism: Clinical and Experimental Research, 11,* 213.

Thomas, E. J., & Santa, C. A. (1982). Unilateral family therapy for alcohol abuse: A working conception. *American Journal of Family Therapy, 10,* 49–58.

Weiner, S., Tamerin, J. S., Steinglass, P., & Mendelson, J. H. (1971). Familial patterns in chronic alcoholism: A study of a father and son during experimental intoxication. *American Journal of Psychiatry, 127,* 1646–1651.

Weiss, R. (1978). The conceptualization of marriage from a behavioral perspective. In T. J. Paolino, Jr., & B. S. McCrady (Eds.), *Marriage and marital therapy* (pp. 165–239). New York: Brunner/Mazel.

Zuckerman, M. & Lubin, B. (1965). *Manual for the Multiple Affect Adjective Check List.* San Diego, CA: Educational and Testing Service.

14

Alcohol-Related Coping Skills in Spouses of Alcoholics: Assessment and Implications for Treatment

ROBERT G. RYCHTARIK

The last decade has seen increasing evidence to suggest that the coping skills of spouses of alcoholics (i.e., how the spouse responds to and copes with the alcoholic's drinking problem) may be predictive of the level of functioning of both the identified alcoholic and the spouse (Finney, Moos, Cronkite, & Gamble, 1983). In the same period, spouse/family programs and self-help groups (e.g., Al-Anon) with the express purpose of improving coping skills have received popular support in the lay and professional literature and have proliferated in the treatment community (Hall, 1984; Howard & Howard, 1978; Johnson, 1973; Maxwell, 1976; Thorne, 1983; Zimberg, 1982). This trend can be seen in the increase of self-help books with such titles as *Getting Them Sober* (Drews, 1980), *How to Live with a Problem Drinker and Survive* (Forrest, 1980), and *Intervention: How to Help Someone Who Doesn't Want Help* (Johnson, 1986). Unfortunately, a similar trend in treatment outcome research with spouses of alcoholics has not occurred. Systematic assessment and experimental evaluation of interventions specifically for spouses of alcoholics has lagged far behind theoretical conceptualizations and clinical practice.

There are at least two reasons for the scarcity of research in this area. The first reason stems from the dominance of Al-Anon in the field and the traditional reluctance of this group and others modeled after it to subject their membership to research investigations. As a result, relatively few data exist regarding the actual efficacy of Al-Anon or the process through which it may promote change. A second, partially related explanation is the absence of an empirical data base upon which systematic methods for assessing and intervening with spouses of alcoholics can be built. For the most part, current spouse interventions have relied heavily on purely clinical data for their content. While the importance of this rich clinical data base cannot be ignored, the additional, more difficult task of transforming clinical knowledge into systematic methods of assessment, intervention, and evaluation has, for the most part, not been undertaken.

In contrast to research on alcohol-related spouse interventions, the past decade *has* seen a noticeable increase in research on marital therapy with alcoholics (e.g., McCrady, Paolino, Longabough, & Rossi, 1979; O'Farrell, Cutter, & Floyd, 1985). Importantly, this marital research received much of its impetus from an already existing empirical data base on assessment and training of marital communication skills in nonalcoholic populations. In fact, the majority of assessment and treatment techniques used in alcoholic marital research have been directly borrowed or adapted from nonalcohol-related marital studies (e.g., the Marital Adjustment Scale, Locke & Wallace, 1959; the Marital Interaction Coding System, Weiss, Hops, & Patterson, 1973). Unfortunately, no such readily available source of tested instruments or techniques exists for use in assessing alcohol-related interventions for spouses of alcoholics. As will be discussed shortly, alcohol-related spouse assessment measures are almost nonexistent and, when present, suffer from important methodological problems. Given this limited availability of assessment methods, it is no wonder that outcome research focusing on spouse interventions and training of alcohol-related coping skills in spouses of alcoholics has also been so scarce. How can alcohol-related coping skills interventions be systematically evaluated in the absence of empirical methods for assessing the very behaviors targeted for change? Indeed, some would even argue that effective interventions cannot even be developed without further empirical knowledge of the behaviors that should be targeted. It would appear then that research on *assessment* of alcohol-related spouse coping skills is an important area of research in its own right and perhaps a necessary precursor to treatment outcome research in this area. As a result, assessment of alcohol-related coping skills will be accorded the primary focus of this chapter.

Before proceeding, several important issues regarding the empirical assessment of coping skills in spouses of alcoholics and corresponding study of interventions for this population should be noted. Perhaps the most complex issue centers on determining the relative efficacy of different coping behaviors. As will be discussed in a later section, the effectiveness of a particular coping skill will vary, in all likelihood, with (1) the situation itself, (2) the individual alcoholic, (3) the characteristics of the spouse, and (4) the strength and cohesiveness of the marital bond. Hence, what may be effective for one spouse may not be effective for another, or an effective response in one situation may be ineffective in another situation. Even if the efficacy of certain coping skills were known, whether spouses can be adequately trained in the use of these skills and whether such training could generalize to the real world is not clear. Also it is not known whether a change in the spouse's way of coping with alcohol-related problems actually results in a positive change in either the alcoholic partner or the spouse.

Central to our ability to address these issues is the development of adequate methods for assessing alcohol-related coping skills. The present chapter briefly reviews research on assessing and training coping skills in spouses of alcoholics. Consistent with the focus of the chapter, particular attention will be given to issues surrounding assessment methods. An alternative, behavioral-analytic model for the assessment of spouse coping skills is then presented, followed by a description of preliminary research evaluating the characteristics of a coping skill measure developed within this framework. Finally, implications of these methods for both basic and applied research on spouse coping skills are discussed.

RESEARCH ON ASSESSMENT AND TRAINING OF COPING SKILLS

Only a handful of controlled evaluations of alcohol-related spouse coping interventions exist in the literature and these studies are primarily small sample, pilot investigations. Also, as already has been noted, research in this area suffers from important methodological problems, chief among them being the absence of adequate measures of spouse coping skills and the failure to assess for changes in coping skills from pre- to posttreatment. For example, McCrady et al. (1986) evaluated, among alcoholic outpatients, the relative efficacy of an alcohol-focused spouse intervention, a minimal spouse intervention, and a combined alcohol-focused intervention/marital therapy condition. Although a detailed description of these different treatment conditions is beyond the scope of the present discussion, it is instructive to note that the alcohol-focused spouse intervention essentially included instructions in how to reinforce abstinence and decrease those behaviors that either cued drinking or protected the drinker from experiencing the consequences of his drinking problem. At 6 and 18 months posttreatment (McCrady, 1986), the study found little differential effect among the three treatment conditions on overall drinking outcomes. Interpretation of the results, however, was difficult since no measure was used to assess whether spouses in the alcohol-focused interventions actually learned new ways of responding to their alcoholic partner. Moreover, even if new skills were acquired, there was no determination of whether these behaviors were maintained at posttreatment. Thus the failure to find differences among the alcohol-focused spouse involvement and other treatment groups, or even the former group's slightly poorer performance on some measures (e.g., time to relapse), may have simply reflected the failure of the intervention to actually change alcohol-specific spouse behaviors.

Other, small sample studies have focused on spouses whose alcoholic partners have refused to seek treatment. Interventions for this population typically have included several components, such as alcohol education, marital relationship enhancement, identification and modification of enabling behaviors, and training in confrontation techniques. Results have been promising. Thomas, Santa, Bronson, and Oyserman (1987), for example, reported a 53% reduction in alcohol consumption from before to after treatment for the alcoholic partners of spouses (treatment and delayed treatment combined, $n = 13$) who received the spouse intervention, with a slight increase in consumption for the alcoholic partners of spouses who did not receive the intervention ($n = 6$). Similar results have been reported by Sisson and Azrin (1986) in a study which also had small samples in the experimental ($n = 7$) and control groups ($n = 5$). As in the McCrady et al. (1986) study no measure of change in actual spouse coping skill was reported in either of these studies.

Even in the one published report where systematic assessment of coping skills has been attempted, measures have been confounded by the drinking status of the alcoholic partner such that cause-and-effect relationships are unclear. Dittrich and Trapold (1984) randomly assigned 23 wives of uncooperative alcoholics to either an 8-week experimental treatment ($n = 10$) or a waiting list control condition ($n = 13$). The experimental treatment included a buddy system, alcohol education, identification of enabling behaviors, training in ways to respond to the alcoholic partner's problem in a rational and assertive manner, and setting of individual goals regardless of the husband's problem. Negative coping behaviors were assessed at pretreatment, posttreatment, 16 weeks posttreatment, and at a 1-year follow-up. The coping behavior measure was the Memphis Enabling Behaviors Inventory (MEBI) which presented subjects with a list of 90 "enabling behaviors" (e.g., "You have done the majority of the alcoholic's household responsibilities," "Bailed the alcoholic out of jail," etc.). The number of behaviors in which the wife indicated that she had engaged during the prior month then served as the inventory score. Results of the treatment program indicated a significant reduction in enabling behaviors at the end of the 8-week treatment for the experimental group relative to the waiting list control group, and a similar reduction in enabling behaviors upon completion of treatment in the latter group. This reduction in enabling behaviors was also maintained at 16-week and 1-year follow-ups. Concurrently, there was a reduction in depression and anxiety and an increase in self-concept in the spouse. Finally, 48% of the husbands had entered some form of treatment for their alcoholism and 39% of the wives had either separated from or had divorced their husbands.

Although the Dittrich and Trapold (1984) results are encouraging, frequency measures such as the MEBI pose special methodological problems in this line of research. Specifically, there is a high level of interdependence between the partner's drinking behavior and how frequently the spouse is put in a position where alcohol-related coping behavior of any type is required. Obviously, the spouse of an abstinent alcoholic has no need to engage in enabling behaviors since there is no drinking to enable. Likewise, the spouse of an individual who has dramatically reduced the frequency of drinking episodes will probably engage in fewer enabling behaviors over time. The question in the Dittrich and Trapold study then becomes whether the reduction in negative coping skills posttreatment was the result of the training program itself, or simply due to the reduction in drinking. Was it really the training in coping skills per se that accounted for the change in the partner's behavior or was it other components in the treatment program that impacted on the alcoholic partner and reduced drinking behavior? In this latter case, a decrease in negative coping by the spouse may have only been an artifact of the changed drinking status of the alcoholic partner.

There is, in fact, considerable evidence to suggest that drinking behavior and the frequency of maladaptive coping behavior in the spouse are highly interrelated. Orford et al. (1975) and Schaffer and Tyler (1979) have reported that a high frequency of coping behavior, regardless of type (i.e., positive or negative), is associated with relatively poor drinking outcome in the alcoholic partner. The few coping behaviors that appear most consistently related to poorer prognosis are those that suggest disengagement or withdrawal from the marital bond (e.g., avoiding, refusing to talk, refusing to sleep together, and contemplating terminating the bond altogether). Though some have speculated that this disengaged style may contribute to the poorer prognosis, it is just as likely that the spouse is disengaging because the alcoholic's behavior is out of control. Clear cause-and-effect relationships, therefore, are not present when total reliance is placed on frequency measures of coping behavior. Indeed, the work of James and Goldman (1971) suggests that coping behaviors in wives of alcoholics *do* change over time and may be highly situation specific. These authors found that wives' coping behaviors varied with the intensity or frequency of the drinking episodes; that all wives engaged in more than one style of coping behavior; and that those styles of coping characterized by withdrawal or attack were more prevalent in wives whose husbands became violent and aggressive. Thus, frequency measures of coping behaviors may only reflect the severity of the partner's drinking problem.

Unfortunately, alternative modes of assessing alcohol-specific coping behavior do not exist. Some research has studied general coping styles in spouses of alcoholics and examined the impact of these on the functioning of the spouse (Finney, Moos, Cronkite, & Gamble, 1983; Moos, Finney, & Gamble, 1982). Although relationships between these general styles of coping and spouse functioning have been found, the extent to which general coping skills are similar to alcohol-related coping skills remains unknown. These measures based on a single event (not necessarily alcohol-related) fail to take into account the temporal variations and situational specificity in coping behavior (Billings & Moos, 1983).

In summary, systematic methods for assessing alcohol-related coping skills in spouses of alcoholics typically have been absent in the literature. In cases where methods have been present, they have suffered from important methodological problems. Until adequate assessment methods are developed which address some of the limitations noted above, research on assessment and treatment of spouses of alcoholics will continue to lag far behind clinical practice. In addition, issues of efficacy and the differential impact of training in relation to alcoholic, spouse, and marital relationship characteristics will remain unknown. The remaining sections of this chapter will focus on the development and preliminary evaluation of an alternative spouse coping skill measure designed to specifically address the assessment problems noted above.

DEVELOPMENT OF THE SPOUSE SITUATION INVENTORY

To avoid limitations of sole reliance on frequency and general coping skill measures, the present author and colleagues developed the Spouse Situation Inventory (SSI; Rychtarik, Carstensen, Alford, Schlundt, & Scott, 1988). The SSI is a situation-specific inventory of alcohol-related problems encountered by spouses of alcoholics. Development of the instrument followed methodological guidelines for constructing behavioral-analytic measures of skill deficits (Goldfried & D'Zurilla, 1969). Whereas traditional conceptualizations of assessment attempt to measure an underlying personality characteristic in order to predict behavior in certain situations, the behavioral-analytic model of Goldfried and D'Zurilla focuses on the importance of situational factors in influencing behavior, and takes the actual behavioral response in the situation as the conceptual unit of measurement. This approach appears particularly appropriate for the assessment of coping skills in spouses of alcoholics given (1) the failure of traditional assessment approaches to find disturbed personality traits which characterize this population (Edwards, Harvey, & Whitehead, 1973), (2) increasing support for the view that spouses of alcoholics are essentially normal people trying to cope with impaired partners (Moos, Finney, & Gamble, 1982), and (3) the variability of alcohol-related spouse behaviors across situations (James & Goldman, 1971).

The behavioral-analytic model under which the SSI was developed specifies five stages of inventory development: (1) an initial situational analysis of representative problem situations; (2) generation of possible solutions or responses to the situations; (3) judgment of responses as to their appro-

priateness and identification of important components of competent responses; (4) generation of a measurement format for scoring responses to
the situations; and (5) evaluation of the instrument using standard criteria
of reliability and validity. Previously, this model of scale development has
been applied successfully to the assessment of various non-alcohol-related
skill deficits in adults (Goldsmith & McFall, 1975; Goldfried & D'Zurilla,
1969; Mathews, Whang, & Fawcett, 1980), adolescents (Freedman,
Rosenthal, Donahoe, Schlundt, & McFall, 1978), and children (Dodge,
McClaskey, & Feldman, 1985). The SSI appears to be the first instrument
of its kind to apply the model to assessment of alcohol-related coping skills
in spouses of alcoholics. Stages in the development of the SSI will be
briefly reviewed below.

Situational Analysis

In the first stage of the inventory's development, a pool of representative
alcohol-related problem situations reportedly encountered by spouses of alcoholics was identified. This was accomplished by systematically gathering
alcohol-related problem situations from three sources: (1) spouses of alcoholics in the inpatient alcohol treatment program and aftercare program of
a Veterans Administration Medical Center; (2) the self-help literature for
spouses of alcoholics; and (3) alcoholism counselors. As a result of these
surveys, 120 problem situations were identified. This initial pool of situations then was reduced further by eliminating redundancies and condens-
ing situations into a single version. To insure that the sample of situations
was typical of those encountered, three alcoholism counselors subsequently
rated the situations as to their representativeness. A situation was eliminated from the sample if there was agreement that it was infrequently encountered or not representative.

The situations remaining after the above elimination process then were
categorized according to content into one of 12 content areas by a clinical psychologist and two clinical psychology residents. Situations were
grouped into content categories since it was hypothesized that an individual spouse's skill could possibly vary with the particular nature of the
situation. These content areas covered a broad range of alcohol-related situations, and included situations requiring the spouse to deal with: (1) a
relapse in the partner; (2) partner's failure to share in household responsibilities; (3) breakdown in the marital relationship; (4) disruption of
family life; (5) partner's drinking-related sexual dysfunction; (6) partner's
denial of the drinking problem; (7) partner's drunken behavior; (8) partner's physical and mental deterioration; (9) violent or potentially violent
behavior in the partner; (10) negative emotional and/or physical reactions
to partner's drinking problem; (11) vocational disruption; and (12) issues
arising from the partner's entering treatment. Those situations in which

there was no agreement in content categorization between the three raters (i.e., all three disagreed on categorization) were eliminated from the sample. A small number of additional situations then were randomly eliminated from some categories so that the final pool consisted of 48 problem situations with four situations within each of the 12 content categories. Finally, situations from each category were randomly assigned to one of four scales, resulting in four inventories of 12 situations each. In this way, each scale was composed of a broad range of situations across the different content areas.

Response Enumeration, Response Evaluation, and Measurement Scoring

To obtain a range of possible responses to the situations selected in the previous step, the scales of the SSI were administered to spouses of alcoholics entering the inpatient alcohol treatment program of a Veterans Administration Medical Center and to spouses of Veterans Administration Medical Center staff, clinical psychology residents, and clinical psychologists. These responses then were judged by three alcoholism counselors for competence, and these same raters noted the specific criteria used to rate competent responses. These criteria subsequently were collated and an independent group of seven alcoholism counselors (all with at least 3 years of counseling experience) rated the importance of the criteria. Criteria upon which there was agreement among the counselors then were incorporated into a scoring manual for rating responses to the 12 situations in each of the four scales.

The above process of scale development has been completed on two of the four 12-item inventories. For the purpose of this chapter, discussion will be limited to the first inventory of this pair. To summarize, the development process for this one inventory resulted in (1) a set of 12 problematic situations encountered by spouses of alcoholics, (2) a list of competent responses for these situations, (3) principles governing effective behaviors in these situations; and (4) a manual for scoring responses. Table 14.1 presents an abbreviated list of the twelve situations incorporated into Form 1 of the SSI. An abridged sample of scoring criteria for Situation 1 of the inventory is shown in Table 14.2.

As the sample scoring criteria in Table 14.2 suggest, each response to a situation was scored on a scale from 0 to 8, with 0 representing the least effective of responses and 8 indicating a very effective or competent response. Although scoring criteria differed depending on the situation, there was some general consistency across the situations with respect to rating criteria. Responses rated as zero reflected, for the most part, a passive or compliant approach to the problem situation (e.g., saying or doing nothing, complying with unreasonable requests). Two-point responses typ-

TABLE 14.1. Abbreviated Content of Situations for SSI, Form 1[a]

Situation	Content
1	Mate lies about drinking in aftercare session
2	Mate is out drinking and spouse is lonely and depressed
3	Mate has hangover and asks spouse to call boss and make excuse for missing work
4	Mate comes in drunk, grabs arm and calls spouse a "no good bitch"
5	Mate relapses, spouse asks mate to call counselor but mate says, "leave me alone"
6	Mate drinking heavily, eating little, has health problems
7	Mate shows up drunk at a meeting at the church
8	Spouse requests mate to stop drinking, mate says, "You knew I drank when you married me."
9	Mate drinking and no longer interested in love-making but spouse is
10	Mate passes out at dinner table in front of family
11	Mate drinking and not providing financial support
12	Mate sulking, spouse fears impending relapse

[a]From Rychtarik, Carstensen, Alford, Schlundt, and Scott (1988). © 1988 Society of Psychologists in Addictive Behaviors. Reprinted by permission.

ically were characterized by the spouse talking to the partner about the problem or verbally confronting the partner without specification of any contingencies or without indicating either compliance or noncompliance with an unreasonable request. Four-point responses represented those in which the consequences to the partner were stated only vaguely by the spouse. Also scored 4 points were responses in which the spouse noted the uselessness of trying to reason with the partner at the time of intoxication but failed to specify what would be said or done when the partner was sober. Six- and 8-point responses typically represented direct refusals to comply with unreasonable requests or verbal responses with contingencies noted and (in the case of the 8-point response) the confrontation occurs when the partner has sobered up (e.g., the next day).

As is evident from the above discussion, the SSI scoring criteria were not based on any empirically derived knowledge about the differential efficacy of coping behaviors. Rather, in the absence of such an empirical data base, the criteria were developed solely on agreed upon clinical experience among individuals in the alcohol treatment field. While the limited empirical foundation of these criteria may pose a problem, the procedures described should be considered only a first step in transforming our clinical knowledge into systematic assessment methods. As is characteristic of the behavioral-analytic approach, the scoring criteria of the SSI also essentially provide the programmatic content necessary for development of skill training interventions for spouses of alcoholics. Evaluation of such systemati-

TABLE 14.2. SSI, Form 1, Situation 1 and Abbreviated Scoring Criteria[a]

Situation	SSI Example Situation
1	Your husband went through an alcohol treatment program. He now attends follow-up sessions once every two weeks. You go with him to these sessions. When the counselor asks your husband about his drinking, your husband lies and says that he hasn't been drinking, but you know he's been drinking pretty heavily for the past week, up until the last couple of days. He told you that if you said anything that he would be furious. What would you say to your spouse and what would you do?
8 Points	Spouse tells the truth in the session
6 Points	Spouse tells the counselor the truth in private
4 Points	Spouse tells the counselor only if directly asked
2 Points	Spouse would have lectured mate before the session, but gives no indication of what he/she would say or do in the session
0 Points	Spouse doesn't say or do anything; agrees with mate's report

[a]From Rychtarik et al. (1988). © 1988 Society of Psychiatrists in Addictive Behaviors. Reprinted by permission.

cally developed programs may finally allow us to assess the accuracy of current clinical thinking which is reflected in SSI scoring criteria. The SSI, however, also could easily be adapted to alternative scoring criteria as our knowledge of effective coping behaviors advances. The inventory may also be well suited for longitudinal research aimed at identifying the efficacy of different spouse coping behaviors with respect to alcoholic partner and spouse functioning. As with any measurement development project, however, initial study of the SSI was directed at reliability and validity issues to be discussed below.

EVALUATION OF THE SSI

Initial evaluation of the SSI centered on assessing the basic psychometric characteristics of the inventory as well as identifying potential valid and extraneous sources of error which could account for variance in the measure. For this purpose generalizability theory (Brennan, 1983; Cronbach, Gleser, Nanda, & Rajaratnam, 1972) was selected. This approach to test construction and evaluation was viewed as most appropriate for several reasons. First, the SSI was not developed according to traditional assessment guidelines in which items are to be selected on the basis of their high intercorrelations with a particular trait. Instead, the SSI was developed to sample a variety of *different* problem situations (i.e., items) encountered by spouses of alcoholics. If we expect considerable situational variability in responding within subjects, then we would expect traditional test theory indices (e.g., coefficient alpha) to be quite low and not applicable. The generalizability method, on the other hand, provides a direct approach to assessing such situational variability in responding.

A second reason for selecting the generalizability approach was its particular usefulness in evaluating behavioral measures such as the SSI where sources of error, such as from raters and situations, have the potential for being quite large. If one were to use classical test theory, only a single source of random error could be identified at any one time. Importantly, generalizability analyses allow for the apportionment of variance to multiple sources. This apportionment is accomplished through a special adaptation of the analysis of variance model which results in estimated variance components for persons, and whatever other sources of error are being evaluated. For example, a generalizability analysis design evaluating the effects of persons, situations, and raters would result in estimated variance components for persons, situations, raters, the person-by-situation interaction, the person-by-rater interaction, a rater-by-situation interaction, and the person-by-situation-by-rater residual term. For the purpose of this discussion, valid sources of variation in the SSI are those attributed to persons and the person-by-situation interaction. That is, we would hope the SSI would be capable of discriminating differences in coping skill level among spouses as well as identifying differences within spouses across different situations. Other sources of variance (i.e., differences between raters or situations) would be considered error.

Finally, the generalizability approach results in an index referred to as the generalizability coefficient. The generalizability coefficient can range from .00 to 1.00 and is essentially a reliability-like correlation coefficient. It provides an indication of the extent to which one can generalize from the present set of situations and raters (as in the above example) to the universe of potential situations and raters when the focus of assessment is discriminating skill level between spouses. The generalizability coefficient is approximately equal to the expected value of the correlation between pairs of randomly parallel SSI inventories. So, whereas optimally we would like to be able to assess a spouse on all possible problem situations that may be encountered, such an assessment could not be accomplished practically. Instead, the generalizability coefficient gives us an indication of the extent to which we can be confident that a similar performance level relative to other spouses would have been obtained had another scale of different problem situations been administered to this population.

In a preliminary generalizability analysis of the SSI (Rychtarik et al., 1988), the inventory was administered in a written, self-report format to 45 spouses of male alcoholics. The subject pool included a wide range of spouses from a Veterans Administration Medical Center Alcohol Treat-

TABLE 14.3. Components and Proportion of Variance for Spouses, Situations, and Raters in Study 1

Source	Variance	Proportion
Spouses	1.56	.18
Situations	2.38	.29
Raters	.00	.00
Spouses × Raters	.13	.02
Spouses × Situations	3.62	.44
Situations × Raters	.00	.00
Spouses × Situations × Raters	.60	.07

*From Rychtarik et al. (1988). © 1988 Society of Psychologists in Addictive Behaviors. Reprinted by permission.

ment Program and from a private chemical dependency treatment unit. The analysis was conducted to isolate the components of variance in the SSI score attributable to differences in spouses, situations, or raters and/or the interactions between these terms. Results of the analysis are shown in Table 14.3. Variations in scores on the SSI largely were accounted for by cross-situational differences within spouses (the spouse-by-situation interaction), differences among situations alone, and differences among spouses. The results attest to the situational specificity of coping skills in spouses of alcoholics and also reflect the nature of the inventory (i.e., a wide collection of different situations). A coefficient of generalizability of .75 was subsequently obtained. Given the early stage of development of the SSI, the generalizability of the instrument appears quite promising.

Another important finding of the Rychtarik et al. (1988) study was that Al-Anon experience had a significant positive effect on spouses' performance on the SSI. Spouses who had experience with Al-Anon scored, on the average, approximately 10 points higher on the SSI ($M = 41.80$, SD = 13.87) than did the inexperienced group ($M = 32.08$, SD = 15.74). The results appear consistent with other research suggesting that Al-Anon experience is associated with fewer counterproductive coping responses in the spouse (Gorman & Rooney, 1979). These results are to be expected given that Al-Anon directly and indirectly provides instruction and support for the reduction of enabling behaviors. The results, therefore, suggest that the SSI may be sensitive to changes in skill level following participation in Al-Anon or other such groups.

The preliminary results of Rychtarik et al. (1988) obviously must be viewed with some caution since only volunteers participated and other variables not assessed may have accounted for the differences obtained. Nevertheless, the results did suggest that the SSI may be capable of discriminating the skill/experience level of spouses and that such skills may be highly situation specific. The results provided the basis for further examination of the instrument in the study to be discussed in some detail in the following section. The intent of this study was to extend in three important areas the previously described work on the SSI. First, the SSI was administered in a role-play, audiotaped format as opposed to the written format of the earlier study. The role-play format was considered optimum for the purposes of SSI administration, since it allowed the spouse to experience the situation more fully and encouraged more spontaneous, first person responses. Although the current SSI scoring system was based primarily on the content of responses, successful application of the SSI in a role-play format would allow for future studies assessing additional SSI response behaviors (e.g., tone of voice, eye contact).

A second aim of the study was to evaluate the differential effect of instructional set (i.e., wives' "best" vs. "actual" responses) on SSI performance. This aspect of the study was intended to provide a test of the vulnerability of the SSI to instructional sets and demand characteristics, and also allowed for some insight into the source of skill deficits identified in this population. Specifically, the investigation addressed the question of whether skill deficits exhibited on the SSI resulted from a lack of knowledge about effective responses or whether the deficits simply reflected fear and anxiety about engaging in what are already known to the spouse as better ways of handling the situations. For example, a wife may know that it is best to allow her alcoholic husband to experience the negative consequences resulting from the drinking problem and therefore recognizes that she should refuse to bail him out of jail should he request that she do so. But, due to her concerns and fear over what he might do should she refuse, she complies with his request. In this case, the wife has the knowledge of the effective response, but fails to engage in it because of other factors. It was hoped that the study would provide some insight into the extent to which this occurs.

The final aim of the study was to examine the relationship of the SSI to other important spouse characteristics and to conduct an initial validity study of the SSI by examining the correspondence between wives' SSI behavior and alcoholic partners' reports of marital conflict in response to drinking. It was hypothesized that low reports of marital conflict over drinking as reported by the husband would be associated with lower SSI total scores or, in other words, more passive responses on the SSI by the wife.

INSTRUCTIONAL SETS AND THE SSI

Participants in the study were wives of 42 married alcoholics consecutively admitted over a 9-month period to a Veterans Administration Medical Center Alcohol Dependence Treatment Program. Of the total sample of 42 wives, five were unable to be contacted or refused to participate in their husband's treatment. An additional five subjects were eliminated from the original sample due to (1) equipment failure during SSI administration (e.g., the tape recorder did not function properly), (2) presence of a major psychiatric disorder in either the alcoholic or the wife, or (3) failure of the spouse to understand the SSI instructions. The final sample of 32 wives represented 76% of the total number of potential participants over the time period of the study. The sample population had a mean age of 44.97 years (SD = 11.92), had on the average 12.32 (SD = 2.26) years of education, and reported they had been married an average of 16.7 years (SD = 14.54). Approximately 61% of the wives were employed full-time, 3% part-time, 26% were unemployed, and 10% were retired. Their alcoholic husbands were of comparable age ($M = 45.77$, SD = 11.42) and educational experience ($M = 12.23$, SD = 2.46), and reported, on the average, a drinking problem duration of 14.03 years (SD = 11.67). In contrast to their wives, approximately 26% of the husbands were employed full-time, 42% were unemployed, 19% were retired, and 13% disabled.

General Procedure

Shortly after the admission of her husband to the treatment program, the wife was scheduled for an assessment interview during which basic demographic information was obtained and the SSI administered. In order to control for possible confounds due to characteristics of the individual administering the SSI, subjects were randomly assigned to one of three SSI administrators: a Ph.D.-level clinical psychologist, a clinical psychology resident, or a masters-level alcoholism counselor. Each subject was administered the SSI twice during the assessment session, once with instructions to respond as they normally or actually would in the presented situations, and once with instructions to respond in what they thought was the best way of handling the situations. The exact order in which subjects received the actual versus best instructions was determined on a random basis.

Instructional Conditions

Subjects assigned to the actual-best presentation order were given the following instructions:

> As part of our efforts to help wives of our patients cope with living with someone who has a drinking problem, and to improve our treatment program, we want to find out how you would react to some real life everyday situations that you or other wives might find themselves in as a result of living with a husband who has a drinking problem. I will read a situation to you. As you listen carefully to the situation, I want you to imagine that it is actually happening to you. Each situation will end with the question, "If you were in this situation how upset would you feel?"

based on this scale [subject is shown a scale ranging from 1 (not upset at all) to 5 (extremely upset)]. Provide me with the number on the scale that indicates how upset you would be in this situation. Then I will ask, "What would you say to your spouse and what would you do?" I want you to say the words you would say if you were in that situation. Right now I'm not interested in what you think you *should* do or what the *best* thing to do is. Rather I'm interested in what you would *really do or actually do*. If you feel the situation requires doing something rather than saying something, then just describe what you would actually do. Remember that we want you to imagine that the situation is actually happening to you while it is being described and that you are to speak as if the situation were happening to you right now, here in this room. Some situations may not seem to fit you too well. They have been obtained from a lot of different people who have been through our program. You may not have had some of these things happen to you, but even if you haven't been in a situation before, do your best to reply to all of them. Do not take more time to respond than you would in real life. There are twelve situations in all. Here's an example.

The wife was then presented with a sample situation, asked for her response, and then provided feedback regarding how well she followed the instructions (e.g., whether she pretended to be in the situation, responded as if talking to husband, etc.). The administrator then answered any procedural questions and made sure that the subject understood the instructions before administering the SSI. The audiotape recorder was turned on and the 12 situations were presented one at a time by the administrator. Following the first presentation of the situations, the same situations were repeated but with the following instructions:

This time around I'd like for you to tell me what you think you *should* be doing, if you feel your previous response was not the *best way* of handling the situation. Sometimes what people *actually* do and what they think they *should be doing* is not the same. If you feel your previous response was the best way you know of handling the situation, fine, just give me that response. If you think there is a better way of handling the situation, a better thing to say or do, then give that to me.

Wives assigned to the best response–actual response instruction sequence were provided instructions identical to those in the actual–best condition, with the exception that initially the wife was asked to respond with what she thought was the *best* way of handling the situation.

Response Ratings

The audiotaped responses subsequently were transcribed, grouped by situation, and randomized within the situation. This arrangement allowed for scoring the randomized responses of all subjects to a particular situation at one time. In this way a particular subject's response to one situation could not influence the scoring of a subsequent response by that subject to another situation. These randomized responses then were scored according to scoring criteria previously developed. Scoring of responses was conducted independently by two raters who were unaware of which participants provided the responses they were scoring. The mean percentage agreement between raters (i.e., number of agreements divided by the number of agreements plus disagreements) across the twelve situations was .90 (SD = .07)

Results

An initial 2 (order of instructions) by 3 (administrator) multivariate analysis of variance was conducted on major demographic and alcoholic partner drinking history variables. No significant effect was found for order or administrator and there was no order by administrator interaction on these variables. Initial analyses on subjects' mean total SSI scores also failed to identify significant main effects or interactions between administrators, order of instructions, and instructional sets. Thus, any differences obtained could not be accounted for by the confounding effects of different demographic characteristics, SSI administrator, or order of instructions. Subsequent analyses were therefore collapsed across administrator and order factors.

Results indicated no significant difference in performance on the SSI between instructional conditions with total score means of 33.38 (SD = 8.32) and 31.62 (SD = 7.64) for the "actual" and "best" conditions, respectively ($t = 1.25$, df = 31, $p > .10$). Results of a subsequent generalizability analysis assessing the effects of persons, situations, and instructions supported these findings and indicated that no more than 1% of the variance could be accounted for by instructional set or interactions between instructions and subjects or instructions and situations. Overall, the lack of differential responding on the SSI under "best" versus "actual" instructions suggested that the low levels of performance exhibited by this group of wives resulted from a lack of knowledge or skill in handling drinking-related situations rather than from fear or anxiety about engaging in a response considered more effective. Moreover, the SSI did not seem to be highly contaminated by demand characteristics.

RELATIONSHIP BETWEEN THE SSI AND OTHER VARIABLES

Several relationships between "actual" responses on the SSI and other wife and alcoholic partner variables were predicted. First, it was expected, based on results of the initial SSI study, that performance on the SSI would be positively correlated with Al-Anon experience. Second, it was hypothesized that SSI performance would be negatively correlated with age, with older wives scoring lower (i.e., exhibiting more passive responses than younger wives), due to generational cohort differences between the age groups or simply to older wives having become desensitized to or emotionally isolated from their partners' drinking problem. Finally, the external validity of the SSI as a measure of actual coping behavior was tested by examining the relationship of wives' SSI performance to their alcoholic partners' reports of marital discord provoked by drinking, as measured by Scale 16 of the Alcohol Use Inventory (AUI; Wanberg, Horn, & Foster, 1977). This latter scale is heavily loaded with items which tap into the alcoholic's perception of the wife's behavior when the partner drinks (e.g., "Does your spouse nag you about your drinking?" or "Does your spouse get angry with you over your drinking?"). High scores on the scale are indicative of higher levels of marital discord over drinking and hence a more active, confrontational role on the part of the wife. It was hypothesized that performance on the SSI, if it is to be reflective of actual behavior in the real world, would correlate significantly with the alcoholic partner's report on this AUI scale. Specifically, more direct, active, confrontational behavior exhibited on the SSI should be positively associated with, and passive SSI behavior negatively associated with, the partner's report on the AUI.

To investigate the above hypotheses, Pearson correlation coefficients were calculated between mean total SSI scores and (1) age of the wife, (2) Al-Anon experience (a dichotomous variable of whether the wife had ever attended Al-Anon), and (3) the husbands' AUI16 raw scores. Results of these analyses, shown in Table 14.4, were in the expected direction with all approaching significance (p's < .10). Subsequently, a more refined analysis of SSI performance and its relationship to the above variables was conducted. This analysis was accomplished by calculating frequency scores for each of the possible response scoring categories (i.e., frequency of 0-, 2-, 4-, and 6- to 8-point responses, respectively). It was hypothesized that

TABLE 14.4. Intercorrelations Between SSI Measures and Wife Age, Al-Anon Experience, Upset Ratings, and Husband's AUI Scale 16[a]

	Age	Al-Anon	AUI16	Upset
SSI total score	−.29[*]	.25[*]	.26[*]	.21
0-point score	.41[**]	−.09	−.35[**]	−.34[**]
2-point score	−.31[**]	−.08	.24	.28[*]
4-point score	.14	−.08	−.14	−.15
6- to 8-point score	−.24[*]	.31[**]	.25[*]	.18

[a]Due to missing data, analyses are based on $N = 31$ except for those on the AUI16 which are based on $N = 30$.
[*]$p < .10$; [**]$p < .05$.

these latter measures would provide a more accurate reflection of the quality of the wives' responses as well as an indication of the consistency with which such responses were used. Pearson correlations were calculated between these frequency measures and Al-Anon, age, and AUI variables. Though the findings from this latter analysis varied with the specific frequency measure examined, the results were in the expected direction and several were significant (see Table 14.4). Specifically, the age of the subject was significantly correlated with the frequency of 0 and 2-point responses. As age increased so too did the frequency of subjects' use of 0-point responses (i.e., passive, compliant responses; $r = .41$, $p = .01$). On the other hand, 2-point responses were used less frequently ($r = .31$, $p = .04$). Also consistent with the above hypotheses was the finding that Al-Anon experienced subjects made use of more 6- and 8-point responses ($r = .31$, $p = .05$). Al-Anon experience did not, however, seem to be associated with higher or lower levels of other SSI frequency measures. Overall, these results supported hypotheses regarding the effects of age, and replicated previous work in showing that individuals with Al-Anon experience, as compared to those without an Al-Anon background, exhibit higher functioning on the SSI.

Support for the external validity of the SSI also was found, as evidenced in the significant, negative correlation between the subjects' 0-point frequency measure and the alcoholic husband's report of the extent to which drinking provokes marital conflict ($r = -.35$, $p = .03$). A higher frequency of zero responses on the SSI (i.e., more passive, compliant responses) was associated with low levels of marital conflict over drinking reported by the husbands. In other words, the more passive an individual was on the SSI (i.e., higher frequency of 0-point responses) the more likely it was that the alcoholic partner would indicate lower levels of marital conflict as a result of drinking (i.e., less nagging by the wife, etc.). This finding suggests that wives' behavior on the SSI may be a representative sample of their behavior in actual drinking-related situations encountered with their husband. It is also interesting to note marital conflict over drinking reported by the husband on the AUI was positively associated with the frequency of 6- and 8-point responses and this association approached significance ($r = .25$, $p = .09$). This finding is consistent with what would be expected since 6- and 8-point responses on the SSI correspond with a more confrontational approach on the part of the wife. More frequent use of these responses would likely result in the husband experiencing more marital conflict over his drinking.

Importantly, a highly significant negative relationship was also noted between wife's age and husband's report of drinking-related marital conflict on the AUI ($r = -.45$, $p < .01$). As the age of the wives increased husbands reported less conflict over drinking in the marriage. Hence, this convergence in findings between the SSI and AUI16 with respect to subject age provided even further support for the notion that behavior on the SSI may be an accurate reflection of actual responding to real world alcohol-related problem situations. Why older wives are perceived as providing less conflict over drinking by their husbands and, consistent with this finding, exhibit more passive, compliant behavior on the SSI is not entirely clear.

It will be recalled that, during SSI administration, each wife was asked to rate how upset she would be if she were in the situation. Upset ratings were given on a scale ranging from 1 (not upset at all) to 5 (extremely upset). To examine the role of this upset variable, mean upset ratings across the 12 situations were computed and included in the correlational analyses (see Table 14.4) The results provided some understanding of older wives' more passive responding on the SSI and their husbands' similar reports of more passive behavior in response to drinking. As the age of the wives increased their reported upset ratings decreased ($r = -.31$, $p = .05$). Likewise, the wives' upset ratings were negatively and significantly correlated with the frequency of zero responses ($r = -.34$, $p = .03$) and positively associated with husbands AUI16 ($r = .32$, $p = .04$). Thus, it can be speculated that older wives appear to become less upset over problem situations and are therefore more likely to respond passively (e.g., doing nothing). Whether this tendency is a result of generational or cohort differences between older and younger women or the result of the older wife somehow emotionally distancing herself from the drinking problem is unclear and will require further research.

CONCLUSIONS AND IMPLICATIONS FOR RESEARCH AND TREATMENT

Overall, the behavioral-analytic assessment model used for the SSI appears to show considerable promise for the development of measures for assessing the coping skills of spouses of alcoholics. Initial evaluations of the SSI suggest that extraneous sources of error such as the rating system and the instructional set contribute little to overall variance in the measure. Importantly, the SSI appears sensitive to differences in skill level between subjects and to differences within subjects across different situations. Moreover, the results of the study presented here suggest that wife behavior on the SSI may be a valid representation of her actual behavior under similar circumstances in the real world.

The SSI, however, is still an instrument under development and is not without its limitations. The scoring system was developed on the basis of only the content of a response and not the manner in which it is presented. Inclusion of behavioral measures such as tone of voice, eye contact, and the like may enhance further the sensitivity of the SSI in differentiating skill level among spouses. A second additional source of variance in SSI scores may be found in wives' cognitions regarding the situations and the consequences of different responses. Assessment of cognitive processes may aid us in understanding better wives' decisions regarding their chosen way of responding to particular situations. An understanding of cognitive processes in younger versus older subjects in the above study, for example, may have helped to explain older subjects' reports of less upset over situations and their subsequent use of more passive responses. Finally, additional factor analytic research is required to determine whether variance from the spouse by situation interaction on the SSI arises from differential performance among 12 situation specific factors (e.g., the different content categories) or whether the situations cluster into two or three factors upon which there is differential performance within subjects and for which there may be differential predictive validity.

Although behavior on the SSI appeared to be a valid representation based on the alcoholic's report (at least for zero responses), validity concerns regarding the SSI remain. As noted earlier, scoring criteria were based only on the current clinical judgment of alcoholism counselors. Whether the skills assessed and scored on the SSI are actually predictive of functioning in the spouse *and/or* the alcoholic is not clear. Specifically, we do not know whether spouses who show a high frequency of 6- to 8-point responses on the SSI also exhibit better psychological adjustment and whether use of these more "effective" responses results in longer periods of abstinence or more rapid resolution of relapses in their alcoholic partners. The higher level of performance on the SSI by individuals with Al-Anon experience is consistent with some limited research showing better drinking outcomes in alcoholics whose spouse has attended Al-Anon (e.g., Wright & Scott, 1978). On the other hand, the correlation between the SSI and Al-Anon experience could be a simple artifact of scoring criteria developed by counselors heavily influenced by the principles of Al-Anon. It is also possible that better outcomes thought to be associated with Al-Anon are attributable to other components of this self-help group (e.g., mutual support) and not to the development of more effective coping skills. Further research addressing these issues is required.

Unfortunately, establishing the validity of measures such as the SSI is a complex task. One might anticipate, for example, that a 6- to 8-point response in which the wife specifies consequences should the partner not seek help for a relapse would be more effective in a cohesive marital relationship in which the alcoholic has a higher investment than in a fragmented relationship in which the alcoholic may be less motivated. Specification of such possible interactions with respect to the effectiveness of spouse coping skills may be important from a treatment standpoint in order to match interventions to particular alcoholics and their families. Future studies differentiating spouses of varying SSI performance on a variety of psychological functioning and partner drinking variables are required, as is longitudinal research evaluating the differential effectiveness of different alcohol-related coping behaviors on alcoholic partner drinking and relapse.

Such research would provide a better empirical foundation upon which to further develop the SSI scoring system. Finally, should further research confirm the validity of the present or revised SSI scoring system, the framework will be in place for systematic evaluation of alcohol-related coping skills interventions for spouses of alcoholics. Such research will assist in addressing whether the results of such interventions generalize to the real world situation, improve the overall psychological functioning of the spouse, or even impact effectively on the drinking behavior of the alcoholic partner.

To date, the SSI remains a research tool in the early stages of development, and its clinical application would be premature. Nevertheless, there are several important implications for treatment should further development and validation of the SSI or similar measures prove successful. First, measures such as these could provide for much needed individualized assessment of spouse coping skills and therefore allow for more effective/efficient interventions tailored to individual need. For example, the inventory could be administered to spouses of individuals admitted for treatment, specific skill deficits noted, individualized treatment goals developed and direct remediation of the deficits provided (e.g., instructions, modeling, behavioral rehearsal). Spouses' progress in learning new skills and their generalization to new situations could then be monitored by readministration of the SSI and appropriate changes in interventions made as indicated. With the use of such measures treatment programs for family members may then become more accountable with respect to meeting their stated goals. It is also hoped that successful development of measures such as the SSI will provide the impetus for the development of comparable assessment inventories for other family members or for families of other populations of alcohol abusers (e.g., husbands of female alcoholics or parents of teenagers with drinking or drug problems).

Although the present chapter has focused on assessment of coping skills in spouses of alcoholics and advocated the empirical development and implementation of individualized assessment and skill training programs for this population, a word of caution must be noted. Simply training spouses or family members in effective coping skills may not be enough to enhance the spouse's/family's adjustment or even impact effectively on the drinking behavior of the partner. A spouse may be able to adequately confront the alcoholic partner and may even specify contingencies but fail to follow through with consequences should they be needed. The emotional support provided by others (e.g., family members, self-help group members, therapist, or clergy) may be an important if not essential element in the behavior change process, at least for some individuals. In other cases, a couple may require training in marital communication skills in addition to specific alcohol-related coping skill intervention. Development of adequate alcohol-related coping skills in the spouse may, therefore, be only one part of effective interventions with this population. Nevertheless, in the absence of adequate assessment tools such as those advocated for development in the present chapter, studies evaluating the relative importance of coping skills training, social support, and marital therapy, and their optimum mix will remain wanting and the basis for our interventions will continue to lack a solid empirical base.

Acknowledgments The author gratefully acknowledges the assistance of Bill Carr, Ceagus Reed, and Armando de Armas in the data collection associated with research reported in this chapter.

REFERENCES

Billings, A. G., & Moos, R. H. (1983). Psychosocial processes of recovery among alcoholics and their families: Implications for clinicians and program evaluators. *Addictive Behaviors, 8,* 205–218.

Brennan, R. L. (1983). *Elements of generalizability theory.* Iowa City, IO: The American College Testing Program.

Cronbach, L. J., Gleser, G. C., Nanda, H., & Rajaratnam, N. (1972). *The dependability of behavioral measurements: Theory of generalizability for scores and profiles.* New York: Wiley.

Dittrich, J. E., & Trapold, M. A. (1984). Wives of alcoholics: A treatment program and outcome study. *Bulletin of the Society of Psychologists in Addictive Behaviors, 3* 91–102.

Dodge, K. A., McClasky, C. L., & Feldman, E. (1985). Situational approach to the assessment of social competence in children. *Journal of Consulting and Clinical Psychology, 3,* 344–353.

Drews, T. R. (1980). *Getting them sober.* Plainfield, NJ: Logos International.

Edwards, P., Harvey, C., & Whitehead, P. C. (1973). Wives of alcoholics: A critical review and analysis. *Quarterly Journal of Studies on Alcohol, 34,* 112–132.

Finney, J. W., Moos, R. H., Cronkite, R. C., & Gamble, W. (1983). A conceptual model of the functioning of married persons with impaired partners: Spouses of alcoholic patients. *Journal of Marriage and the Family, 45,* 23–34.

Forrest, G. G. (1980). *How to live with a problem drinker and survive.* New York, Atheneum.

Freedman, B. J., Rosenthal, L., Donahoe, C. P., Jr., Schlundt, D. G., & McFall, R. M. (1978). A social-behavioral analysis of skill deficits in delinquent and nondelinquent adolescent boys. *Journal of Consulting and Clinical Psychology, 46,* 1448–1462.

Goldfried, M. R., & D'Zurilla, T. J. (1969). A behavioral-analytical model for assessing competence. In C. D. Spielberger (Ed.), *Current topics in clinical and community psychology* (pp. 151–196). New York: Academic Press.

Goldsmith, J. B., & McFall, R. M. (1975). Development and evaluation of an interpersonal skill-training program for psychiatric inpatients. *Journal of Abnormal Psychology, 84,* 51–58.

Gorman, J. M., & Rooney, J. F. (1979). The influence of Al-Anon on the coping behavior of wives of alcoholics. *Journal of Studies on Alcohol, 40,* 1030–1038.

Hall, S. M. (1984). The abstinence phobias: Links between substance abuse and anxiety. *International Journal of the Addictions, 19,* 613–631.

Howard, D. P., & Howard, N. T. (1978). Treatment of the significant other. In S. Zimberg, J. Wallace, & S. B. Blume (Eds.), *Practical approaches to alcoholism psychotherapy.* New York: Plenum.

James, J. E., & Goldman, M. (1971). Behavior trends of wives of alcoholics. *Quarterly Journal of Studies on Alcohol, 32,* 373–381.

Johnson, V. E. (1973). *I'll quit tomorrow.* New York: Harper.

Johnson, V. E. (1986). *Intervention: How to help someone who doesn't want help.* Minneapolis, MN: Johnson Institute Books.

Locke, H. J., & Wallace, K. M. (1959). Short marital-adjustment and prediction tests: Their reliability and validity. *Journal of Marriage and Family Living, 21,* 251–255.

Mathews, R. M., Whang, P. L., & Fawcett, S. B. (1980). Development and validation of an occupational skills assessment instrument. *Behavioral Assessment, 2,* 71–85.

Maxwell, R. (1976). *The booze battle.* New York: Ballantine Books.

McCrady, B. S. (1986). The family in the change process. In W. R. Miller, & N. Heather (Eds.), *Treating addictive behaviors: Processes of change* (pp. 305–318). New York: Plenum.

McCrady, B. S., Noel, N. E., Abrams, D. B., Stout, R. L., Nelson, H. F., & Hay, W. M. (1986). Comparative effectiveness of three types of spouse involvement in outpatient behavioral alcoholism treatment. *Journal of Studies on Alcohol, 47,* 459–467.

McCrady, B. S., Paolino, T. J., Jr., Longabaugh, R., & Rossi, J. (1979). Effects of joint hospital admission and couples treatment for hospitalized alcoholics: A pilot study. *Addictive Behaviors, 4,* 155–165.

Moos, R. H., Finney, J. W., & Gamble, W. (1982). The process of recovery from alcoholism: II. Comparing spouses of alcoholic patients and matched community controls. *Journal of Studies on Alcohol, 43,* 888–909.

O'Farrell, T. J., Cutter, H. S. G., & Floyd, F. J. (1985). Evaluating behavioral marital therapy for male alcoholics: Effects on marital adjustment and communication from before to after treatment. *Behavior Therapy, 16,* 147–167.

Orford, J., Guthrie, S., Nicholls, P., Oppenheimer, E., Egert, S., & Hensman, C. (1975). Self-reported coping behavior of wives of alcoholics and its associations with drinking outcome. *Journal of Studies on Alcohol, 36,* 1254–1267.

Rychtarik, R. G., Carstensen, L. L., Alford, G. S., Schlundt, D. G., & Scott, W. O. (1988). Situational assessment of alcohol-related coping skills in wives of alcoholics. *Psychology of Addictive Behaviors, 2,* 66–73.

Schaffer, J. B., & Tyler, J. D. (1979). Degree of sobriety in male alcoholics and coping styles used by their wives. *British Journal of Psychiatry, 135,* 431–437.

Sisson, R. W., & Azrin, N. H. (1986). Family-member involvement to initiate and promote treatment of problem drinkers. *Journal of Behavior Therapy & Experimental Psychiatry, 17,* 15–21.

Thomas, E. J., Santa, C., Bronson, D., & Oyserman, D. (1987). Unilateral family therapy with the spouses of alcoholics. *Journal of Social Service Research, 10,* 145–162.

Thorne, D. R. (1983). Techniques for use in intervention. *Journal of Alcohol and Drug Education, 28,* 46–50.

Wanberg, K. W., Horn, J. L., & Foster, F. M. (1977). A differential assessment model for alcoholism. *Journal of Studies on Alcohol, 38,* 512–543.

Weiss, R. L., Hops, H., & Patterson, G. R. (1973). A framework for conceptualizing marital conflict: A technology for altering it, some data for evaluating it. In L. A. Hamerlynck, L. C. Handy, & E. J. Mash (Eds.), *Behavior change: Methodology concepts, and practice* (pp. 309–342). Champaign, IL: Research Press.

Wright, K. D., & Scott, T. B. (1978). The relationship of wives treatment to the drinking status of alcoholics. *Journal of Studies on Alcohol, 9,* 1577–1581.

Zimberg, S. (1982). *The clinical management of alcoholism.* New York: Brunner/ Mazel.

Index